NANDA International, Inc.
NURSING DIAGNOSES:
DEFINITIONS & CLASSIFICATION
2015–2017

NANDA International, Inc.
NURSING DIAGNOSES:
DEFINITIONS & CLASSIFICATION
2015–2017

Tenth Edition

Edited by

T. Heather Herdman, PhD, RN, FNI

and

Shigemi Kamitsuru, PhD, RN, FNI

WILEY Blackwell

This edition first published 2014
© 2014, 2012, 2009, 2007, 2005, 2003, 2001, 1998, 1996, 1994 by NANDA International, Inc.

Registered Office
John Wiley & Sons, Ltd., The Atrium, Southern Gate, Chichester, West Sussex, PO19 8SQ, UK

Editorial Offices
9600 Garsington Road, Oxford, OX4 2DQ, UK
The Atrium, Southern Gate, Chichester, West Sussex, PO19 8SQ, UK
1606 Golden Aspen Drive, Suites 103 and 104, Ames, Iowa 50010, USA

For details of our global editorial offices, for customer services and for information about how to apply for permission to reuse the copyright material in this book please see our website at www.wiley.com/wiley-blackwell

ISBN 9781118914939
ISSN 1943-0728

A catalogue record for this book is available from the Library of Congress and the British Library.

Wiley also publishes its books in a variety of electronic formats. Some content that appears in print may not be available in electronic books.

Cover image: iStockphoto / © alvarez

Set in 10/12pt Meridien by SPi Publisher Services, Pondicherry, India
Printed and bound in Malaysia by Vivar Printing Sdn Bhd

1   2014

Correct citation of this text (APA Format, based on the 6th Edition):

Herdman, T.H. & Kamitsuru, S. (Eds.). (2014). *NANDA International Nursing Diagnoses: Definitions & Classification, 2015–2017*. Oxford: Wiley Blackwell.

Contents

NANDA International, Inc. Guidelines for Copyright Permission   *xix*
Preface   *xxii*
Introduction   *xxvi*
About the Companion Website   *xxviii*

PART 1   CHANGES TO THE NANDA INTERNATIONAL TERMINOLOGY   1

Introduction   **3**
T. Heather Herdman, RN, PhD, FNI

What's New in the 2015–2017 Edition of *Diagnoses and Classification?*

Acknowledgments   4
Chapter authors   4
Chapter reviewers   5
Reviewer for standardization of diagnostic terms   5
Changes to health promotion and risk diagnoses   5
New nursing diagnoses, 2015–2017   5
Table 1.1   New NANDA-I Nursing Diagnoses, 2015–2017   6
Revised nursing diagnoses, 2015–2017   7
Table 1.2   Revised NANDA-I Nursing Diagnoses, 2015–2017   8
Changes to slotting of current diagnoses within the NANDA-I Taxonomy II, 2015–2017   11
Table 1.3   Slotting Changes to NANDA-I Nursing Diagnoses, 2015–2017   11
Revisions to nursing diagnosis labels within the NANDA-I Taxonomy II, 2015–2017   11
Nursing diagnoses removed from the NANDA-I Taxonomy II, 2015–2017   11
Table 1.4   Revisions to Nursing Diagnosis Labels of NANDA-I Nursing Diagnoses, 2015–2017   12
Standardization of diagnostic indicator terms   12

Table 1.5   Nursing Diagnoses Removed from the
    NANDA-I Taxonomy II, 2015–2017   13
Other changes made in the 2015–2017 edition   15

PART 2   NURSING DIAGNOSIS   17

Chapter 1   Nursing Diagnosis Basics   21
Susan Gallagher-Lepak, RN, PhD

Figure 1.1   Example of a Collaborative Healthcare Team   22
How does a nurse (or nursing student) diagnose?   23
Figure 1.2   The Modified Nursing Process   23
Understanding nursing concepts   24
Assessment   24
Nursing diagnosis   25
Table 1.1   Parts of a Nursing Diagnosis Label   25
Table 1.2   Key Terms at a Glance   26
Planning/intervention   27
Evaluation   28
Use of nursing diagnosis   28
Brief chapter summary   29
Questions commonly asked by new learners
    about nursing diagnosis   29
References   30

Chapter 2   From Assessment to Diagnosis   31
T. Heather Herdman, RN, PhD, FNI and
Shigemi Kamitsuru, RN, PhD, FNI

What happens during nursing assessment?   31
Figure 2.1   Steps in Moving from Assessment
    to Diagnosis   32
Why do nurses assess?   32
The screening assessment   33
Not a simple matter of "filling in the blanks"   34
Assessment framework   35
Should we use the NANDA-I taxonomy
    as an assessment framework?   35
Data analysis   35
Figure 2.2   Converting Data to Information   36
Subjective versus objective data   37
Clustering of information/seeing a pattern   38
Figure 2.3   The Modified Nursing Process   39
Identifying potential nursing diagnoses
    (diagnostic hypotheses)   39
In-depth assessment   41
Figure 2.4   In-Depth Assessment   42

Confirming/refuting potential nursing diagnoses 43
Eliminating possible diagnoses 43
Potential new diagnoses 44
Differentiating between similar diagnoses 44
    Table 2.1   The Case of Caroline: A Comparison
    of Identified Defining Characteristics and
    Related Factors 45
    Table 2.2   The Case of Caroline: A Comparison
    of Domains and Classes of Potential
    Diagnoses 47
    Figure 2.5   SEA TOW: A Thinking Tool for
    Diagnostic Decision-Making 48
Making a diagnosis/prioritizing 49
Summary 50
References 50

Chapter 3   An Introduction to the NANDA-I Taxonomy   52

T. Heather Herdman, RN, PhD, FNI

Taxonomy: Visualizing a taxonomic structure 52
    Figure 3.1   Domains and Classes of *Classified
    Groceries, Inc.* 54
    Figure 3.2   Classes and Concepts of *Classified
    Groceries, Inc.* 55
Classification in nursing 56
    Figure 3.3   NANDA-I Taxonomy II Domains
    and Classes 58
    Figure 3.4   NANDA-I Domain 1, *Health Promotion*,
    with Classes and Nursing Diagnoses 60
Using the NANDA-I taxonomy 60
Structuring nursing curricula 60
    Figure 3.5   NANDA-I Taxonomy II Activity/Rest
    Domain 61
Identifying a nursing diagnosis outside your area
of expertise 62
    Figure 3.6   Use of the NANDA-I Taxonomy II and
    Terminology to Identify and Validate a Nursing
    Diagnosis Outside the Nurse's Area of Expertise 63
    Case Study: Mrs. Lendo 64
    Figure 3.7   Diagnosing Mrs. Lendo 65
The NANDA-I nursing diagnosis taxonomy:
A short history 65
    Table 3.1   Domains, Classes, and Nursing Diagnoses
    in the NANDA-I Taxonomy II 66

Figure 3.8   Seven Domains of the Proposed
   Taxonomy III   79
Figure 3.9   Proposed Taxonomy III Domains
   and Classes   80
Table 3.2   Proposed Taxonomy III Domains, Classes,
   and Nursing Diagnoses   81
References   90

Chapter 4   NANDA-I Taxonomy II: Specifications and Definitions   91
T. Heather Herdman, RN, PhD, FNI

Structure of Taxonomy II   91
Figure 4.1   The ISO Reference Terminology Model
   for a Nursing Diagnosis   92
A multiaxial system for constructing diagnostic concepts   92
Figure 4.2   The NANDA-I Model of a Nursing
   Diagnosis   93
Definitions of the axes   94
Axis 1 The focus of the diagnosis   94
Table 4.1   Foci of the NANDA-I Nursing Diagnoses   95
Axis 2 Subject of the diagnosis   97
Axis 3 Judgment   97
Axis 4 Location   97
Table 4.2   Definitions of Judgment Terms
   for Axis 3, NANDA-I Taxonomy II   98
Table 4.3   Locations in Axis 4, NANDA-I Taxonomy II   100
Axis 5 Age   100
Axis 6 Time   100
Axis 7 Status of the diagnosis   100
Developing and submitting a nursing diagnosis   101
Figure 4.3   A NANDA-I Nursing Diagnosis Model:
   (Individual) Impaired Standing   101
Figure 4.4   A NANDA-I Nursing Diagnosis Model:
   Risk for Disorganized Infant Behavior   102
Figure 4.5   A NANDA-I Nursing Diagnosis Model:
   Readiness for Enhanced Family Coping   102
Further development   103
References   103
Other recommended reading   104

Chapter 5   Frequently Asked Questions   105
T. Heather Herdman, RN, PhD, FNI and
Shigemi Kamitsuru, RN, PhD, FNI

Basic questions about standardized nursing languages   105
Basic questions about NANDA-I   106

Basic questions about nursing diagnoses 110
Questions about defining characteristics 116
Questions about related factors 117
Questions about risk factors 118
Differentiating between similar nursing diagnoses 119
Questions regarding the development of a treatment plan 121
Questions about teaching/learning nursing diagnoses 123
Questions about using NANDA-I in electronic health
  records 126
Questions about diagnosis development and review 127
Questions about the *NANDA-I Definitions and
  Classification* text 127
References 129

PART 3   THE NANDA INTERNATIONAL
NURSING DIAGNOSES 131

**International Considerations on the use
of the *NANDA-I Nursing Diagnoses*** 133
T. Heather Herdman, RN, PhD, FNI

Domain 1: Health Promotion 137

Class 1. Health awareness 139
Deficient **diversional activity** – 00097 139
Sedentary **lifestyle** – 00168 140
Class 2. Health management 141
Frail elderly syndrome – 00257 141
Risk for **frail elderly syndrome** – 00231 142
Deficient community **health** – 00215 144
Risk-prone **health behavior** – 00188 145
Ineffective **health maintenance** – 00099 146
Ineffective **health management** – 00078 147
Readiness for enhanced **health management** – 00162 148
Ineffective family **health management** – 00080 149
Non**compliance** – 00079 150
Ineffective **protection** – 00043 152

Domain 2: Nutrition 153

Class 1. Ingestion 155
Insufficient **breast milk** – 00216 155
Ineffective **breastfeeding** – 00104 156
Interrupted **breastfeeding** – 00105 158
Readiness for enhanced **breastfeeding** – 00106 159

Ineffective infant **feeding pattern** – 00107 160
Imbalanced **nutrition**: less than body
   requirements – 00002 161
Readiness for enhanced **nutrition** – 00163 162
Obesity – 00232 163
Overweight – 00233 165
Risk for **overweight** – 00234 167
Impaired **swallowing** – 00103 169
Class 2. Digestion
None at present time
Class 3. Absorption
None at present time
Class 4. Metabolism 171
Risk for unstable **blood glucose level** – 00179 171
Neonatal **jaundice** – 00194 172
Risk for neonatal **jaundice** – 00230 173
Risk for impaired **liver function** – 00178 174
Class 5. Hydration 175
Risk for **electrolyte** im**balance** – 00195 175
Readiness for enhanced **fluid balance** – 00160 176
Deficient **fluid volume** – 00027 177
Risk for deficient **fluid volume** – 00028 178
Excess **fluid volume** – 00026 179
Risk for imbalanced **fluid volume** – 00025 180

Domain 3: Elimination and Exchange **181**

Class 1. Urinary function 183
Impaired urinary **elimination** – 00016 183
Readiness for enhanced urinary
   elimination – 00166 184
Functional urinary **incontinence** – 00020 185
Overflow urinary **incontinence** – 00176 186
Reflex urinary **incontinence** – 00018 187
Stress urinary **incontinence** – 00017 188
Urge urinary **incontinence** – 00019 189
Risk for urge urinary **incontinence** – 00022 190
Urinary retention – 00023 191
Class 2. Gastrointestinal function 192
Constipation – 00011 192
Risk for **constipation** – 00015 194
Chronic functional **constipation** – 00235 196
Risk for chronic functional **constipation** – 00236 198
Perceived **constipation** – 00012 199
Diarrhea – 00013 200

Dysfunctional **gastrointestinal motility** – 00196   201
Risk for dysfunctional **gastrointestinal**
    motility – 00197   202
Bowel **incontinence** – 00014   203
Class 3. Integumentary function
None at this time
Class 4. Respiratory function   204
Impaired **gas exchange** – 00030   204

Domain 4: Activity/Rest   **205**

Class 1. Sleep/rest   209
Insomnia – 00095   209
Sleep deprivation – 00096   210
Readiness for enhanced **sleep** – 00165   212
Disturbed **sleep pattern** – 00198   213
Class 2. Activity/exercise   214
Risk for **disuse syndrome** – 00040   214
Impaired bed **mobility** – 00091   215
Impaired physical **mobility** – 00085   216
Impaired wheelchair **mobility** – 00089   218
Impaired **sitting** – 00237   219
Impaired **standing** – 00238   220
Impaired **transfer ability** – 00090   221
Impaired **walking** – 00088   222
Class 3. Energy balance   223
Fatigue – 00093   223
Wandering – 00154   224
Class 4. Cardiovascular/pulmonary responses   225
Activity in**tolerance** – 00092   225
Risk for **activity** in**tolerance** – 00094   226
Ineffective **breathing pattern** – 00032   227
Decreased **cardiac output** – 00029   228
Risk for decreased **cardiac output** – 00240   230
Risk for impaired **cardiovascular function** – 00239   231
Risk for ineffective **gastrointestinal**
    perfusion – 00202   232
Risk for ineffective **renal perfusion** – 00203   233
Impaired **spontaneous ventilation** – 00033   234
Risk for decreased cardiac **tissue perfusion** – 00200   235
Risk for ineffective cerebral **tissue**
    perfusion – 00201   236
Ineffective peripheral **tissue perfusion** – 00204   237
Risk for ineffective peripheral **tissue**
    perfusion – 00228   238

Dysfunctional **ventilatory weaning response** – 00034   239

Class 5. Self-care   241

Impaired **home maintenance** – 00098   241
Bathing self-care deficit – 00108   242
Dressing self-care deficit – 00109   243
Feeding self-care deficit – 00102   244
Toileting self-care deficit – 00110   245
Readiness for enhanced **self-care** – 00182   246
Self-neglect – 00193   247

Domain 5: Perception/Cognition   **249**

Class 1. Attention   251
Unilateral neglect – 00123   251
Class 2. Orientation
None at this time
Class 3. Sensation/perception
None at this time
Class 4. Cognition   252
Acute **confusion** – 00128   252
Risk for acute **confusion** – 00173   253
Chronic **confusion** – 00129   254
Labile **emotional control** – 00251   255
Ineffective **impulse control** – 00222   256
Deficient **knowledge** – 00126   257
Readiness for enhanced **knowledge** – 00161   258
Impaired **memory** – 00131   259
Class 5. Communication   260
Readiness for enhanced **communication** – 00157   260
Impaired **verbal communication** – 00051   261

Domain 6: Self-Perception   **263**

Class 1. Self-concept   265
Readiness for enhanced **hope** – 00185   265
Hopelessness – 00124   266
Risk for compromised **human dignity** – 00174   267
Disturbed **personal identity** – 00121   268
Risk for disturbed **personal identity** – 00225   269
Readiness for enhanced **self-concept** – 00167   270
Class 2. Self-esteem   271
Chronic low **self-esteem** – 00119   271
Risk for chronic low **self-esteem** – 00224   272
Situational low **self-esteem** – 00120   273

Risk for situational low **self-esteem** – 00153   274
Class 3. Body image   275
Disturbed **body image** – 00118   275

Domain 7: Role Relationships   **277**

Class 1. Caregiving roles   279
Caregiver **role strain** – 00061   279
Risk for caregiver **role strain** – 00062   282
Impaired **parenting** – 00056   283
Readiness for enhanced **parenting** – 00164   286
Risk for impaired **parenting** – 00057   287
Class 2. Family relationships   289
Risk for impaired **attachment** – 00058   289
Dysfunctional **family processes** – 00063   290
Interrupted **family processes** – 00060   293
Readiness for enhanced **family processes** –
00159   294
Class 3. Role performance   295
Ineffective **relationship** – 00223   295
Readiness for enhanced **relationship** – 00207   296
Risk for ineffective **relationship** – 00229   297
Parental **role conflict** – 00064   298
Ineffective **role performance** – 00055   299
Impaired **social interaction** – 00052   301

Domain 8: Sexuality   **303**

Class 1. Sexual identity
None at present time
Class 2. Sexual function   305
Sexual dysfunction – 00059   305
Ineffective **sexuality pattern** – 00065   306
Class 3. Reproduction   307
Ineffective **childbearing process** – 00221   307
Readiness for enhanced **childbearing process** –
00208   309
Risk for ineffective **childbearing process** –
00227   310
Risk for disturbed **maternal–fetal dyad** – 00209   311

Domain 9: Coping/Stress Tolerance   **313**

Class 1. Post-trauma responses   315
Post-trauma syndrome – 00141   315
Risk for **post-trauma syndrome** – 00145   317
Rape-trauma syndrome – 00142   318

Relocation stress syndrome – 00114   319
Risk for **relocation stress syndrome** – 00149   320
Class 2. Coping responses   321
Ineffective **activity planning** – 00199   321
Risk for ineffective **activity planning** – 00226   322
Anxiety – 00146   323
Defensive **coping** – 00071   325
Ineffective **coping** – 00069   326
Readiness for enhanced **coping** – 00158   327
Ineffective community **coping** – 00077   328
Readiness for enhanced community **coping** – 00076   329
Compromised family **coping** – 00074   330
Disabled family **coping** – 00073   332
Readiness for enhanced family **coping** – 00075   333
Death anxiety – 00147   334
Ineffective **denial** – 00072   335
Fear – 00148   336
Grieving – 00136   338
Complicated **grieving** – 00135   339
Risk for complicated **grieving** – 00172   340
Impaired **mood regulation** – 00241   341
Readiness for enhanced **power** – 00187   342
Powerlessness – 00125   343
Risk for **power**lessness – 00152   344
Impaired **resilience** – 00210   345
Readiness for enhanced **resilience** – 00212   346
Risk for impaired **resilience** – 00211   347
Chronic **sorrow** – 00137   348
Stress overload – 00177   349
Class 3. Neurobehavioral stress   350
Decreased intracranial **adaptive capacity** – 00049   350
Autonomic dysreflexia – 00009   351
Risk for **autonomic dysreflexia** – 00010   352
Disorganized infant **behavior** – 00116   354
Readiness for enhanced **organized** infant
   behavior – 00117   356
Risk for **disorganized** infant **behavior** – 00115   357

Domain 10: Life Principles   **359**
Class 1. Values
None at this time
Class 2. Beliefs   361
Readiness for enhanced **spiritual well-being** –
   00068   361

Class 3. Value/belief/action congruence   363

Readiness for enhanced **decision-making** – 00184   363

Decisional conflict – 00083   364

Impaired **emancipated decision-making** – 00242   365

Readiness for enhanced **emancipated decision-making** – 00243   366

Risk for impaired **emancipated decision-making** – 00244   367

Moral distress – 00175   368

Impaired **religiosity** – 00169   369

Readiness for enhanced **religiosity** – 00171   370

Risk for impaired **religiosity** – 00170   371

Spiritual distress – 00066   372

Risk for **spiritual** distress – 00067   374

Domain 11: Safety/Protection   **375**

Class 1. Infection   379

Risk for **infection** – 00004   379

Class 2. Physical injury   380

Ineffective **airway clearance** – 00031   380

Risk for **aspiration** – 00039   381

Risk for **bleeding** – 00206   382

Risk for **dry eye** – 00219   383

Risk for **falls** – 00155   384

Risk for **injury** – 00035   386

Risk for corneal **injury** – 00245   387

Risk for perioperative **positioning injury** – 00087   388

Risk for **thermal injury** – 00220   389

Risk for urinary tract **injury** – 00250   390

Impaired **dentition** – 00048   391

Impaired oral **mucous membrane** – 00045   392

Risk for impaired oral **mucous membrane** – 00247   394

Risk for peripheral neurovascular **dysfunction** – 00086   395

Risk for **pressure ulcer** – 00249   396

Risk for **shock** – 00205   398

Impaired **skin integrity** – 00046   399

Risk for impaired **skin integrity** – 00047   400

Risk for **sudden infant death syndrome** – 00156   401

Risk for **suffocation** – 00036   402

Delayed **surgical recovery** – 00100   403

Risk for delayed **surgical recovery** – 00246   404
Impaired **tissue integrity** – 00044   405
Risk for impaired **tissue integrity** – 00248   406
Risk for **trauma** – 00038   407
Risk for vascular **trauma** – 00213   409
Class 3. Violence   410
Risk for **other-directed violence** – 00138   410
Risk for **self-directed violence** – 00140   411
Self-mutilation – 00151   412
Risk for **self-mutilation** – 00139   414
Risk for **suicide** – 00150   416
Class 4. Environmental hazards   418
Contamination – 00181   418
Risk for **contamination** – 00180   420
Risk for **poisoning** – 00037   421
Class 5. Defensive processes   422
Risk for adverse **reaction to iodinated
contrast media** – 00218   422
Risk for **allergy response** – 00217   423
Latex allergy response – 00041   424
Risk for **latex allergy response** – 00042   425
Class 6. Thermoregulation   426
Risk for imbalanced **body temperature** – 00005   426
Hyperthermia – 00007   427
Hypothermia – 00006   428
Risk for **hypothermia** – 00253   430
Risk for perioperative **hypothermia** – 00254   432
Ineffective **thermoregulation** – 00008   433

Domain 12: Comfort   **435**
Class 1. Physical comfort   437
Impaired **comfort** – 00214   437
Readiness for enhanced **comfort** – 00183   438
Nausea – 00134   439
Acute **pain** – 00132   440
Chronic **pain** – 00133   442
Labor **pain** – 00256   444
Chronic **pain syndrome** – 00255   445
Class 2. Environmental comfort   437
Impaired **comfort** – 00214   437
Readiness for enhanced **comfort** – 00183   438
Class 3. Social comfort   437
Impaired **comfort** – 00214   437

Readiness for enhanced **comfort** – 00183   438
Risk for **loneliness** – 00054   446
Social isolation – 00053   447

Domain 13: Growth/Development   **449**

Class 1. Growth   451
Risk for disproportionate **growth** – 00113   451
Class 2. Development   452
Risk for delayed **development** – 00112   452

**Nursing Diagnoses Accepted for Development
and Clinical Validation 2015–2017**   **455**
Disturbed **energy field** – 00050   455

**PART 4   NANDA INTERNATIONAL, INC.
2015–2017**   **457**

NANDA International Position Statements   **459**
The use of Taxonomy II as an assessment
framework   459
The structure of the Nursing Diagnosis statement
when included in a care plan   459

**NANDA International Processes and Procedures
for Diagnosis Submission and Review**   **461**
NANDA-I Diagnosis Submission: Level
of evidence criteria   461

Glossary of Terms   **464**
Nursing diagnosis   464
Diagnostic axes   465
Components of a nursing diagnosis   467
Definitions for classification of nursing diagnoses   468
References   469

An Invitation to Join NANDA International   **470**
NANDA International: A Member-Driven Organization   470
Our vision   470
Our mission   470
Our purpose   470
Our history   471

NANDA International's Commitment   471
Involvement Opportunities   472
Why join NANDA-I?   472
Who is using the NANDA International Taxonomy?   473

Index   *475*

Visit the companion website for this book at www.wiley.com/ go/nursingdiagnoses

NANDA International, Inc. Guidelines for Copyright Permission

The materials presented in this book are copyrighted and all copyright laws apply. For any usage other than reading or consulting the book in the English language, a licence is required from Wiley.

Examples of such reuse include but are not restricted to:

- A publishing house, other organization, or individual wishing to translate the entire book, or parts thereof.
- An author or publishing house wishing to use the entire nursing diagnosis taxonomy, or parts thereof, in a commercially available textbook or nursing manual.
- An author or company wishing to use the nursing diagnosis taxonomy in audio-visual materials.
- A software developer or computer-based patient record vendor wishing to use the nursing diagnosis taxonomy in English in a software program or application (for example, an electronic health record, an e-learning course, or an electronic application for a smartphone or other electronic device).
- A nursing school, researcher, professional organization, or health-care organization wishing to use the nursing diagnosis taxonomy in an educational program.
- A researcher wishing to use the taxonomy for non-commercial academic research purposes. Please be aware that the proposal will be submitted by Wiley to NANDA-I for approval before permission is granted. Researchers are encouraged to submit the outcomes of their research to the *International Journal of Nursing Knowledge*, and to present the results at a NANDA-I conference, as appropriate.
- A hospital wishing to integrate the nursing diagnosis taxonomy into their own electronic health records.
- Any of the usages outlined above in a language other than English.

Please send all requests by e-mail to: **nanda@wiley.com** or by post to:

NANDA International Copyright Requests
Global Rights Department
John Wiley & Sons, Ltd
The Atrium
Southern Gate
Chichester
West Sussex
PO19 8SQ
UK

Translations Terms and Conditions

Terms and conditions for translations will be as follows:

- There will be no buy-back by Wiley or NANDA-I of unsold copies of any translations at the time that the next edition is released.
- Publishers cannot add or remove any content from the original version provided by Wiley. This includes the addition of forewords, new prefaces or comments by translators or other parties. The only exception to this is the addition, under the name of the editor, of names of the translators in each language, who should be identified as translators (not as authors or editors).
- Publishers will be required to submit the name, qualifications and résumé of the chief translator for approval prior to commencing any translation work.
- Publishers must also submit both the cover design and the manuscript of the translation to Wiley for approval by NANDA-I prior to printing the translation. NANDA-I requires up to 12 weeks to complete this approval process, so it should be built into the production schedule.
- Any and all changes requested by NANDA-I must be included in the translation, and publishers shall be required to submit page proofs for a final check before printing the translation.

Publishers will also be required to grant Wiley the right to re-use and license the translation to third parties in electronic format. To this end, a customized version of the following Clause will be included in all translation licenses:

> The Proprietor shall have the non-exclusive right to use the Translation in any form of electronic media now known or later developed ("Electronic Rights"), to update or arrange for others to update the

electronic version of the Translation when new editions of the Work become available and to sublicense such rights to third parties. The Publisher shall notify the Proprietor of any suitable third parties who may be interested in licensing the Electronic Rights from the Proprietor. The Publisher shall provide the digital files for the Translation to the Proprietor in a format to be agreed, as soon as reasonably practicable, but not later than xx months after signature of this Agreement. In consideration of the foregoing rights in this clause 1(e), the Proprietor shall pay to the Publisher an annual royalty to be agreed.

For the avoidance of doubt, we wish to make clear that this does not include e-book rights (unabridged verbatim electronic copies of the print Translation), and is only intended, for example, for software development usages.

Preface

The 2015–2017 edition of the classic NANDA International, Inc. text, *Nursing Diagnoses: Definitions & Classification*, provides more clinically applicable diagnoses as a result of the Diagnostic Development Committee's attentiveness to the potential translations of the diagnostic label, definition, defining characteristics, related factors, and risk factors. In the past, a number of nurses asked about the applicability of our work in their own countries and jurisdiction. Changes within the 2015–2017 edition have been implemented to incorporate the diversity and practice differences across the world. The latest edition is not only considered a language, but, truthfully, it is a body of nursing knowledge. These new and revised diagnoses are based on the state of evidence around the world, and they are submitted by nurses, reviewed and revised by nurses, and approved by expert nurse diagnosticians, researchers, and educators. The latest edition enhances the cultural applicability with 25 new nursing diagnoses and 13 revised diagnoses. Additionally, the text includes changes to the official NANDA-I nursing diagnosis category definitions (problem-focused, risk, health promotion), and the overall nursing diagnosis definition.

NANDA International, Inc. (NANDA-I) is a not-for-profit membership organization. This means that with the exception of our business management and administration functions, all of our work is accomplished by volunteers. Some of the world's most talented nurse scientists and scholars are or have been NANDA-I volunteers. Contrary to most business entities, there is not an office somewhere with nurse researchers working on nursing diagnoses. The volunteers are people like you and me who give their time and expertise to NANDA-I, because of their strongly held beliefs about the importance of patient care and the contributions that nursing and nurses can and do make to society.

With the publication of each new edition of our work, more translations are added. I am delighted that the work is published in numerous languages for this international membership organization. Our relationship with our publishing partner, Wiley Blackwell, has evolved over the past five years. One of the arrangements is to ensure that each and every translation is accurate and exact. Together with our publishers, we now have a robust quality assurance mechanism in place to ensure the accuracy of each translation. The source document for each translation is always this, the American English version. We are deeply committed to ensuring the integrity of our work worldwide and invite you to support us in this quest in order to improve patient safety and the consistency of high-quality evidence-based care. As a not-for-profit organization, we obviously need an income to run the organization, facilitate meetings of our committees and Board of Directors, sponsor our website and knowledge base, and support educational offerings and conferences throughout the world, and this comes from the licenses we sell for the publishing and use of our work in electronic form. For the first time this year, we will be offering an electronic application of the NANDA-I terminology, complete with an assessment feature and decision support for some of the most commonly used diagnoses. This type of work, too, requires funding for development and testing.

As an international organization, we truly value cultural diversity and practice differences. However, as the provider of the world's most successful standardized nursing diagnostic language and knowledge, we have a duty to provide you with exactly that: standardized nursing diagnostic knowledge. We do not support changing diagnoses at the request of translators or clinical specialists in just one edition in a particular language, when diagnosis lacks applicability in that particular culture. This is because we are deeply committed to realizing the clinical benefits of nursing diagnostic knowledge content for diverse cultures and specialties. We do not believe that we should be supporting the censorship of clinical information in this text. As a registered nurse you are accountable for appropriate diagnosis, and the use of appropriate terms, within your practice. Clearly, it would be inappropriate for all of us to use each and every one of the diagnoses in this edition, because none of us could claim competence in every sphere of nursing practice simultaneously. Clinically safe nurses are reflective practitioners; a central component to safe practice is to thoroughly understand one's own clinical competence. It is highly likely that there are numerous diagnoses in this edition that you will never use in your own practice; others you may use daily. This also links to the issue of cultural applicability because if, when studying this edition, you find a diagnosis that is not applicable to your practice or culture, it is within your gift simply not to use it. However, based on my own varied clinical experiences as a registered nurse, I would implore you to not ignore completely those diagnoses that might at first seem culturally awkward. We live in a transcultural and highly mobile society, and exploring those diagnoses that might initially seem unusual can challenge your thinking and open up new possibilities and understanding. This is all part of being a reflective and life-long learning practitioner.

Each diagnosis has been the product of one or more of our NANDA-I volunteers or NANDA-I users, and most have a defined evidence base. Each and every new and revised diagnosis will have been refined and debated by our DDC members before finally being submitted to NANDA-I members for a vote of approval. Only if our members vote positively for the inclusion of a new or refined diagnosis does the work "make it" into the published edition. However, if you feel that a particular diagnosis is incorrect and requires revision, we welcome your views. You should contact the chair of the DDC through our website. Please provide as much evidence as possible to support your views. By working in this way, rather than changing just one translation or edition, we can ensure that our nursing diagnostic knowledge continues to have integrity and consistency, and that all benefit from the wisdom and work of individual scholars. We welcome you to submit new diagnoses, as well as revisions to current diagnoses, by using the submission guidelines found on our website.

One of the key membership developments in the past few years has been educational content published by Artmed/Panamericana Editora Ltda. (Porto Alegre, Brazil), which compiles educational modules, published in Portuguese, known as PRONANDA. A similar offering will soon be provided in Spanish. Other developments are the NANDA-I database for researchers and others needing to design electronic content. The Educational and Research Committee is preparing new educational materials to help with the educational process. The aim of this new edition of our book is to support those learning to diagnose, and to enable decision-makers to have access to information about diagnoses that describe the problems, risks, and health promotion needs of persons, families, groups, and communities. I personally was very interested in membership of NANDA-I because the body of nursing knowledge content is essential in the design of clinical decision support logic for electronic health record systems and for data analysis.

I want to commend the work of all NANDA-I volunteers, committee members, chairpersons, and members of the Board of Directors for their time, commitment and enthusiasm, and ongoing support. I want to thank our staff, led by our CEO/Executive Director, Dr. T. Heather Herdman, for its efforts and support. I appreciate the publishing partnership with Wiley-Blackwell as well as our translation and global publishing partners, which support the dissemination of knowledge content and the database developed by NANDA-I.

My special thanks to the members of the Diagnosis Development Committee for their outstanding and timely efforts to review and edit the diagnoses that are the core portion of this book, and especially for the leadership of the DDC by our Chair since 2010, Dr. Shigemi Kamitsuru. This wonderful committee, with representation from North and Latin America, Europe, and Asia, is the true "power house" of the NANDA-I knowledge content, and I am deeply impressed and pleased by the astonishingly comprehensive work of these volunteers over the years.

Finally, when I first learned about and learned to use nursing diagnoses 30 years ago, I never imagined that I would one day be the President of NANDA-I, setting the agenda for this incredible body of nursing knowledge. I welcomed the opportunity to volunteer for NANDA-I, because I found value in supporting the advancement of meaningful and useful knowledge to support nurses and students of nursing. All registered nurses and advanced practice nurses are making clinical decisions within practice, education, administration of critical thinking processes, and informatics clinical decision support system designs. For these reasons, NANDA International, Inc. has had, and continues to have, a role in improving the quality of evidence-based care and the safety of patient care, and remains the core base of knowledge for nursing professionals.

Jane M. Brokel, PhD, RN, FNI
President, NANDA International, Inc.

Introduction

This book is divided into four parts:

- **Part 1** provides the introduction to the NANDA International, Inc. (NANDA-I) Taxonomy of Nursing Diagnoses. Taxonomy II organizes the diagnoses into domains and classes. Information is provided on diagnoses that are new to, or were removed from, the taxonomy during the past review cycle.
- **Part 2** provides chapters on the basics of nursing diagnosis, assessment, and clinical judgment. These chapters are primarily written for students, clinicians, and educators. The accompanying website includes educational materials designed to support students and faculty in understanding and teaching this material. Changes to the chapters were made based on incredibly helpful feedback received from readers around the world, and questions that we receive on a daily basis at NANDA International, Inc.
- **Part 3** provides the core contents of the *NANDA International Nursing Diagnoses: Definitions & Classification* book: the 235 diagnoses themselves, including definitions, defining characteristics, risk factors, and related factors, as appropriate. The diagnoses are categorized using Taxonomy II, and ordered by Domain first, then Class, and then alphabetically within each class (in the English language) by the focus of each diagnosis. We recommend that all translations maintain this order, (Domain, class, alphabetic order in their own language), to facilitate ease of discussion between inter-language groups.
- **Part 4** includes information that relates specifically to NANDA International. Information on processes and procedures related to review of NANDA-I diagnoses, the submission process, and level of evidence criteria are provided. A glossary of terms is given. Finally, information specific to the organization and the benefits of membership are outlined.

How to Use This Book

As noted above, the nursing diagnoses are listed by Domain first, then by Class, and then alphabetically within each class (in the English language) by the focus of each diagnosis. For example, *Impaired standing* is listed under Domain 4 (Activity / Rest), Class 2 (Activity / Exercise):

Domain 4: Activity / Rest
    Class 2: Activity / Exercise
        Impaired **standing** (00238)

It is our hope that the organization of *NANDA-I Nursing Diagnoses: Definitions & Classification, 2015–2017* will make it efficient and effective to use. We welcome your feedback. If you have suggestions, please send them by email to: execdir@nanda.org.

About the Companion Website

This book is accompanied by a companion website:

www.wiley.com/go/nursingdiagnoses

The website includes:

- Videos
- References
- Weblinks

Part 1
Changes to the NANDA International Terminology

Introduction   **3**

What's New in the 2015–2017 Edition of *Diagnoses*
and *Classification*?   **4**
  Acknowledgments   4
  Changes to Health Promotion and Risk Diagnoses   5
  New Nursing Diagnoses, 2015–2017   5
  Revised Nursing Diagnoses, 2015–2017   7
  Changes to Slotting of Current Diagnoses within
    the NANDA-I Taxonomy II, 2015–2017   11
  Revisions to Nursing Diagnosis Labels within
    the NANDA-I Taxonomy II, 2015–2017   11
  Nursing Diagnoses Removed from the NANDA-I
    Taxonomy II, 2015–2017   11
  Standardization of Diagnostic Indicator Terms   12
  Other Changes Made in the 2015–2017 Edition   15

NANDA International, Inc. Nursing Diagnoses: Definitions & Classification 2015–2017,
Tenth Edition. Edited by T. Heather Herdman and Shigemi Kamitsuru.
© 2014 NANDA International, Inc. Published 2014 by John Wiley & Sons, Ltd.
Companion website: www.wiley.com/go/nursingdiagnoses

Introduction

T. Heather Herdman, RN, PhD, FNI

In this section, introductory information on the new edition of the *NANDA International Taxonomy, 2015–2017* is presented. This includes an overview of major changes to this edition: new and revised diagnoses, changes to slotting within the taxonomy, changes to diagnostic labels, and diagnoses that were removed or retired.

Those individuals and groups who submitted new or revised diagnoses for approval are identified. A historical perspective on submitters to the complete NANDA-I terminology, which was developed by Betty Ackley for the previous edition of this book, has been updated to include this information, and is now available on our website, at www.nanda.org.

A description of editorial changes is also provided; readers will note that nearly every diagnosis has some changes as we have worked to increase the standardization of the terms used within our diagnostic indicators (defining characteristics, related factors, risk factors).

I would like to offer a particularly significant note of appreciation to Dr. Susan Gallagher-Lepak, of the University of Wisconsin – Green Bay College of Professional Studies, who worked with me over a period of several months to standardize these terms. Additional thanks go to my co-editor, Dr. Shigemi Kamitsuru, who further reviewed and revised our work, which then came full circle back to us for consensus. This process has been a daunting one, with more than 5,600 individual terms requiring review! However, the standardization of these terms has now enabled the coding of all of the diagnostic indicator terms, facilitating their use as assessment data within electronic health records, leading to the development within those records of critical clinical decision support tools for professional nurses. These codes are now available on the NANDA-I website.

NANDA International, Inc. Nursing Diagnoses: Definitions & Classification 2015–2017, Tenth Edition. Edited by T. Heather Herdman and Shigemi Kamitsuru.
© 2014 NANDA International, Inc. Published 2014 by John Wiley & Sons, Ltd.
Companion website: www.wiley.com/go/nursingdiagnoses

What's New in the 2015–2017 Edition of *Diagnoses and Classification*?

Changes have been made in this edition based on feedback from users, to address the needs of both students and clinicians, as well as to provide additional support to educators. All of the chapters are new for this edition, with the exception of the chapter *NANDA-I Taxonomy: Specifications and Definitions*, which provides a revision of that found in the previous edition. There are corresponding web-based presentations available for teachers and students that augment the information found within the chapters; icons appear in chapters that have these accompanying support tools.

A new chapter, focusing on *Frequently Asked Questions*, is included. These questions represent the most common questions we receive through the NANDA-I website, and when we present at conferences around the globe.

Acknowledgments

It goes without saying that the dedication of several individuals to the work of NANDA International, Inc. (NANDA-I) is evident in their donation of time and effort to the improvement of the NANDA-I terminology and taxonomy. This text represents the culmination of the tireless volunteer work of a group of very dedicated, extremely talented individuals who have developed, revised, and studied nursing diagnoses for more than 40 years.

Additionally, we would like to take the opportunity to acknowledge and personally thank the following individuals for their contributions to this particular edition of the NANDA-I text.

Chapter Authors

■ The Basics of Nursing Diagnosis – Susan Gallagher-Lepak, PhD, RN

NANDA International, Inc. Nursing Diagnoses: Definitions & Classification 2015–2017,
Tenth Edition. Edited by T. Heather Herdman and Shigemi Kamitsuru.
© 2014 NANDA International, Inc. Published 2014 by John Wiley & Sons, Ltd.
Companion website: www.wiley.com/go/nursingdiagnoses

Chapter Reviewers

◼ An introduction to the NANDA-I taxonomy – Kay Avant, PhD, RN, FNI, FAAN; Gunn von Krogh, RN, PhD

Reviewer for Standardization of Diagnostic Terms

◼ Susan Gallagher-Lepak, PhD, RN

Please contact us at execdir@nanda.org if you have questions on any of the content or if you find errors, so that these may be corrected for future publication and translation.

T. Heather Herdman, PhD, RN, FNI
Shigemi Kamitsuru, PhD, RN, FNI
Editors
NANDA International, Inc.

Changes to Health Promotion and Risk Diagnoses

The overall definitions for nursing diagnoses were changed during this cycle. These changes had impacts on the way in which current risk and health promotion diagnoses should be defined, so you will note changes to every definition of these diagnoses. These changes were presented to the NANDA-I membership, and approved via online voting.

The risk diagnoses were changed to eliminate "risk" from the definition, which has now been replaced by the use of the word "vulnerable."

The health promotion diagnoses were changed to ensure that the definitions reflected that these diagnoses are appropriate for use at any stage in the health–illness continuum, and that a state of balance or health is not required. Similarly, defining characteristics of these diagnoses needed to change, as in many cases they represented healthy, stable states. All of the defining characteristics now begin with the phrase "Expresses the desire to enhance," because health promotion requires the willingness of the patient to improve upon his current status, whatever that might be.

New Nursing Diagnoses, 2015–2017

A significant body of work representing new and revised nursing diagnoses was submitted to the NANDA-I Diagnosis Development Committee, with a substantial portion of that work being presented to the NANDA-I membership for consideration in this review cycle. NANDA-I would like to take this opportunity to congratulate those submitters who successfully met the level of evidence criteria with their submissions and/or revisions. Twenty-five new diagnoses were approved by the Diagnosis Development Committee, the NANDA-I Board of Directors, and the NANDA-I membership (Table I.1).

Table I.1   *New NANDA-I Nursing Diagnoses, 2015–2017*

Approved diagnosis (New)	Submitter(s)
Domain 1. Health Promotion	
Frail elderly syndrome	Margarita Garrido Abejar; Mª Dolores Serrano Parra; Rosa Mª Fuentes Chacón
Risk for **frail elderly syndrome**	Margarita Garrido Abejar; Mª Dolores Serrano Parra; Rosa Mª Fuentes Chacón
Domain 2. Nutrition	
Risk for **overweight**	T. Heather Herdman, PhD, RN, FNI
Overweight	T. Heather Herdman, PhD, RN, FNI
Obesity	T. Heather Herdman, PhD, RN, FNI
Domain 3. Elimination and Exchange	
Chronic **functional constipation**	T. Heather Herdman, PhD, RN, FNI
Domain 4. Activity / Rest	
Impaired **sitting**	Christian Heering, EdN, RN
Impaired **standing**	Christian Heering, EdN, RN
Risk for decreased **cardiac output**	Eduarda Ribeiro dos Santos, PhD, RN; Vera Lúcia Regina Maria, PhD, RN; Mariana Fernandes de Souza, PhD, RN; Maria Gaby Rivero de Gutierrez, PhD, RN; Alba Lúcia Bottura Leite de Barros, PhD, RN
Risk for impaired **cardiovascular function**	María Begoña Sánchez Gómez PhD(c), RN; Gonzalo Duarte Clíments PhD(c), RN
Domain 9. Coping / Stress Tolerance	
Impaired **mood regulation**	Heidi Bjørge, MnSc, RN
Domain 10. Life Principles	
Impaired **emancipated decision-making**	Ruth Wittmann-Price, PhD, RN
Readiness for enhanced **emancipated decision-making**	Ruth Wittmann-Price, PhD, RN
Risk for impaired **emancipated decision-making**	Ruth Wittmann-Price, PhD, RN

Table I.1   *Continued*

Approved diagnosis (New)	Submitter(s)
Domain 11. Safety / Protection	
Risk for **corneal injury**	Andreza Werli-Alvarenga, PhD, RN; Tânia Couto Machado Chianca, PhD, RN; Flávia Falci Ercole, PhD, RN
Risk for **impaired oral mucous membrane**	Emilia Campos de Carvalho, PhD, RN; Cristina Mara Zamarioli, RN; Ana Paula Neroni Stina, RN; Vanessa dos Santos Ribeiro, undergraduate student; Sheila Ramalho Coelho Vasconcelos de Morais, MNSc, RN
Risk for **pressure ulcer**	T. Heather Herdman, PhD, RN, FNI; Cássia Teixeira dos Santos MSN, RN; Miriam de Abreu Almeida PhD, RN; Amália de Fátima Lucena PhD, RN
Risk for **delayed surgical recovery**	Rosimere Ferreira Santana, PhD, RN; Dayana Medeiros do Amaral, BSN; Shimmenes Kamacael Pereira, MSN, RN; Tallita Mello Delphino, MSN, RN; Deborah Marinho da Silva, BSN; Thais da Silva Soares, BSN
Risk for **impaired tissue integrity**	Katiucia Martins Barros MS, RN; Daclé Vilma Carvalho, PhD, RN
Risk for **urinary tract injury**	Danielle Cristina Garbuio, MS; Elaine Santos, MS, RN; Emília Campos de Carvalho, PhD, RN; Tânia Couto Machado Chianca, PhD, RN; Anamaria Alves Napoleão, PhD, RN
Labile **emotional control**	Gülendam Hakverdioğlu Yönt, PhD, RN; Esra Akın Korhan, PhD, RN; Leyla Khorshid, PhD, RN
Risk for **hypothermia**	T. Heather Herdman, PhD, RN, FNI
Risk for **perioperative hypothermia**	Manuel Schwanda, BSc.,RN; Prof. Marianne Kriegl, Mag.; Maria Müller Staub, PhD, EdN, RN, FEANS
Domain 12. Comfort	
Chronic pain syndrome	T. Heather Herdman, PhD, RN, FNI
Labor pain	Simone Roque Mazoni, PhD, RN; Emilia Campos de Carvalho, PhD, RN

Revised Nursing Diagnoses, 2015–2017

Thirteen diagnoses were revised during this cycle; five were approved by the DDC through the expedited review process and eight were revised through the standard review process. Table I.2 shows those

Table I.2   *Revised NANDA-I Nursing Diagnoses, 2015–2017*

Approved diagnosis (Revised)	Revision					Comment	Submitter(s)
	DC removed	DC added	ReF/RiF removed	ReF/RiF added	Definition revised		
Domain 2. Nutrition							
Ineffective **breastfeeding**	1	1	1	10	X	■ Definition reflects change in focus from the attachment/ bonding process to that of nutrition ■ 2 defining characteristics reassigned to related factors	T. Heather Herdman, RN, PhD, FNI
Interrupted **breastfeeding**	6	1		1	X	■ Definition reflects change in focus from attachment/bonding process to that of nutrition ■ 1 defining characteristic reassigned to related factor	T. Heather Herdman, RN, PhD, FNI
Readiness for enhanced **breastfeeding**	1	2			X	■ Definition reflects change in focus from attachment/bonding process to that of nutrition	T. Heather Herdman, RN, PhD, FNI
Excess fluid **volume**		2					Eneida Rejane Rabelo da Silva ScD, RN; Quenia Camille Soares Martins ScD, RN; Graziella Badin Aliti ScD, RN

Table 1.2 Continued

Approved diagnosis (Revised)	Revision					Comment	Submitter(s)
	DC removed	DC added	ReF/RiF removed	ReF/RiF added	Definition revised		
Domain 4. Activity / Rest							
Impaired physical mobility		1					Eneida Rejane Rabelo da Silva ScD, RN; Angelita Paganin MSc, RN
Domain 7. Role Relationships							
Risk for caregiver role strain					X	▪ Definition revised to be consistent with the problem-focused definition	
Domain 10. Life Principles							
Spiritual distress	4	7		11	X		Silvia Caldeira PhD, RN; Emilia Campos de Carvalho PhD, RN; Margarida Vieira PhD, RN
Domain 11. Safety / Protection							
Risk for imbalanced body temperature				10		▪ Diagnosis revised to incorporate neonatal characteristics	T. Heather Herdman, RN, PhD, FNI
Hyperthermia		9	1	3	X	▪ Diagnosis revised to incorporate neonatal characteristics	T. Heather Herdman, RN, PhD, FNI
Hypothermia		24	4	8	X	▪ Diagnosis revised to incorporate neonatal characteristics	T. Heather Herdman, RN, PhD, FNI

Continued

Table 1.2 *Continued*

Approved diagnosis (Revised)	Revision				Definition revised	Comment	Submitter(s)
	DC removed	DC added	ReF/RiF removed	ReF/RiF added			
Delayed **surgical recovery**	6	4	1	8			Rosimere Ferreira Santana, Associate PhD, RN; Shimmenes Kamacael Pereira, MSN, RN; Tallita Mello Delphino, MSN, RN; Dayana Medeiros do Amaral, BSN; Deborah Marinho da Silva, BSN; Thais da Silva Soares, BSN; Marcos Venicius de Oliveira Lopes, PhD, RN
Impaired **tissue integrity**			3	10	X		Katiucia Martins Barros MS, RN; Daclé Vilma Carvalho PhD, RN
Domain 12. Comfort							
Acute **pain**	6	6	1	3	X		T. Heather Herdman, RN, PhD, FNI
Chronic **pain**	10	5	2	35	X		T. Heather Herdman, RN, PhD, FNI

DC, defining characteristic; ReF, related factor; RiF, risk factor.

diagnoses, highlights the revisions that were made for each of them, and identifies the submitters.

Changes to Slotting of Current Diagnoses within the NANDA-I Taxonomy II, 2015–2017

A review of the current taxonomic structure, and slotting of diagnoses within that structure, led to some changes in the way some diagnoses are now classified within the NANDA-I taxonomy. Five nursing diagnoses were reslotted within the NANDA-I taxonomy; these are noted in Table I.3 with their previous and new places in the taxonomy noted.

Table I.3   *Slotting Changes to NANDA-I Nursing Diagnoses, 2015–2017*

Nursing diagnosis	Previous slotting		New slotting	
	Domain	Class	Domain	Class
Noncompliance	Life Principles	Value/Belief/ Action Congruence	Health Promotion	Health Management
Ineffective **breastfeeding**[1]	Role Relationship	Caregiving Roles	Nutrition	Ingestion
Interrupted **breastfeeding**[1]	Role Relationship	Caregiving Roles	Nutrition	Ingestion
Readiness for enhanced **breastfeeding**[1]	Role Relationship	Caregiving Roles	Nutrition	Ingestion
Readiness for enhanced **hope**	Life Principles	Values	Self-Perception	Self-Concept
Risk for **loneliness**	Self-Perception	Self-Concept	Comfort	Social Comfort

[1] Reslotting due to diagnosis revision, including definition change.

Revisions to Nursing Diagnosis Labels within the NANDA-I Taxonomy II, 2015–2017

Changes were made in five diagnosis labels. These changes, and their rationale, are shown in Table I.4.

Nursing Diagnoses Removed from the NANDA-I Taxonomy II, 2015–2017

Seven nursing diagnoses were removed from the taxonomy, either because they were slotted for removal if they were not updated to bring them to a level of evidence of 2.1, due to a change in the classification

Table I.4 *Revisions to Nursing Diagnosis Labels of NANDA-I Nursing Diagnoses, 2015–2017*

Previous diagnostic label	New diagnostic label	Rationale
Ineffective **self-health management**	Ineffective **health management**	There is no need to include the "self" in the diagnostic label, as the focus of the diagnosis is assumed to be the individual unless otherwise stated.
Readiness for enhanced **self-health management**	Readiness for enhanced **health management**	There is no need to include the "self" in the diagnostic label, as the focus of the diagnosis is assumed to be the individual unless otherwise stated.
Ineffective family **therapeutic regimen management**	Ineffective family **health management**	Definition is consistent with the individual health management diagnoses, therefore the diagnostic label should reflect the same diagnostic focus.
Impaired individual **resilience**	Impaired **resilience**	There is no need to include "individual" in the diagnostic label, as the focus of the diagnosis is assumed to be the individual unless otherwise stated.
Risk for compromised **resilience**	Risk for impaired **resilience**	The problem-focused diagnosis carries the diagnostic label, Impaired resilience, and the definition of the risk diagnosis is consistent with that diagnosis.

of level of evidence supporting the diagnosis, or because new diagnoses replaced them. Table I.5 provides information on each of the diagnoses that were removed from the taxonomy.

Standardization of Diagnostic Indicator Terms

For the past two cycles of this book, work has been slowly underway to decrease variation in the terms used for defining characteristics, related factors, and risk factors. This work was undertaken in earnest during this cycle of the book, with several months being dedicated for the review, revision, and standardization of terms being used. This was no easy task, and it involved many hours of review, literature searches, discussion, and consultation with clinical experts in different fields.

The process we used included individual review of assigned domains, followed by a second reviewer independently reviewing the current

Table I.5   *Nursing Diagnoses Removed from the NANDA-I Taxonomy II, 2015–2017*

Retired diagnostic label	New diagnostic label	Rationale
Disturbed **energy field** (00050)	–	Removed from taxonomy, but reassigned to level of evidence (LOE) 1.2, Theoretical Level, for Development and Validation (LOE 1.2 is not accepted for publication and inclusion in the taxonomy; all literature support currently provided for this diagnosis is regarding intervention rather than for the nursing diagnosis itself)
Adult **failure to thrive** (00101)	**Frail elderly syndrome**	New diagnosis replaced previous diagnosis
Readiness for enhanced **immunization status** (00186)	–	Diagnosis was indicated for retirement in the 2012–2014 edition. Additionally, this content is currently covered within the diagnosis, Readiness for enhanced **health management**
Imbalanced **nutrition**: more than body requirements (00001)	**Overweight Obesity**	New diagnoses replaced previous diagnosis
Risk for imbalanced **nutrition**: more than body requirements (00003)	Risk for **overweight**	New diagnosis replaced previous diagnosis
Impaired **environmental interpretation syndrome** (00127)	–	Diagnosis was indicated for removal in the 2012–2014 edition unless additional work was completed to bring it into compliance with the definition of syndrome diagnoses. This work was not completed.
Delayed **growth and development** (00111)		Diagnosis was indicated for removal in the 2012–2014 edition, unless additional work was completed to separate the foci of (1) growth and (2) development into separate diagnostic concepts. This work was not completed.

and newly recommended terms. The two reviewers then met together, either in person or via web-based video conferencing, and reviewed each and every line a third time, together. Once consensus was reached, the third reviewer then took the current terms and recommended terms, and independently reviewed these. Any discrepancies were discussed until consensus was reached. After the entire process was completed for every diagnosis, including new and revised diagnoses, a process of filtering for similar terms was begun. For example, every term with the stem "pulmo-" was searched, to ensure that consistency was maintained. Common phrases were also used to filter, such as verbalizes, reports, states; lack of; insufficient; inadequate; excess, etc. This process continued until the team was unable to find additional terms that had not previously been reviewed.

That said, we know the work is not done, it is not perfect, and there may be disagreements with some of the changes that were made. We can tell you that there are more than 5,600 diagnostic indicators within the terminology, and we believe that we have made a good first effort at standardization of the terms.

The benefits of this are many, but three are perhaps the most notable:

1. **Translations should be improved**. There have been multiple questions over the last two editions that were difficult to answer. Some examples include:

    (a) When you say *lack* in English, does that mean *absence of* or *insufficient*? The answer is often "Both!" Although the duality of this word is well accepted in English, the lack of clarity does not support the clinician in any language, and it makes it very difficult to translate into languages in which a different word would be used depending on the intended meaning.

    (b) Is there a reason why some defining characteristics are noted in the singular and yet in another diagnosis the same characteristic is noted in the plural (e.g., absence of significant other(s), absence of significant other, absence of significant others)?

    (c) There are many terms that are similar, or that are examples of other terms used in the terminology. For example, what is the difference between: *abnormal skin color (e.g., pale, dusky), color changes, cyanosis, pale, skin color changes, slight cyanosis*? Are the differences significant? Could these be combined into one term? Some of the translations are almost the same (e.g., *abnormal skin color, color changes, skin color changes*) can we use the same term or must we translate exactly as in the English?

    Decreasing the variation in these terms should now facilitate translation, as one term/phrase will be used throughout the terminology for similar diagnostic indicators.

2. **Clarity for clinicians should be improved**. It is confusing to students and practicing nurses alike when they see similar but slightly different terms in different diagnoses. Are they the same? Is there some subtle difference they don't understand? Why can't NANDA-I be more clear? And what about all of those "e.g.s" in the terminology? Are they there to teach, to clarify, to list every potential example? There seems to be a mixture of all of these appearing within the terminology.

   You will notice that many of the "e.g.s" have been removed, unless it was felt that they were truly needed to clarify intent. "Teaching tips" that were present in some parentheses are gone, too – the terminology is not the place for these. And we have done our best to condense terms and standardize them, whenever possible.

3. **This work has enabled the coding of the diagnostic indicators**, which will facilitate their use for populating assessment databases within electronic health records, and increase the availability of decision support tools regarding accuracy in diagnosis and linking diagnosis to appropriate treatment plans. Although we did not include the phrase codes within this edition of the taxonomy, a list of all diagnostic indicators, and their codes, is available at the NANDA-I website. It is strongly recommended that these codes be used in all publications to ensure accuracy in translation.

Other Changes Made in the 2015–2017 Edition

The list of diagnostic indicators has been shortened in a couple of other ways. First, because defining characteristics are identified as those things that can be observed, which includes what can be seen and heard, we have removed terms such as "observed" and "verbalizes," so that it is no longer necessary to have two terms that relate to the same data. For example, previously there would have been two separate defining characteristics relate to pain, *reports pain* and *observed evidence of pain*; in this edition you will simply see *pain*, which can either be observed or reported.

Secondly, some of the subcategories of terms have been deleted (e.g., objective/subjective) because they are no longer necessary. Other deletions include lists of pharmaceutical agents, categorized under the subcategory of pharmaceutical agents.

Part 2
Nursing Diagnosis

Chapter 1: Nursing Diagnosis Basics   21

Chapter 2: From Assessment to Diagnosis   31

Chapter 3: An Introduction to the NANDA-I Taxonomy   52

**Chapter 4: NANDA-I Taxonomy II: Specifications
and Definitions**   91

Chapter 5: Frequently Asked Questions   105

NANDA International, Inc. Nursing Diagnoses: Definitions & Classification 2015–2017,
Tenth Edition. Edited by T. Heather Herdman and Shigemi Kamitsuru.
© 2014 NANDA International, Inc. Published 2014 by John Wiley & Sons, Ltd.
Companion website: www.wiley.com/go/nursingdiagnoses

In this section, we present chapters that are aimed at the student, educator, and nurse in clinical practice. The accompanying website features presentation materials to supplement the information provided in these chapters.

Chapter 1 Nursing Diagnosis Basics

Susan Gallagher-Lepak, RN, PhD

This chapter provides a brief review of nursing diagnosis terms and the process of diagnosing. It serves as a basic introduction to nursing diagnosis: what it is, its role within the nursing process, an introduction to the link between assessment and diagnosis, and usage of nursing diagnosis.

Chapter 2 From Assessment to Diagnosis

T. Heather Herdman, RN, PhD, FNI and Shigemi Kamitsuru, RN, PhD, FNI

This chapter, relates to the importance of nursing assessment for accurate diagnosis within nursing practice.

Chapter 3 An Introduction to the NANDA-I Taxonomy

T. Heather Herdman, RN, PhD, FNI

Written primarily for students and nurses in practice, this chapter explains the purpose of a taxonomy, and how to use the taxonomy within practice and education. Table 3.1 presents the 235 NANDA-I nursing diagnoses that are found within the NANDA-I Taxonomy II, and their placement within its 13 domains and 47 classes. Table 3.2 provides the nursing diagnoses as they are placed within the *proposed* Taxonomy III.

Chapter 4 NANDA-I Taxonomy II: Specifications and Definitions

T. Heather Herdman, RN, PhD, FNI (revised from 2012–2014)

This chapter provides more detailed information on the structure of the NANDA-I taxonomy, including the multiaxial system for construction of nursing diagnoses during diagnostic development. Each axis is described and defined. The nursing diagnoses and their foci are provided, and each nursing diagnosis is shown as it is placed (slotted) within the NANDA-I Taxonomy II, and the *proposed* Taxonomy III. A clear link is made between the use of standardized nursing language that permits diagnostic accuracy and the aspect of patient safety;

point-of-care "creation" of terms to describe clinical reasoning is strongly discouraged due to the lack of standardization, which can lead to inappropriate plans of care, poor outcomes, and the inability to accurately research or demonstrate the impact of nursing care on human responses.

Chapter 5 Frequently Asked Questions

T. Heather Herdman, RN, PhD, FNI and Shigemi Kamitsuru, RN, PhD, FNI

This chapter provides answers to some of the most frequently asked questions that we receive from students, educators, and nurses in practice around the world through the NANDA-I website, and when members of the Board of Directors travel to present at a variety of conferences internationally.

Chapter 1

Nursing Diagnosis Basics

Susan Gallagher-Lepak, RN, PhD

Healthcare is delivered by various types of healthcare professionals, including nurses, physicians, and physical therapists, to name just a few. This is true in hospitals as well as other settings across the continuum of care (e.g., clinics, home care, long-term care, churches, prisons). Each healthcare discipline brings its unique body of knowledge to the care of the client. In fact, a unique body of knowledge is often cited as a defining characteristic of a profession.

Collaboration, and at times overlap, occurs between professionals in providing care (Figure 1.1). For example, a physician in a hospital setting may write an order for the client to walk twice per day. Physical therapy focuses on core muscles and movements necessary for walking. Nursing has a holistic view of the patient, including balance and muscle strength related to walking, as well as confidence and motivation. Social work may have involvement with insurance coverage for necessary equipment.

Each health profession has a way to describe "**what**" the profession knows and "**how**" it acts on what it knows. This chapter is primarily focused on the "what." A profession may have a common language that is used to describe and code its knowledge. Physicians treat disease and use the International Classification of Disease taxonomy, ICD-10, to represent and code the medical problems they treat. Psychologists, psychiatrists, and other mental health professionals treat mental health disorders and use the Diagnostic and Statistical Manual of Mental Disorders, DSM-V. Nurses treat human responses to health problems and/or life processes and use the NANDA International, Inc. (NANDA-I) nursing diagnosis taxonomy. The nursing diagnosis taxonomy, and the process of diagnosing using this taxonomy, will be further described.

NANDA International, Inc. Nursing Diagnoses: Definitions & Classification 2015–2017,
Tenth Edition. Edited by T. Heather Herdman and Shigemi Kamitsuru.
© 2014 NANDA International, Inc. Published 2014 by John Wiley & Sons, Ltd.
Companion website: www.wiley.com/go/nursingdiagnoses

Figure 1.1   *Example of a Collaborative Healthcare Team*

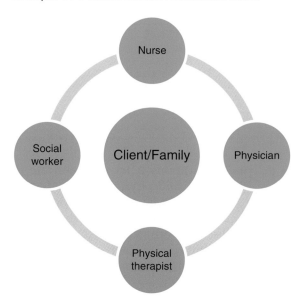

The NANDA-I taxonomy provides a way to classify and categorize areas of concern to nursing (i.e., foci of the diagnoses). It contains 235 nursing diagnoses grouped into 13 domains and 47 classes. A domain is a "sphere of knowledge; examples of domains in the NANDA-I taxonomy include: Nutrition, Elimination/Exchange, Activity/Rest, or Coping/Stress Tolerance (Merriam-Webster, 2009). Domains are divided into classes (groupings that share common attributes).

Nurses deal with responses to health conditions/life responses among individuals, families, groups, and communities. Such responses are the central concern of nursing care and fill the circle ascribed to nursing in Figure 1.1. A nursing diagnosis can be problem-focused, or a state of health promotion or potential risk (Herdman, 2012):

- **Problem-focused diagnosis** – a clinical judgment concerning an *undesirable human response* to a health condition/life process that exists in an individual, family, group, or community
- **Risk diagnosis** – a clinical judgment concerning the *vulnerability of an individual, family, group or community for developing an undesirable human response* to health conditions/life processes
- **Health promotion diagnosis** – a clinical judgment concerning *motivation and desire* to increase well-being and to actualize human health potential. These responses are expressed by a readiness to enhance specific health behaviors, and can be used in any heath state. Health promotion responses may exist in an individual, family, group, or community

Although limited in number in the NANDA-I taxonomy, a **syndrome** can be present. A syndrome is a clinical judgment concerning a specific *cluster of nursing diagnoses* that occur together, and are best addressed together and through similar interventions. An example of a syndrome is *chronic pain syndrome* (00255). Chronic pain is recurrent or persistent pain that has lasted at least three months and that significantly affects daily functioning or well-being. This syndrome is differentiated from chronic pain in that additionally the chronic pain has a significant impact on other human responses and thus includes other diagnoses, such as *disturbed sleep pattern* (00198), *social isolation* (00053), *fatigue* (00093), or *impaired physical mobility* (00085).

How Does a Nurse (or Nursing Student) Diagnose?

The nursing process includes assessment, nursing diagnosis, planning, outcome setting, intervention, and evaluation (Figure 1.2). Nurses use assessment and clinical judgment to formulate hypotheses, or explanations, about presenting actual or potential problems, risks, and/or

Figure 1.2 *The Modified Nursing Process*
From T.H. Herdman (2013). Manejo de casos empleando diagnósticos de enfermería de la NANDA Internacional. [Case Management using NANDA International nursing diagnosis] XXX CONGRESO FEMAFEE 2013. Monterrey, Mexico. (Spanish).

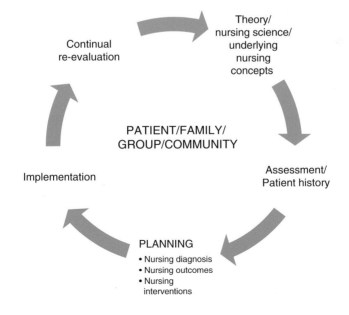

health promotion opportunities. All of these steps require knowledge of underlying concepts of nursing science before patterns can be identified in clinical data or accurate diagnoses can be made.

Understanding Nursing Concepts

Knowledge of key concepts, or nursing diagnostic foci, is necessary before beginning an assessment. Examples of critical concepts important to nursing practice include breathing, elimination, thermoregulation, physical comfort, self-care, and skin integrity. Understanding such concepts allows the nurse to identify patterns in the data and diagnose accurately. Key areas to understand with the concept of pain, for example, include manifestations of pain, theories of pain, populations at risk, related pathophysiological concepts (e.g., fatigue, depression), and management of pain. Full understanding of key concepts is needed as well to differentiate diagnoses. For example, in order to understand hypothermia or hyperthermia, a nurse must first understand the core concepts of thermal stability and thermoregulation. In looking at problems that can occur with *thermoregulation*, the nurse will be faced with the diagnoses of *hypothermia* (00006) (or risk for), *hyperthermia* (00007) (or risk for), but also *risk for imbalanced body temperature* (00005) and *ineffective thermoregulation* (00008). The nurse may collect a significant amount of data, but without a sufficient understanding of the core concepts of thermal stability and thermoregulation, the data needed for accurate diagnosis may have been omitted and patterns in the assessment data go unrecognized.

Assessment

Assessment involves the collection of subjective and objective information (e.g., vital signs, patient/family interview, physical exam) and review of historical information in the patient chart. Nurses also collect information on strengths (to identify health promotion opportunities) and risks (areas that nurses can prevent or potential problems they can postpone). Assessments can be based on a particular nursing theory such as one developed by Sister Callista Roy, Wanda Horta, or Dorothea Orem, or on a standardized assessment framework such as Marjory Gordon's Functional Health Patterns. These frameworks provide a way of categorizing large amounts of data into a manageable number of related patterns or categories of data.

The foundation of nursing diagnosis is clinical reasoning. Clinical reasoning is required to distinguish normal from abnormal data, cluster related data, recognize missing data, identify inconsistencies in data, and make inferences (Alfaro-Lefebre, 2004). Clinical judgment is "an interpretation or conclusion about a patient's needs, concerns, or health problems, and/or the decision to take action (or not)" (Tanner, 2006, p. 204). Key issues, or foci, may be evident early in the assessment (e.g., altered skin integrity, loneliness) and allow the nurse to begin the diagnostic process. For example, a patient may report pain and/or show agitation while holding a body part. The nurse will recognize the client's discomfort based on client report and/or pain behaviors. Expert nurses can quickly identify clusters of clinical cues from assessment data and seamlessly progress to nursing diagnoses. Novice nurses take a more sequential process in determining appropriate nursing diagnoses.

Nursing Diagnosis

A nursing diagnosis is a clinical judgment concerning a human response to health conditions/life processes, or vulnerability for that response, by an individual, family, group, or community. A nursing diagnosis typically contains two parts: 1) descriptor or modifier, and 2) focus of the diagnosis, or the key concept of the diagnosis (Table 1.1). There are some exceptions in which a nursing diagnosis is only one word such as *fatigue* (00093), *constipation* (00011), and *anxiety* (00146). In these diagnoses, the modifier and focus are inherent in the one term.

Nurses diagnose health problems, risk states, and readiness for health promotion. Problem-focused diagnoses should not be viewed as more important than risk diagnoses. Sometimes a risk diagnosis can be the diagnosis with the highest priority for a patient. An example may be a patient who has the nursing diagnoses of *chronic pain* (00133), *overweight* (00233), *risk for impaired skin integrity* (00047), and *risk for falls* (00155), and who has been newly admitted to a skilled nursing facility. Although *chronic pain* and *overweight* are her problem-focused diagnoses, her *risk for falls* may be her number one priority diagnosis, especially as she adjusts to a new environment. This may be especially true when related risk factors are identified in the assessment

Table 1.1 *Parts of a Nursing Diagnosis Label*

Modifier	Diagnostic Focus
Ineffective	Airway Clearance
Risk for	Overweight
Readiness for Enhanced	Knowledge
Impaired	Memory
Ineffective	Coping

Table 1.2 *Key Terms at a Glance*

Term	Brief Description
Nursing Diagnosis	Problem, strength, or risk identified for a client, family, group, or community
Defining Characteristic	Sign or symptom (objective or subjective cue)
Related Factor	Cause or contributing factor (etiological factor)
Risk Factor	Determinant (increase risk)

(e.g., poor vision, difficulty with gait, history of falls, and heightened anxiety with relocation).

Each nursing diagnosis has a label, and a clear definition. It is important to state that merely having a label or a list of labels is insufficient. It is critical that nurses know the definitions of the diagnoses they most commonly use. In addition, they need to know the "diagnostic indicators" – the data that are used to diagnose and to differentiate one diagnosis from another. These diagnostic indicators include defining characteristics and related factors or risk factors (Table 1.2). **Defining characteristics** are observable cues/inferences that cluster as manifestations of a diagnosis (e.g., signs or symptoms). An assessment that identifies the presence of a number of defining characteristics lends support to the accuracy of the nursing diagnosis. **Related factors** are an integral component of all problem-focused nursing diagnoses. Related factors are etiologies, circumstances, facts, or influences that have some type of relationship with the nursing diagnosis (e.g., cause, contributing factor). A review of client history is often where related factors are identified. Whenever possible, nursing interventions should be aimed at these etiological factors in order to remove the underlying cause of the nursing diagnosis. **Risk factors** are influences that increase the vulnerability of an individual, family, group, or community to an unhealthy event (e.g., environmental, psychological, genetic).

A nursing diagnosis does not need to contain all types of diagnostic indicators (i.e., defining characteristics, related factors, and/or risk factors). Problem-focused nursing diagnoses contain defining characteristics and related factors. Health promotion diagnoses generally have only defining characteristics, although related factors may be used if they might improve the understanding of the diagnosis. It is only risk diagnoses that have risk factors.

A common format used when learning nursing diagnosis includes _____ [nursing diagnosis] related to _____ [cause/related factors] as evidenced by _____ [symptoms/defining characteristics]. For example, *ineffective airway clearance* related to *excessive mucus and asthma* as evidenced by *decreased breath sounds bilaterally, crackles over left lobe and persistent, ineffective coughing*. Depending on the electronic health record in a particular healthcare institution, the "related to" and "as evidenced by" components may not be included within the electronic system. This information, however, should be recognized in the assessment data collected and recorded in the patient chart in order to provide support for the nursing diagnosis. Without this data, it is impossible to verify diagnostic accuracy, which puts the quality of nursing care into question.

Planning/Intervention

Once diagnoses are identified, prioritizing of selected nursing diagnoses must occur to determine care priorities. High-priority nursing diagnoses need to be identified (i.e., urgent need, diagnoses with a high level of congruence with defining characteristics, related factors, or risk factors) so that care can be directed to resolve these problems, or lessen the severity or risk of occurrence (in the case of risk diagnoses).

Nursing diagnoses are used to identify intended outcomes of care and plan nursing-specific interventions sequentially. A nursing outcome refers to a measurable behavior or perception demonstrated by an individual, family, group, or community that is responsive to nursing intervention (Center for Nursing Classification [CNC], n.d.). The Nursing Outcome Classification (NOC) is a system that can be used to select outcome measures related to nursing diagnosis. Nurses often, and incorrectly, move directly from nursing diagnosis to nursing intervention without consideration of desired outcomes. Instead, outcomes need to be identified before interventions are determined. The order of this process is similar to planning a road trip. Simply getting in a car and driving will get a person somewhere, but that may not be the place the person really wanted to go. Better is to first have a clear location (outcome) in mind, and then choose a route (intervention) to get to a desired location.

An intervention is defined as "any treatment, based upon clinical judgment and knowledge, that a nurse performs to enhance patient/ client outcomes" (CNC, n.d.). The Nursing Interventions Classification (NIC) is a comprehensive, evidence-based taxonomy of interventions that nurses perform across various care settings. Using nursing knowledge, nurses perform both independent and interdisciplinary interventions. These interdisciplinary interventions overlap with care provided by other healthcare professionals (e.g., physicians, respiratory and physical therapists). For example, blood glucose management is a concept important to nurses, *risk for unstable blood glucose* (00179) is a nursing diagnosis, and nurses implement nursing interventions to treat this condition. *Diabetes mellitus*, in comparison, is a medical diagnosis, yet nurses provide both independent and inter-disciplinary interventions to clients with diabetes who have various types of problems or risk states. Refer to the Kamitsuru's Tripartite Model of Nursing Practice (Figure 5.2) on p. 121.

Evaluation

A nursing diagnosis "provides the basis for selection of nursing interven-tions to achieve outcomes for which nursing has accountability" (Herdman, 2012). The nursing process is often described as a stepwise process, but in reality a nurse will go back and forth between steps in the process. Nurses will move between assessment and nursing diagnosis, for example, as additional data is collected and clustered into meaningful patterns, and the accuracy of nursing diagnoses is evaluated. Similarly, the effectiveness of interventions and achievement of identified outcomes is continuously evaluated as the client status is assessed. Evaluation should ultimately occur at each step in the nursing process, as well as once the plan of care has been implemented. Several questions to consider include: "What data might I have missed? Am I making an inappropriate judgment? How confident am I in this diagnosis? Do I need to consult with someone with more experience? Have I confirmed the diagnosis with the patient/family/group/community? Are the outcomes established appropriate for this patient in this setting, given the reality of the client's condition and resources available? Are the interventions based on research evidence or tradition (e.g., "what we always do")?

Use of Nursing Diagnosis

This description of nursing diagnosis basics, although aimed primarily at nursing students and beginning nurses learning nursing diagnosis, can benefit all nurses in that it highlights critical steps in using nursing diagnosis and provides examples of areas in which inaccurate diagnos-ing can occur. An area that needs continued emphasis, for example, includes the process of linking knowledge of underlying nursing concepts to assessment, and ultimately nursing diagnosis. The nurse's understanding of key concepts (or diagnostic foci) directs the assess-ment process and interpretation of assessment data. Relatedly, nurses diagnose problems, risk states, and readiness for health promotion. Any of these types of diagnoses can be the priority diagnosis (or diagnoses), and the nurse makes this clinical judgment.

In representing knowledge of nursing science, the taxonomy pro-vides the structure for a standardized language in which to communi-cate nursing diagnoses. Using the NANDA-I terminology (the diagnoses themselves), nurses can communicate with each other as well as professionals from other healthcare disciplines about "what" nursing is uniquely. The use of nursing diagnoses in our patient/family interactions can help them to understand the issues on which nurses will be focusing, and can engage them in their own care. The terminology provides a shared language for nurses to address health problems, risk states, and readiness for health promotion. NANDA International's nursing diagnoses are used internationally, with translation into 16 languages. In an increasingly global and electronic world, NANDA-I also allows nurses involved in scholarship to communicate about phenomena of concern to nursing in manuscripts and at conferences in a standardized way, thus advancing the science of nursing.

Nursing diagnoses are peer reviewed, and submitted for acceptance/ revision to NANDA-I by practicing nurses, nurse educators, and nurse researchers around the world. Submissions of new diagnoses and/or revisions to existing diagnoses have continued to grow in number over the 40 plus years of the NANDA-I terminology. Continued submissions (and revisions) to NANDA-I will further strengthen the scope, extent, and supporting evidence of the terminology.

Brief Chapter Summary

This chapter describes types of nursing diagnoses (i.e., problem-focused, risk, health promotion, syndrome) and steps in the nursing process. The nursing process begins with an understanding of underlying concepts of nursing science. Assessment follows, and involves collection and clustering of data into meaningful patterns. Nursing diagnosis, a subsequent step in the nursing process, involves clinical judgment about a human response to a health condition or life process, or vulnerability for that response by an individual, family, group, or community. The nursing diagnosis components were reviewed in this chapter, including the label, definition, and diagnostic indicators (i.e., defining characteristics and related factors, or risk factors). Given that a patient assessment will typically generate a number of nursing diagnoses, prioritization of nursing diagnoses is needed and this will direct care delivery. Critical next steps in the nursing process include identification of nursing outcomes and nursing interventions. Evaluation occurs at each step of the nursing process and at its conclusion.

Questions Commonly Asked by New Learners About Nursing Diagnosis*

- Are nursing diagnoses different than medical diagnoses? (p. 112)
- How many defining characteristics do I need to make a nursing diagnosis? (p. 117)

- How many related factors do I need to use when diagnosing? (p. 118)
- How many nursing diagnoses do I need for each patient? (p. 124)
- How do I know which nursing diagnosis is most accurate? (p. 119)
- How are nursing diagnoses revised or added within NANDA-I? (p. 461)

*For answers to these and other questions, see Chapter 5, Frequently Asked Questions (pp. 105–130).

References

Alfaro-Lefebre, R. (2004). *Critical thinking and clinical judgment: A practical approach to outcome-focused thinking* (4th ed.). St. Louis: Saunders Elsevier.

American Psychiatric Association (2013). Diagnostic and Statistical Manual of Mental Disorders (5th Ed.). Arlington, VA: American Psychiatric Association, accessed from dsm.psychiatryonline.org

Center for Nursing Classification & Clinical Effectiveness (CNC), University of Iowa College of Nursing (n.d.) Overview: Nursing Interventions Classification (NIC). Retrieved from http://www.nursing.uiowa.edu/cncce/nursing-interventions-classification-overview, accessed March 13, 2014.

Center for Nursing Classification & Clinical Effectiveness (CNC), University of Iowa College of Nursing (n.d.). Overview: Nursing Outcome Classification (NOC). Retrieved from http://www.nursing.uiowa.edu/cncce/nursing-outcomes-classification-overview, accessed March 13, 2014.

Herdman, T. H. (ed.) (2012) *NANDA International. Nursing diagnoses: Definitions and classification, 2012–2014.* Ames, IA: Wiley-Blackwell.

Herdman, T. H. (2013). Manejo de casos empleando diagnósticos de enfermería de la NANDA Internacional. [Case management using NANDA International nursing diagnoses]. XXX CONGRESO FEMAFEE 2013. Monterrey, Mexico. (Spanish)

Merriam-Webster (2009). *Merriam-Webster's collegiate dictionary* (11th ed.). Springfield, MA: Merriam-Webster.

Tanner, C.A. (2006). Thinking like a nurse: A research-based model of clinical judgment in nursing. *Journal of Nursing Education*, 45(6), 204–211.

Chapter 2

From Assessment to Diagnosis

T. Heather Herdman, RN, PhD, FNI and Shigemi Kamitsuru, RN, PhD, FNI

Assessment is the first and the most critical step in the nursing process. If this step is not handled well, nurses will lose control over the subsequent steps of the nursing process. Without proper nursing assessment, there can be no nursing diagnosis, and without nursing diagnosis, there can be no independent nursing interventions. Assessment should not be performed merely to fill in the blank spaces on a form or computer screen. If this rings a bell for you, it's time to take a new look at the purpose of assessment!

What Happens during Nursing Assessment?

During the assessment and diagnosis steps of the nursing process, nurses collect data from a patient (or family/group/community), process that data into information, and then organize that information into meaningful categories of knowledge, also known as nursing diagnoses. Assessment provides the best opportunity for nurses to establish an effective therapeutic relationship with the patient. In other words, assessment is both an intellectual and an interpersonal activity.

As you can see in Figure 2.1, assessment involves multiple steps, with the goal being to diagnose and prioritize these diagnoses, which then become the basis for nursing treatment. Now, this probably sounds like a long, involved process and, frankly, who has time for all of that? In the real world, however, some of these steps happen in the blink of an eye. For instance, if a nurse sees a patient who is holding her lower abdomen and grimacing, he might immediately suspect that the patient is experiencing *acute pain* (00132). Thus, the movement from data collection (observation of the patient's behavior) to determining potential diagnoses (e.g., *acute pain*) occurs in a split second. However, this

NANDA International, Inc. Nursing Diagnoses: Definitions & Classification 2015–2017,
Tenth Edition. Edited by T. Heather Herdman and Shigemi Kamitsuru.
© 2014 NANDA International, Inc. Published 2014 by John Wiley & Sons, Ltd.
Companion website: www.wiley.com/go/nursingdiagnoses

Figure 2.1 *Steps in Moving from Assessment to Diagnosis*

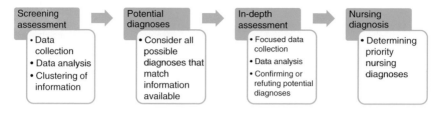

Screening assessment		Potential diagnoses		In-depth assessment		Nursing diagnosis
• Data collection • Data analysis • Clustering of information	➡	• Consider all possible diagnoses that match information available	➡	• Focused data collection • Data analysis • Confirming or refuting potential diagnoses	➡	• Determining priority nursing diagnoses

quickly determined diagnosis might not be the right one – or it may not be the highest priority for your patient. Getting there does take time.

So, how do you accurately diagnose? Only by continuing to the further step of in-depth assessment – and the proper use of the data collected during that assessment – can you ensure accuracy in diagnosis. The patient may indeed be experiencing *acute pain*, but without in-depth assessment, there is no way for the nurse to know that the pain is related to intestinal cramping and diarrhea. This chapter provides foundational knowledge for what to do with all of that data you have collected. After all, why bother collecting it if you aren't going to use it?

In the next section, we will go through each of the steps in the process that takes us from assessment to diagnosis. But first, let's spend a few minutes discussing the purpose – because assessment is not simply a task that nurses complete, we need to really understand its purpose so we can understand how it applies to our professional role as nurses.

Why Do Nurses Assess?

Nurses need to assess patients from the viewpoint of the nursing discipline to diagnose accurately and to provide effective care. What is the "nursing discipline"? Simply put, it is the body of knowledge that comprises the science of nursing. Diagnosing a patient based on his/her medical diagnosis or medical information is neither a recommended nor a safe diagnostic process. Such an overly simplified conclusion could lead to inappropriate interventions, prolonged length of stay, and unnecessary readmissions.

Remember that nurses diagnose actual or potential human responses to health conditions/life processes, or a vulnerability for that response – the focus here is "human responses." Human beings are complicated – we just don't all respond to one situation in the same way. Those responses are based on many factors: genetics, physiology, health condition, and past experience with illness/injury. However, they are also influenced by the patient's culture, ethnicity, religion/spiritual beliefs, gender, and family upbringing. This means that human responses are not so easily identified. If we simply assume that every patient with a particular medical diagnosis will respond in a certain way, we may treat conditions (and therefore use the nurse's time and other resources) that do not exist while missing others that truly need our attention.

It is possible that there may be close relationships between some nursing diagnoses and medical conditions; however, to date we do not have sufficient scientific evidence to definitively link all nursing diagnoses to particular medical diagnoses. For instance, there is no way to identify the patient's ability for independent daily living or the availability/quality of family support, based on a medical diagnosis of myocardial infarction or osteoporosis. Nor can one assume that every patient with a medical diagnosis will respond in the same way: every patient who has experienced a mastectomy does not experience *disturbed body image* (00118), for example. Therefore, nursing assessment and diagnosis should be driven from the viewpoint of the nursing discipline.

Unfortunately, in your practice, you will probably observe nurses who assign or "pick" a diagnosis before they have assessed the patient. What is wrong with this pathway to diagnosis? As an example, a nurse may begin to complete a plan of care based on the nursing diagnosis of *anxiety* (00146) for a patient undergoing surgery, before the patient has even arrived on the unit or been evaluated. Nurses working in surgical units encounter many preoperative patients, and those patients are often very anxious. Those nurses may know that preoperative teaching is an effective intervention in reducing anxiety.

So, assuming a relationship between preoperative patients and anxiety could be useful in practice. However, the statement "preoperative patients have anxiety" may not apply to every patient (it is a hypothesis), and so it must be validated with each and every patient. This is especially true because anxiety is a subjective experience – although we may think the patient seems anxious, or we may expect him to be anxious, only he can really tell us if he *feels* anxious. In other words, the nurse can understand how the patient feels only if the patient tells the nurse about his feelings, so *anxiety* is a problem-focused nursing diagnosis which requires subjective data from the patient. What appears to be *anxiety* may actually be *fear* (00148) or *ineffective coping* (00069); we simply cannot know until we assess and validate our findings. Thus, before nurses diagnose a patient, a thorough assessment is absolutely necessary.

The Screening Assessment

There are two types of assessment: screening and in-depth assessment. While both require data collection, they serve different purposes. The screening assessment is the initial data collection step, and is probably the easiest to complete. The in-depth assessment is more focused, enabling the nurse to explore information that was identified in the initial screening assessment, and to search for additional cues that might support or refute potential nursing diagnoses.

Not a Simple Matter of "Filling in the Blanks"

Most schools and healthcare organizations provide nurses with a standardized form – on paper or in the electronic health record – that must be completed for each patient within a specified period of time. For example, patients who are admitted to the hospital may need to have this assessment completed within 24 hours of admission. Patients seen in an ambulatory clinic may have a required assessment prior to being seen by the primary care provider (a physician or nurse practitioner, for example). Some organizations will have tools that enable completion of an assessment based on a particular nursing theory or model (e.g., Roy Adaptation Model), body system review, or some other method of organizing the data to be collected.

The performance of the screening assessment requires specific competences for the accurate completion of various procedures to obtain data, and it requires a high level of skill in interpersonal communication. Patients must feel safe and trust the nurse before they will feel comfortable answering personal questions or providing answers, especially if they feel that their responses might not be "normal" or "accepted."

We say that the initial screening assessment may be the easiest step because, in some ways, it is initially a process of "filling in the blanks." The form requires the patient's temperature, so the nurse takes the temperature and inputs that data into the assessment form. The form requires that information is collected about the patient's cardiac system, and the nurse completes all of the blank spaces on the form that deal with this system (heart rate, rhythm, presence of a murmur, pedal pulses, etc.).

However, appropriate nursing assessment requires far more than this initial screening. Obviously, when the nurse reviews data collected during her assessment, and starts to recognize potential diagnoses, she will need to collect further data that can help her determine if there are other human responses occurring that are of concern, that indicate risks for the patient, or that suggest health promotion opportunities. The nurse will also want to identify the etiology or precipitating factors of areas of concern. It is quite possible that these in-depth questions are not included in the organization's assessment form, because there is simply no way to include every possible question that might need to be asked for every possible human response!

Assessment Framework

Let's take a moment to consider the type of framework that supports a thorough nursing assessment. An evidence-based assessment framework should be used for accurate nursing diagnosis as well as safe patient care. It should also represent the discipline of the professional using it: in this case, the assessment form should represent knowledge from the nursing discipline.

Should we use the NANDA-I taxonomy as an assessment framework?

There is sometimes confusion over the difference between the NANDA-I Taxonomy II of nursing diagnoses and Gordon's Functional Health Patterns (FHP) assessment framework (1994). The NANDA-I taxonomy was developed based on Gordon's work; that is why the two frameworks look similar. However, their purposes and functions are entirely different. (See Chapters 3 and 4 for more specific information on the NANDA-I taxonomy.)

The NANDA-I Taxonomy serves its intended purpose of sorting/categorizing nursing diagnoses. Each domain and class is defined, so the framework helps nurses to locate a nursing diagnosis within the taxonomy. On the other hand, the FHP framework was scientifically developed to standardize the structure for nursing assessment (Gordon, 1994). It guides the history-taking and physical examination by nurses, providing items to assess and a structure for organizing assessment data. In addition, the sequence of 11 patterns provides an efficient and effective flow for the nursing assessment.

As stated in the NANDA-I Position Statement (2010), use of an evidence-based assessment framework, such as Gordon's FHP, is highly recommended for accurate nursing diagnosis and safe patient care. It is not intended that the NANDA-I Taxonomy should be used as an assessment framework.

Data Analysis

The second step in the process is the conversion of data to information. Its purpose is to help us to consider what the data we collected in the screening assessment might mean, or to help us identify additional data that need to be collected. The terms "information" and "data" are sometimes used interchangeably, but the actual characteristics of data and information are quite different. In order to have a better understanding of assessment and nursing diagnosis, it is useful to take a moment to differentiate data from information.

Figure 2.2   Converting Data to Information: The Case of Caroline, a 14-year-old Female Seen in Ambulatory Clinic

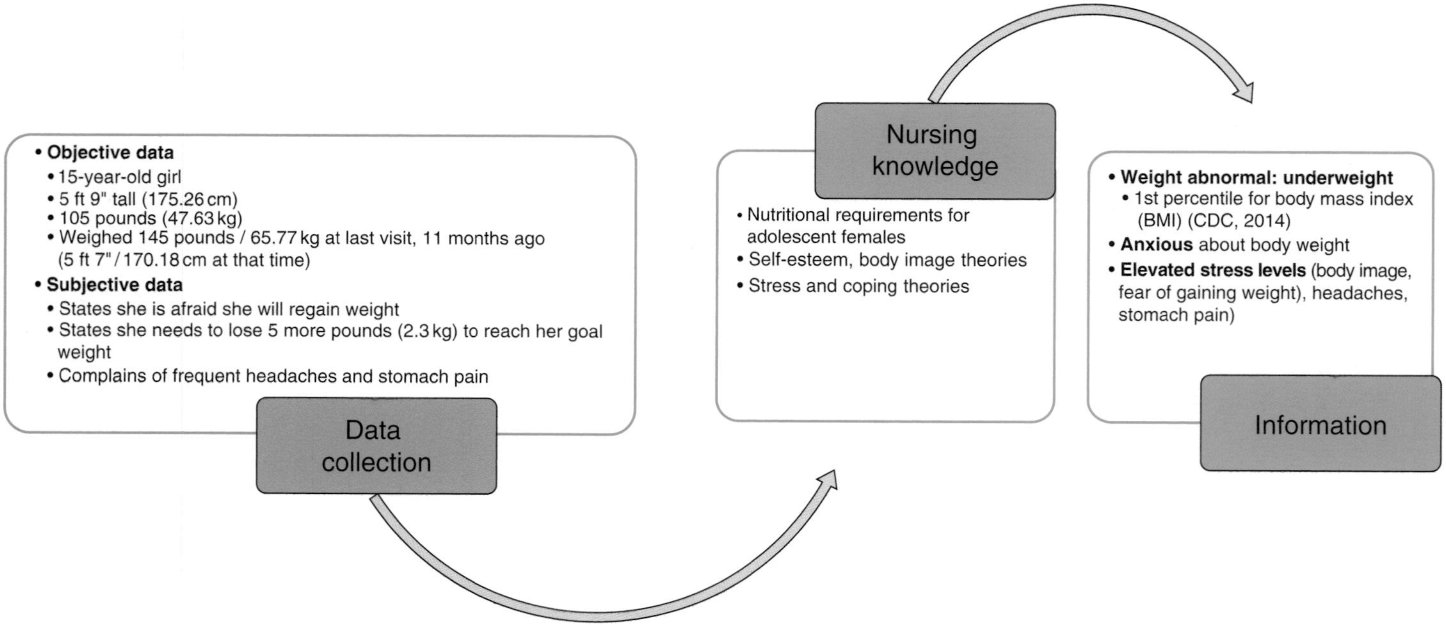

Data collection

- **Objective data**
  - 15-year-old girl
  - 5 ft 9" tall (175.26 cm)
  - 105 pounds (47.63 kg)
  - Weighed 145 pounds / 65.77 kg at last visit, 11 months ago (5 ft 7" / 170.18 cm at that time)
- **Subjective data**
  - States she is afraid she will regain weight
  - States she needs to lose 5 more pounds (2.3 kg) to reach her goal weight
  - Complains of frequent headaches and stomach pain

Nursing knowledge

- Nutritional requirements for adolescent females
- Self-esteem, body image theories
- Stress and coping theories

Information

- **Weight abnormal: underweight**
  - 1st percentile for body mass index (BMI) (CDC, 2014)
- **Anxious** about body weight
- **Elevated stress levels** (body image, fear of gaining weight), headaches, stomach pain

Data are the raw facts collected by nurses through their observations. Nurses collect data from a patient (or family/group/community) and then, using their nursing knowledge, they transform those data into information. Information can be seen as data with an assigned judgment or meaning, such as "high" or "low," "normal" or "abnormal," and "important" or "unimportant." Figure 2.2 provides an example of how objective and subjective data can be converted to information through the application of nursing knowledge.

It is important to note that the same data can be interpreted differently depending on the context, or the gathering of new data. For example, let's suppose that a nurse checks the body temperature of Mr. W who was just admitted to the hospital with an infected surgical wound and difficulty breathing. The thermometer indicates his temperature is 37.5 °C/99.5 °F, via the axillary route. This plain fact is given meaning by comparing it to accepted normal values, as the nurse processes data into information: Mr. W has a slight fever. However, what if the nurse learns that when Mr. W was seen in the ambulatory clinic two hours ago, his temperature was 39.0 °C/102.2 °F? With this new piece of data, the current temperature data can be reinterpreted: Mr. W's temperature has decreased (it is improving).

When documenting assessment, therefore, it is important to include both data and information. Information cannot be validated by others if original data are not provided. For example, simply indicating "Mr. W had a fever" is not clinically useful. How severe was the fever? How were data gathered (oral, axillary, core temperature)? Documentation that shows that Mr. W had a fever of 37.5 °C/ 99.5 °F, via the axillary method, enables another nurse to compare new temperature readings against the previous ones, and to identify if the patient is improving.

Subjective versus Objective Data

Nurses collect and document two types of data related to a patient: subjective and objective data. While physicians value objective over subjective data for medical diagnoses, nurses value both types of data for nursing diagnoses (Gordon, 2008).

What is the difference between subjective and objective data? The dictionary (Merriam-Webster, 2014) defines *subjective* as "based on feelings or opinions rather than facts"; *objective* means "based on facts rather than feelings or opinions." One thing you should be careful of here is that when these terms are used in the context of nursing assessment, they have a slightly different meaning from this general dictionary definition. Although the basic idea remains the same, "subjective" does not mean the *nurse's* feelings or opinions, but that of the subject of nursing care: the patient/family/group/community.

Moreover, "objective" signifies those facts observed by the nurse or other healthcare professionals.

In other words, the *subjective data* come from verbal reports from the patient regarding perceptions and thoughts on his/her health, daily life, comfort, relationships, and so on. For instance, a patient may report "I have had severe back pain for a week," or "I don't have anyone in my life with whom I can share my feelings." Sometimes, however, the patient is unable to provide subjective data, and so we must rely on other sources, such as family members/close friends. Parents may provide useful information about their child's behavior based on their daily observations and knowledge. An example might be a parent telling the nurse that "She usually curls up in a ball and rocks herself when she hurts." Nurses can use this information to validate the baby's behavior, and such behavior can be used as subjective data.

Nurses collect these subjective data through the process of history-taking or interview. History-taking is not merely asking the patient one question after another using a routine format. In order to obtain accurate data from a patient, nurses must incorporate active listening skills, and use open-ended questions as much as possible, especially as follow-up questions when potentially abnormal data are identified.

The *objective data* are those things that nurses observe about the patient. Objective data are collected through physical examinations and diagnostic test results. Here, "to observe" does not only mean the use of eyesight: it requires the use of all senses. For example, nurses look at the patient's general appearance, listen to his lung sounds, they may smell foul wound drainage, and feel the skin temperature using touch. Additionally, nurses use various instruments and tools with the patient to collect numerical data (e.g., body weight, blood pressure, oxygen saturation, pain level). In order to obtain reliable and accurate objective data, nurses must have appropriate knowledge and skills to perform physical assessment and to use standardized tools or monitoring devices.

Ask yourself: Do these data signify:

- A problem?
- A strength?
- A vulnerability?

Clustering of Information/Seeing a Pattern

Once the nurse has collected data and transformed it into information, the next step is to begin to answer the question: What are my patient's human responses (nursing diagnoses)? This requires the knowledge of

Figure 2.3 *The Modified Nursing Process (Herdman, 2013)*

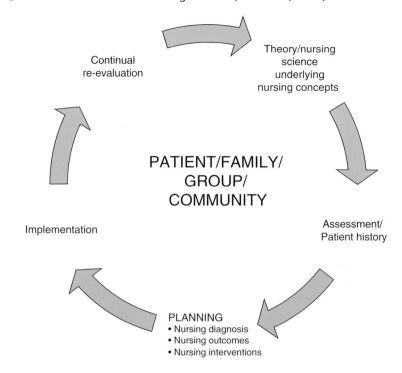

a variety of theories and models from nursing as well as several related disciplines. It also requires knowledge about the concepts that underlie the nursing diagnoses themselves. Do you remember the modified nursing process diagram introduced in Chapter 1 (Figure 1.2)? In this diagram, Herdman (2013) identifies the importance of theory/nursing science underlying nursing concepts. Assessment techniques are mean- ingless if we do not know how to use the data!

If the nurse who assessed the adolescent, Caroline (Figure 2.3), did not know the normal BMIs in that age group, he might not have been able to interpret that patient's weight as being underweight. If he did not understand theories related to child development, self-esteem, body image, stress, and coping in this age group, then he might not identify other vulnerabilities or problem responses exhibited by Caroline.

Identifying Potential Nursing Diagnoses (Diagnostic Hypotheses)

At this step in the process, the nurse looks at the information that is coming together to form a pattern; it provides him with a way of seeing what human responses the patient may be experiencing. Initially, the nurse considers all potential diagnoses that may come to mind. In the expert nurse, this can happen in seconds – for novice or student nurses, it may take support from more expert nurses or faculty members to guide their thinking.

Ask yourself, now that you have collected your assessment data and converted it into information, how do you know what's important and what's irrelevant for this particular patient?

Seeing patterns in the data requires an understanding of the concept that supports each diagnosis. For example, if you have assessed Ms. K and you note that she is having difficulty breathing, her pulse oximeter shows her oxygenation is 88%, she is using accessory muscles to breathe, and she has supraclavicular retractions, what does this tell you? Unless you have a good understanding of normal breathing patterns, normal gas exchange, and ventilation, it may not tell you very much at all. You may know that Ms. K has some problem with her breathing, but not enough to know what you should look for to identify a cause (related factors) or even what other data (defining characteristics) you should look for to determine an accurate diagnosis. This situation can lead to the nurse just "picking a diagnosis" from a list, or trying to use the medical diagnosis as the basis for the nursing diagnosis. Conceptual knowledge of each nursing diagnosis allows the nurse to give accurate meanings to the data collected from the patient, and prepares her to perform the in-depth assessment.

When you have this conceptual knowledge, you will begin to look at the data you collected in a different way. You will turn that data into information, and start to observe how that information starts to group together to form patterns, or to "paint a picture" of what might be happening with your patient. Take another look at Figure 2.2. With conceptual nursing knowledge of nutrition, self-esteem, stress, coping, and adolescent development, you might begin to see the information as possible nursing diagnoses, such as:

- Imbalanced nutrition, less than body requirements (00002)
- Disturbed body image (00118)
- Situational low self-esteem (00120).

Unfortunately, this step is often where nurses stop: they develop a list of diagnoses and either launch directly into action (determining interventions), or they simply "pick" one of the diagnoses that sounds most appropriate, based on the diagnosis label, and then move on to selecting interventions for those diagnoses. This is, quite simply, the wrong thing to do. For diagnoses to be accurate, they must be validated – and that requires additional, in-depth assessment to confirm or to refute, or "rule out," a diagnosis.

By combining basic nursing knowledge and nursing diagnosis knowledge, the nurse can now move from identifying potential diagnoses based on the screening assessment to an in-depth assessment, and then to determining the accurate nursing diagnosis(es).

In-Depth Assessment

At this stage, you have reviewed the information resulting from the screening assessment to determine if it was normal or abnormal, or if it represented a risk (vulnerability) or a strength. Those items that were not considered normal, or were seen as a vulnerability, should have been considered in relation to a problem-focused or risk diagnosis. Areas in which the patient indicated a desire to improve something (for example, to enhance nutrition) should be considered as a potential health promotion diagnosis.

If some data are interpreted as abnormal, further in-depth assessment is crucial in order to diagnose the patient accurately. However, if nurses simply collect data without paying much attention to them, critical data may be overlooked. Take another look at Figure 2.2. The nurse could have stopped his assessment here, and simply moved on to a diagnosis of *impaired nutrition, less than body requirements* (00002). He could have provided education about proper nutrition and normal weight ranges for Caroline's age and height. He could have developed a nutrition plan or made a referral to a dietitian. However, while all of those things might be appropriate, he would have neglected to identify some major issues that are probably significant, which, if not addressed, will lead to continued issues with Caroline's weight and nutritional status.

Through the in-depth assessment, however, Caroline's nurse was able to identify peer pressure, bullying, and high stress levels regarding school performance, her desire to "fit in" at school, her goal of attending a top university, and the need to win an academic scholarship to afford tuition (Figure 2.4). He learned that Caroline had vulnerabilities consistent with a stressful social environment (peers who focused on weight/appearance, threat of bullying, and a best friend with self-injurious behavior). However, he also identified that Caroline had a strength in the support she received from her parents and brother – a very important thing to build in to any plan of care. So, with this additional in-depth assessment, the nurse could now revise his potential diagnoses:

- Imbalanced nutrition, less than body requirements (00002)
- Stress overload (00177)
- Ineffective coping (00069)
- Anxiety (00146)
- Disturbed body image (00118)
- Situational low self-esteem (00120)

Figure 2.4   *In-Depth Assessment: The Case of Caroline, a 14-year-old Female Seen in Ambulatory Clinic*

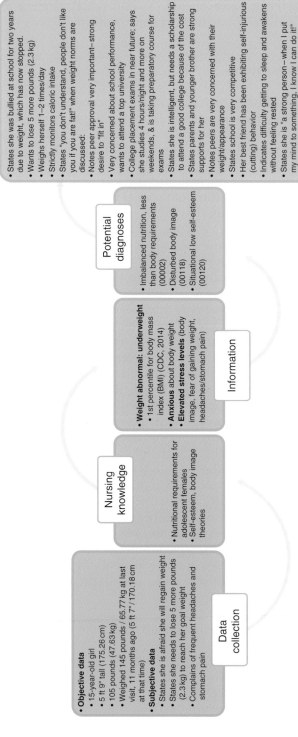

Data collection

Objective data
- 15-year-old girl
- 5 ft 9" tall (175.26 cm)
- 105 pounds (47.63 kg)
- Weighed 145 pounds / 65.77 kg at last visit, 11 months ago (5 ft 7"/170.18 cm at that time)

Subjective data
- States she is afraid she will regain weight
- States she needs to lose 5 more pounds (2.3 kg) to reach her goal weight
- Complains of frequent headaches and stomach pain

Nursing knowledge
- Nutritional requirements for adolescent females
- Self-esteem, body image theories

Information
- **Weight abnormal: underweight**
  - 1st percentile for body mass index (BMI) (CDC, 2014)
- **Anxious** about body weight
- **Elevated stress levels** (body image, fear of gaining weight, headaches/stomach pain)

Potential diagnoses
- Imbalanced nutrition, less than body requirements (00002)
- Disturbed body image (00118)
- Situational low self-esteem (00120)

In-depth assessment
- States she was bullied at school for two years due to weight, which has now stopped.
- Wants to lose 5 more pounds (2.3 kg)
- Weighs herself 1–2 times/day
- Strictly monitors caloric intake
- States "you don't understand, people don't like you if you are fat!" when weight norms are discussed:
- Notes peer approval very important – strong desire to "fit in"
- Very concerned about school performance, wants to attend a top university
- College placement exams in near future; says she studies 4 hours/night and more on weekends, & is taking preparatory course for exams
- States she is intelligent, but needs a scholarship to attend a good college because of the cost
- States parents and younger brother are strong supports for her
- Notes peers are very concerned with their weight/appearance
- States school is very competitive
- Her best friend has been exhibiting self-injurious (cutting) behavior
- Indicates difficulty getting to sleep and awakens without feeling rested
- States she is "a strong person – when I put my mind to something, I know I can do it!" Smiles when she talks about the strength of her determination.

Confirming/Refuting Potential Nursing Diagnoses

Whenever new data are collected and processed into information, it is time to reconsider previous potential or determined diagnoses. In this step, there are three primary things to consider:

- Did the in-depth assessment provide new data that would rule out or eliminate one or more of your potential diagnoses?
- Did the in-depth assessment point toward new diagnoses that you had not previously considered?
- How can you differentiate between similar diagnoses?

It is also important to remember that other nurses will need to be able to continue to validate the diagnosis you make, and to understand how you arrived at your diagnosis. It is for this reason that it is important to use standardized terms, such as the NANDA-I nursing diagnoses, which provide not only a label (e.g., *ineffective coping* (00069)), but also a definition and assessment criteria (defining characteristics and related factors, or risk factors), so that other nursing professionals can continue to validate – or perhaps refute – the diagnosis as new data become available for the patient. Terms that are simply constructed by nurses at the bedside, without these validated definitions and assessment criteria, have no consistent meaning and cannot be clinically validated or confirmed. When a NANDA-I nursing diagnosis does not exist that fits a pattern you identify in a patient, it is safer to describe the condition in detail rather than to make up a term that will have different meanings to different nurses. Remember that patient safety depends on good communication – so use only standardized terms that have clear definitions and assessment criteria so that they can be easily validated.

Eliminating Possible Diagnoses

One of the goals of in-depth assessment is to eliminate, or "rule out," one or more of the potential diagnoses you were considering. You do this by reviewing the information you have obtained and comparing it to what you know about the diagnoses. It is critical that the assessment data support the diagnosis(es). Diagnoses that are not well supported through the assessment criteria provided by NANDA-I (defining characteristics, related factors, or risk factors) and/or that are not supported by etiological factors (causes or contributors to the diagnoses) are not appropriate for a patient.

> **Ask Yourself: When I look at the patient information:**
>
> Is it consistent with the definition of the potential diagnosis?
> Are the objective/subjective data identified in the patient defining characteristics or risk factors of the diagnosis?
> Does it include causes (related factors) of the potential problem-focused diagnosis?

As we look at Figure 2.4 and consider the potential diagnoses that Caroline's nurse identified, we can begin to eliminate some of these as valid diagnoses. Sometimes it is helpful to do a side-to-side comparison of the diagnoses, focusing on those defining characteristics and related factors that were identified throughout the assessment and patient history (Table 2.1).

For example, after reflection, Caroline's nurse quickly eliminates from considation the diagnosis, *situational low self-esteem*. The definition of this diagnosis simply does not fit Caroline's confidence in her intelligence, her ability to achieve what she puts her mind to, and her pride in her strength of determination. Although she does have some related factors for this diagnosis, she does not have the signs/symptoms of someone with this diagnosis and, in fact, she has strengths that are quite contrary to it. The nurse also eliminates *anxiety*. Although Caroline does have some defining characteristics and related factors for this diagnosis, she does not refer to herself as anxious, nor does she identify a feeling of dread or apprehension. Rather, she clearly states stressors that exist in her life, and sees these as a challenge to be overcome.

Potential New Diagnoses

It is very possible, such as in the case of Caroline (Figure 2.4), that new data will lead to new information and, in turn, to new diagnoses. The same questions that you used to eliminate potential diagnoses should be used as you consider these diagnoses.

Differentiating between Similar Diagnoses

It is helpful to narrow down your potential diagnoses by considering those that are very similar, but that have a distinctive feature making one more relevant to the patient than the other. Let's take another

Table 2.1 The Case of Caroline: A Comparison of Identified Defining Characteristics and Related Factors

	Imbalanced nutrition, less than body requirements (00002)	Stress overload (00177)	Ineffective coping (00069)	Anxiety (00146)	Disturbed body image (00118)	Situational low self-esteem (00120)
Definition	Intake of nutrients insufficient to meet metabolic needs	Excessive amounts and types of demands that require action	Inability to form a valid appraisal of the stressors, inadequate choices of practiced responses, and/or inability to use available resources	Vague, uneasy feeling of discomfort or dread accompanied by an autonomic response (the source is often nonspecific or unknown to the individual); a feeling of apprehension caused by anticipation of danger. It is an alerting sign that warns of impending danger and enables the individual to take measures to deal with that threat	Confusion in mental picture of one's physical self	Development of a negative perception of self-worth in response to a current situation
Defining characteristics	▪ Body weight 20% or more below ideal weight range ▪ Food intake less than recommended daily allowance (RDA) ▪ Misperception	▪ Excessive stress ▪ Feeling of pressure ▪ Negative impact from stress ▪ Tension	▪ Alteration in sleep pattern ▪ Ineffective coping strategies	**Behavioral** ▪ Insomnia **Affective** ▪ Distress ▪ Fear ▪ Self-focused ▪ Uncertainty ▪ Worried **Sympathetic** ▪ Anorexia **Parasympathetic** ▪ Alteration in sleep pattern **Cognitive** ▪ Fear ▪ Preoccupation ▪ Rumination	▪ Alteration in view of one's body ▪ Behavior of monitoring one's body ▪ Fear of reaction by others ▪ Focus on past appearance ▪ Negative feeling about body ▪ Perceptions that reflect an altered view of one's body appearance ▪ Preoccupation with change	

Continued

Table 2.1 Continued

	Imbalanced nutrition, less than body requirements (00002)	Stress overload (00177)	Ineffective coping (00069)	Anxiety (00146)	Disturbed body image (00118)	Situational low self-esteem (00120)
Related factors	■ Insufficient dietary intake ■ Psychological disorder	■ Excessive stress ■ Repeated stressors	■ Gender differences in coping strategies ■ Ineffective tension release strategies ■ Insufficient sense of control ■ Insufficient social support ■ Maturational crisis ■ Situational crisis ■ Uncertainty	■ Maturational crisis ■ Situational crisis ■ Stressors	■ Alteration in self-perception ■ Cultural incongruence ■ Developmental transition ■ Impaired psychosocial functioning	■ Alteration in body image ■ Developmental transition ■ History of rejection

Table 2.2 *The Case of Caroline: A Comparison of Domains and Classes of Potential Diagnoses*

Diagnosis	Domain	Class
Imbalanced nutrition, less than body requirements (00002)	Nutrition	Ingestion
Stress overload (00177)	Coping/stress tolerance	Coping responses
Ineffective coping (00069)	Coping/stress tolerance	Coping responses
Disturbed body image (00118)	Self-perception	Body image

look at our patient, Caroline. After the in-depth assessment, the nurse had six potential diagnoses; two diagnoses were eliminated, leaving four potential diagnoses. One way to start the process of differentiation is to look at where the diagnoses are located within the NANDA-I taxonomy. This gives you a clue about how the diagnoses are grouped together into the broad area of nursing knowledge (domain) and the subcategories, or group of diagnoses with similar attributes (class).

A quick review of Table 2.2 shows only one diagnosis within the nutrition domain, and one within the self-perception domain. However, two diagnoses are found within the coping/stress tolerance domain; these diagnoses are also located in the same class, that of coping responses. This suggests that some differentiation could support a narrowing of potential diagnoses within those sharing similar attributes.

> ***Ask Yourself: When I look at the patient information in light of similar nursing diagnoses:***
>
> Do the diagnoses share a similar focus, or is it different?
> If the diagnoses share a similar focus, is one more focused/specific than the other?
> Does one diagnosis potentially lead to another that I have identified? That is, could it be the causative factor of that other diagnosis?

As the nurse considers what he knows about Caroline, he can look at the coping responses he identified as potential diagnoses in light of these questions. The diagnoses do not share a similar diagnostic focus: one focuses on stress and one focuses on coping. *Stress overload* is fairly specific: there are excessive amounts and types of demands requiring

Figure 2.5 *SEA TOW: A Thinking Tool for Diagnostic Decision-Making (adapted from Rencic, 2011)*

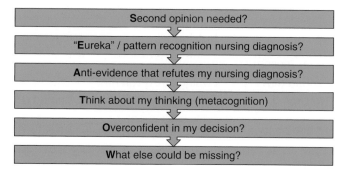

Second opinion needed?
"**E**ureka" / pattern recognition nursing diagnosis?
Anti-evidence that refutes my nursing diagnosis?
Think about my thinking (metacognition)
Overconfident in my decision?
What else could be missing?

action by the patient. Caroline has clearly identified stressors (bullying, peer pressure, desire to "fit in," college entrance exams, need for a scholarship to attend college, a good friend exhibiting cutting behavior, etc.). *Ineffective coping* looks at how the individual evaluates stressors, and the choices she makes to respond to them, and/or how she accesses available resources to respond to them.

It is easy to see how *stress overload* could lead to *ineffective coping*: elimination of stressors, or a reframing of how Caroline perceives those stressors, could then have an impact how the patient copes with the situation. The nurse might take some time to consider if it is possible for the patient to eliminate or reframe the stressors, or if the priority is to focus on the ineffective coping in response to the stressors. This should, if possible, be a discussion and a decision that are made together with the patient. After all, Caroline is the one living this experience, so her focus and prioritization should help drive the nurse's plan of care.

A thinking tool (Figure 2.5) used by our colleagues in medicine can be useful as a review prior to determining your final diagnosis(es): it uses the acronym SEA TOW (Rencic, 2011). This tool can easily be adapted for nursing diagnosis, too.

It is always a good idea to ask a colleague, or an expert, for a *second opinion* if you are unsure of the appropriate diagnosis. Is the diagnosis you are considering the result of a "*Eureka*" moment? Did you recognize a pattern in the data from your assessment and patient interview? Did you confirm this pattern by reviewing the diagnostic indicators (defining characteristics, related factors or risk factors)? Did you collect *anti-evidence*: data that seem to refute this diagnosis? Can you justify the diagnosis even with these data, or do the data suggest you need to look deeper? *Think about your thinking*: was it logical, reasoned, built on your knowledge of nursing science and the human response that you are diagnosing? Do you need additional information about the response before you are ready to confirm it? Are you *overconfident*? This can happen when you are accustomed to patients presenting with particular diagnoses, and so you "jump" to a diagnosis, rather than truly applying clinical reasoning skills. Finally, *what else could be missing*? Are there other data you need to collect or review in order to validate, confirm, or rule out a potential nursing diagnosis? Use of the SEA TOW acronym can help you validate your clinical reasoning process and increase the likelihood of accurate diagnosis.

Making a Diagnosis/Prioritizing

The final step is to determine the diagnosis(es) that will drive nursing intervention for your patient. After reviewing everything he learned about his patient, Caroline, the nurse may have determined three key diagnoses, one of which is new:

- Imbalanced nutrition, less than body requirements (00002)
- Disturbed body image (00118)
- Readiness for enhanced coping (00158)

The *imbalanced nutrition* diagnosis must be addressed to prevent potential consequences of malnutrition, especially during Caroline's phase of adolescence (puberty) in which she needs to ensure good nutrition for growth and healthy development. This may be the primary, or high priority, diagnosis. *Disturbed body image* continues as a diagnosis, because Caroline currently feels that she needs to be "really thin," and despite the fact that she is underweight, she continues to express the desire to lose additional weight. Her consistent reference to her history of being overweight, her daily or twice daily monitoring of her weight, and her fear of gaining weight all indicate that this issue must be addressed together with the nutrition diagnosis in order for the intervention to be successful.

In discussion with Caroline, the stressors she is experiencing are real and probably cannot be modified; unfortunately, bullying and the cultural pressure in adolescence regarding weight are very real. For Caroline, her desire for a university education places stress on her to perform well on entrance exams and in her high school courses in order to have the possibility for financial support through an academic scholarship. Therefore, a focus on stress overload might not be effective for this patient. However, as the nurse talked with her about the concerns with how she coped with these stresses, Caroline indicated a desire to enhance her own knowledge of stress management techniques, to better manage the stressors in her life, and to learn to reach out to others to enhance her social support. This further data showed the nurse that, in regard to coping strategies, there was a health promotion opportunity for Caroline, and so *readiness for enhanced coping* was a more appropriate diagnosis for Caroline than *ineffective coping.*

Remember that the nursing process, which includes evaluation of the diagnosis, is an ongoing process and as more data become available, or as the patient's condition changes, the diagnosis(es) may also change – or the prioritization may change. Think back for a moment to the initial screening assessment that the nurse performed on Caroline. Do you see that, without further follow-up, he would have missed the health promotion opportunity for Caroline (*readiness for enhanced coping*), and he might have designed a plan to address self-esteem issues that would not have been appropriate for her?

Can you see why the idea of just "picking" a nursing diagnosis to go along with the medical diagnosis simply isn't the way to go? The in-depth, ongoing assessment provided so much more information about Caroline, which can be used to determine not only the appropriate diagnoses, but realistic outcomes and interventions that will best meet her individual needs.

Summary

Assessment is a critical role of professional nurses, and requires an understanding of nursing concepts on which nursing diagnoses are developed. Collecting data for the sole purpose of completing some mandatory form or computer screen is a waste of time, and it certainly does not support individualized care for our patients. Collecting data with the intent of identifying critical information, considering nursing diagnoses, and then driving in-depth assessment to validate and prioritize diagnosis – this is the hallmark of professional nursing.

So, although it may seem to be a simple way to proceed, standardizing nursing diagnoses without assessment can and often does lead to inaccurate diagnoses, inappropriate outcomes, and ineffective and/or unnecessary interventions for diagnoses that are not relevant to the patient – and may lead to completely missing the most important nursing diagnosis for your patient.

References

Bellinger, G., Casstro, D., & Mills, A., Date, Information, Knowledge, and Wisdom. http://otec.uoregon.edu/data-wisdom.htm, accessed January 29, 2014.

Bergstrom, N., Braden, B. J., Laguzza, A., & Holman, V. (1987). The Braden Scale for predicting pressure sore risk. *Nursing Research*, 36(4), 205–210.

Centers for Disease Control & Prevention (2014). BMI Percentile Calculator for Child and Teen. http://apps.nccd.cdc.gov/dnpabmi/Result.aspx?&dob=2/9/2000&dom=1/29/2014&age=167&ht=69&wt=105&gender=2&method=0&inchtext=0&wttext=0, accessed January 29, 2014.

Gordon, M. (1994). Nursing diagnosis: process and application (Vol. 3). St. Louis, MI: Mosby.

Gordon, M. (2008). *Assess Notes: Nursing assessment and diagnostic reasoning.* Philadelphia, PA: F.A. Davis.

Herdman, T. H. (2013). Manejo de casos empleando diagnósticos de enfermería de la NANDA Internacional. [Case management using NANDA International nursing diagnoses]. XXX CONGRESO FEMAFEE 2013. Monterrey, Mexico. (Spanish).

Merriam-Webster.com. Merriam-Webster, n.d. http://www.merriam-webster.com/dictionary/subjective, accessed January 29, 2014.

NANDA-I. (2010). Position statement. http://www.nanda.org/nanda-international-use-of-taxonomy-II-assessment-framework.html, accessed March 20, 2014.

Rencic, J. (2011). Twelve tips for teaching expertise in clinical reasoning. *Medical Teacher, 33*(11), 887–892.

Chapter 3

An Introduction to the NANDA-I Taxonomy

T. Heather Herdman, RN, PhD, FNI

NANDA International, Inc. provides a standardized *terminology* of nursing diagnoses, and it presents all of its diagnoses in a classification scheme, more specifically a *taxonomy*. It is important to understand a little bit about a taxonomy, and how taxonomy differs from terminology. So, let's take a moment to talk about what taxonomy actually represents. A definition of the NANDA-I taxonomy might be: "a systematic ordering of phenomena that define the knowledge of the nursing discipline." That is quite a statement! More simply put, the NANDA–I taxonomy of nursing diagnoses is a classification schema to help us to organize the concepts of concern for nursing practice.

Taxonomy: Visualizing a Taxonomic Structure

A *taxonomy* is a way of classifying or ordering things into categories; it is a hierarchical classification scheme of main groups, subgroups, and items. For example, the current biological taxonomy originated with Carl Linnaeus in 1735. He originally identified three kingdoms (animal, plant, mineral), which were then divided into classes, orders, families, genera, and species (Quammen, 2007). You probably learned about the revised biological taxonomy in a basic science class in your high school or university setting. *Terminology*, on the other hand, is the language that is used to describe a specific thing; it is the language used within a particular discipline to describe its knowledge. Therefore, the nursing diagnoses form a language of the discipline, so when we want to talk about the diagnoses themselves, we are talking about the *terminology* of nursing knowledge. When we want to talk about the way in which we structure or categorize the NANDA-I diagnoses, then we are talking about the *taxonomy*. The word taxonomy comes from two Greek words: *taxis*, meaning arrangement, and *nomos*, meaning law.

NANDA International, Inc. Nursing Diagnoses: Definitions & Classification 2015–2017,
Tenth Edition. Edited by T. Heather Herdman and Shigemi Kamitsuru.
© 2014 NANDA International, Inc. Published 2014 by John Wiley & Sons, Ltd.
Companion website: www.wiley.com/go/nursingdiagnoses

Let's think about taxonomy as it relates to something we all have to deal with in our daily lives. When you need to buy food, you go to the grocery store. Suppose that there's a new store in your neighborhood, Classified Groceries, Inc., so you decide to go there to do your shopping. When you enter the store, you notice that the layout seems very different from your regular store, but the person greeting you at the door hands you a diagram to help you learn your way around (Figure 3.1).

You can see that this store has organized all of the grocery items into eight main categories or grocery store aisles: proteins, grain products, vegetables, fruits, processed foods, snack foods, deli foods, and beverages. These categories/aisles could also be called "domains" – they are broad levels of classification that divide phenomena into main groups. In this case, the phenomena represent "groceries."

You may also have noticed that the diagram doesn't just show the eight aisles; each aisle has a few key phrases identified that further help us to understand what types of foods would be found in each aisle. For example, in the aisle (domain) entitled "Proteins," we see six subcategories: "Cheese products," "Egg products," "Fish products," "Meat products," "Meat substitutes," and "Milk products." Another way of saying this would be that these subcategories are "Classes" of foods that are found under the "Domain" of Proteins.

One of the rules people try to follow when they develop a taxonomy is that the classes should be mutually exclusive – in other words, one type of food should not be found in multiple classes. This isn't always possible, but this should still be the goal, because it makes it much clearer for people who want to use the structure. If you find black beans in the protein aisle, but the pinto and navy beans are in the vegetable aisle, it makes it hard for people to understand the classification system that is being used.

Looking back at our store diagram, you notice there is additional information on the other side of the paper you've been given (Figure 3.2). Each of the grocery aisles is further explained, providing a more detailed level of information about the groceries that are found in different cases located in that aisle. As an example, Figure 3.2 shows the information provided on the "Proteins" Aisle. You note that now you have the six "classes," along with additional detail below those classes. These represent various types (or concepts) of foods, all of which share similar properties that cluster them together into one group.

Given the information we have been provided, we could easily manage our shopping list. If we needed goat milk, we would pretty quickly be able to find the aisle marked "Proteins," the case marked "Milk products," and we could confirm that goat milk would be found there. Likewise, if we wanted chicken and ham, we would again look at the

Figure 3.1 *Domains and Classes of Classified Groceries, Inc.*

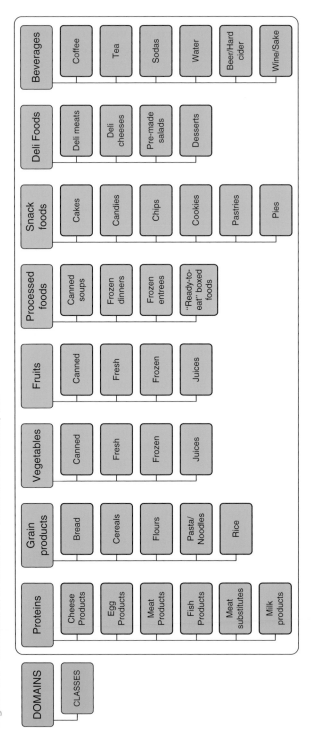

Figure 3.2 *Classes and Concepts of Classified Groceries, Inc.*

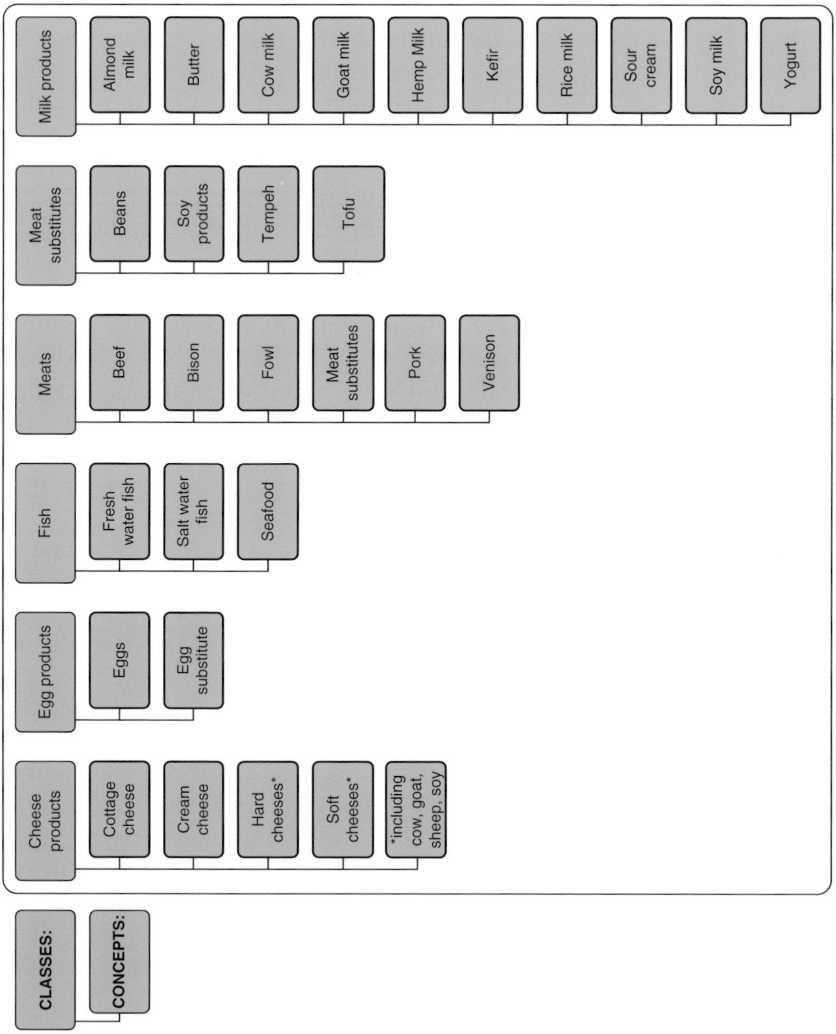

CLASSES:

CONCEPTS:

Cheese products	Egg products	Fish	Meats	Meat substitutes	Milk products
Cottage cheese	Eggs	Fresh water fish	Beef	Beans	Almond milk
Cream cheese	Egg substitute	Salt water fish	Bison	Soy products	Butter
Hard cheeses*		Seafood	Fowl	Tempeh	Cow milk
Soft cheeses*			Meat substitutes	Tofu	Goat milk
*including cow, goat, sheep, soy			Pork		Hemp Milk
			Venison		Kefir
					Rice milk
					Sour cream
					Soy milk
					Yogurt

aisle marked "Proteins," find the case marked "Meat Products," and then see "Fowl" – for our chicken – and "Pork" – for our ham.

The purpose of this grocery taxonomy, then, is to help shoppers quickly determine what section of the store contains the grocery supplies that they want to buy. Without this, shoppers would have to walk up and down each aisle and try to make sense of what products were in which aisles – depending on the size of the store, this could be a very frustrating and confusing experience! So, the diagram being provided by the store personnel provides a "concept map," or a guide for shoppers to understand quickly how the groceries have been classified into locations within the store, with the goal of improving the shopping experience.

This example of a grocery taxonomy may not meet the goal of avoiding overlap between concepts and classes in a way that is logical for all shoppers. For example, juices are found in the domain *Fruits* (fruit juices) and in the domain *Vegetables* (vegetable juices), but *not* in the domain *Beverages*. Although one group of individuals might find this categorization logical and clear, others might suggest that all beverages should be together. What is important is that the distinction between the domains is well defined; that is, that all fruit and fruit products are found within the fruit domain, whereas the beverage domain contains beverages that are not fruit or vegetable based. The problem with this distinction might be that we could argue that wine and hard cider should then be in the fruit aisle, and beer and sake should be in the grains aisle!

By now, you're probably getting a good idea of the difficulty of developing a taxonomy that reflects the concepts it is trying to classify in a clear, concise, and consistent manner. Thinking about our grocery store example, can you imagine different ways in which items in the store might have been grouped together?

Taxonomies are works in progress: they continue to grow, evolve, and even dramatically change as more knowledge is developed about the area of study. There is often a lot of debate about what structure is best for categorizing phenomena of concern to different disciplines. There are many different ways of categorizing things and, truly, there is no "absolutely right" way. The goal is to find a logical, consistent way to categorize similar things while avoiding overlap between the concepts and the classes. For users of taxonomies, the goal is to understand how it classifies similar concepts into its domains and classes, in order to identify particular concepts quickly as needed.

Classification in Nursing

According to Abbott (1988), professions develop abstract, formal knowledge from the original origin of that knowledge. Professions organize their formal knowledge into consistent, logical, conceptualized dimensions so that it reflects the professional domain, and makes it relevant for clinical practice. For professionals in healthcare the knowledge of diagnosis is a significant part of professional knowledge and is essential for clinical practice. Knowledge of nursing diagnoses must therefore be organized in a way that legitimizes professional practice, and consolidates the nursing profession's jurisdiction (Abbott, 1988).

Within the NANDA-I nursing diagnostic taxonomy, we use a hierarchical graphic to show our domains and classes (Figure 3.3). The diagnoses themselves aren't actually depicted in this graphic, although they could be. The primary reason we don't include the diagnoses is that there are 235 of them, and that would make the graphic very large – and very hard to read!

Classification is a way of understanding reality by naming and ordering items, objects, and phenomena into categories (von Krogh, 2011). In healthcare, terminologies denote disciplinary knowledge, and demonstrate how a specific group of professionals perceive the significant areas of knowledge of the discipline. A taxonomy in healthcare therefore has multiple functions, including to:

- provide a view of the knowledge and practice area of a specific profession
- organize phenomena in a way that refers to changes in health, processes, and mechanisms that are of concern to the professional
- show the logical connection between factors that can be controlled or manipulated by professionals in the discipline (von Krogh, 2011)

Within nursing, what is most important is that the diagnoses are classified in a way that makes sense clinically, so that when a nurse is trying to identify a diagnosis that he may not see very often in practice, he can logically use the taxonomy to find appropriate information on possible related diagnoses. Although the NANDA-I Taxonomy II (Figure 3.3) is *not* intended to function as a nursing assessment framework, it does provide a structure for classifying nursing diagnoses into domains and classes, each of which is clearly defined.

To provide an example of what it would look like if we did include the nursing diagnoses in the graphic representation of the taxonomy, Figure 3.4 shows just one domain with its classes and nursing diagnoses. As you can see, this is a lot of information!

Nursing knowledge includes individual, family, group, and community responses (healthy and unhealthy), risks, and strengths. The NANDA-I taxonomy is meant to function in the following ways – it should:

- provide a model, or cognitive map, of the knowledge of the nursing discipline
- communicate that knowledge, perspectives, and theories

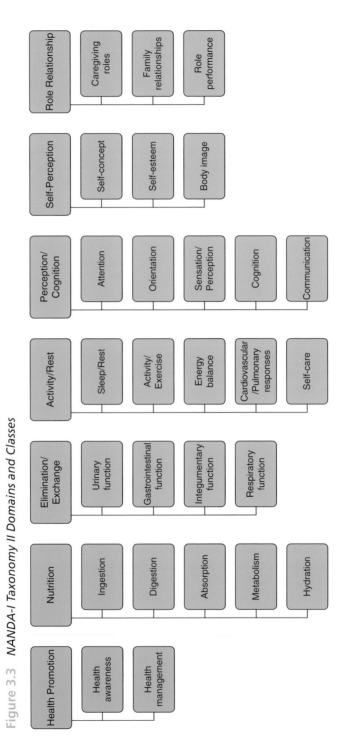

Figure 3.3 *NANDA-I Taxonomy II Domains and Classes*

Figure 3.3 *Continued*

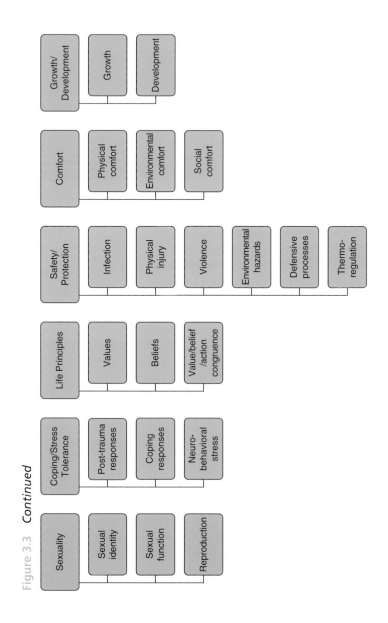

Figure 3.4 *NANDA-I Domain 1,* Health Promotion, *with Classes and Nursing Diagnoses*

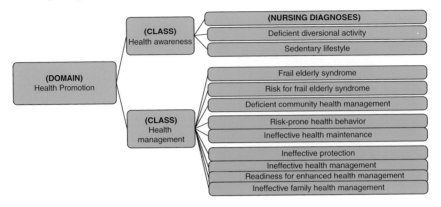

- provide structure and order for that knowledge
- serve as a support tool for clinical reasoning
- provide a way to organize nursing diagnoses within an electronic health record (adapted from von Krogh, 2011).

Using the NANDA-I Taxonomy

Although the taxonomy provides a way of categorizing nursing phenomena, it can also serve other functions. It can help faculty to develop a nursing curriculum, for example. And it can help a nurse identify a diagnosis, perhaps one that he may not use frequently, but that he needs for a particular patient. Let's look at both of these ideas.

Structuring Nursing Curricula

Although the NANDA-I nursing taxonomy is not intended to be a nursing assessment framework, it can support the organization of undergraduate education. For example, curricula can be developed around the domains and classes, allowing courses to be taught that are based on the core concepts of nursing practice, which are categorized in each of the NANDA-I domains.

A course might be built around the Activity/Rest domain (Figure 3.5), with units based on each of the classes. In Unit 1, the focus could be on sleep/rest, and the concept of sleep would be explored in depth. What is sleep? What impact does it have on individual and family health? What are some of the common sleep-related problems that our patients encounter? In what types of patients might we be most likely to identify

Figure 3.5 *NANDA-I Taxonomy II Activity/Rest Domain*

Sleep/Rest	Activity/Exercise	Energy Balance	Cardiovascular/Pulmonary Responses	Self-care
Insomnia	Risk for disuse syndrome	Fatigue	Activity intolerance	Impaired home maintenance
Sleep deprivation	Impaired bed mobility	Wandering	Risk for activity intolerance	Readiness for enhanced self-care
Readiness for enhanced sleep	Impaired physical mobility		Ineffective breathing pattern	Bathing self-care deficit
Disturbed sleep pattern	Impaired wheelchair mobility		Decreased cardiac output	Dressing self-care deficit
	Impaired sitting		Risk for decreased cardiac output	Feeding self-care deficit
	Impaired standing		Risk for impaired cardiovascular function	Toileting self-care deficit
	Impaired transfer ability		Risk for ineffective gastrointestinal perfusion	Self-neglect
	Impaired walking		Risk for ineffective renal perfusion	
			Impaired spontaneous ventilation	
			Risk for decreased cardiac tissue perfusion	
			Risk for ineffective cerebral tissue perfusion	
			Ineffective peripheral tissue perfusion	
			Risk for ineffective peripheral tissue perfusion	
			Dysfunctional ventilatory weaning response	

these conditions? What are the primary etiologies? What are the consequences if these conditions go undiagnosed and/or untreated? How can we prevent, treat, and/or improve these conditions? How can we manage the symptoms?

Building a nursing curriculum around these key concepts of nursing knowledge enables students to truly understand and build expertise in the knowledge of nursing science, while also learning about and understanding related medical diagnoses and conditions that they will also encounter in everyday practice.

Designing nursing courses in this way enables students to learn a lot about the disciplinary knowledge of nursing. Activity tolerance, breathing pattern, cardiac output, mobility, self-care, and tissue perfusion are some of the key concepts of Domain 4 (Figure 3.5) – they are the "neutral states" that we must understand before we can identify potential or actual problems with these responses.

Understanding *tissue perfusion*, for example, as a core concept of nursing practice requires a strong understanding of anatomy, physiology, and pathophysiology (including related medical diagnoses), as well as responses from other domains that might coincide with problems in tissue perfusion. Once you truly understand the concept of tissue perfusion (the "normal" or neutral state), identifying the abnormal state is much easier because you know what you should be seeing if tissue perfusion were normal, and if you are not seeing those data, you start to suspect that there might be a problem (or a risk may exist for a problem to develop). So, developing nursing courses around these core concepts enables nursing faculty to focus on the knowledge of the nursing discipline, and then to incorporate related medical diagnoses and/or interdisciplinary concerns in a way that allows nurses to focus first on nursing phenomena, and then to bring their specific knowledge to an interdisciplinary view of the patient to improve patient care. This then moves into content on realistic patient outcomes, and evidence-based interventions that nurses will utilize (dependent and independent nursing interventions) to provide the best possible care to the patient to achieve outcomes for which nurses have accountability.

Identifying a Nursing Diagnosis Outside Your Area of Expertise

Nurses build expertise in those nursing diagnoses that they most commonly see in their clinical practice. If your area of interest is perinatal nursing practice, then your expertise may include such key concepts as the childbearing process, health management, nutrition, fatigue, resilience, parenting, breastfeeding – just to name a few! But you will deal with patients who, despite being primarily in your care because of the

Figure 3.6 *Use of the NANDA-I Taxonomy II and Terminology to Identify and Validate a Nursing Diagnosis Outside the Nurse's Area of Expertise*

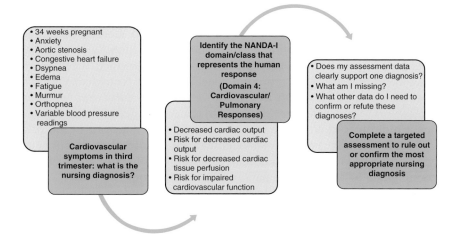

impending birth of a baby, will also have other issues that require your attention. The NANDA-I taxonomy can help you to identify potential diagnoses for these patients, while the NANDA-I terminology (the diagnoses themselves) can support your clinical reasoning skills by clarifying what assessment data/diagnostic indicators are necessary for quickly, but accurately, diagnosing your patients.

Perhaps your patient is discovered to have a congenital heart defect that was undetected until her circulating volume expanded to meet the needs of her growing fetus – a perfectly normal occurrence during pregnancy, but one that, with her condition, has put her health, and that of her fetus, at significant risk. You know that your patient is not tolerating the normal hemodynamic changes associated with pregnancy (increased heart rate, cardiac output, and blood volume), but you aren't sure which nursing diagnosis is the most accurate for her condition. By looking at the taxonomy, you can quickly form a "cognitive map" that can help you to find more information on diagnoses of relevance to this patient (Figure 3.6).

You know you are looking at a cardiovascular response, and a quick review of the taxonomy leads you to Domain 4 (Activity/Rest), Class 4 (Cardiovascular/Pulmonary Responses). You then see that there are four diagnoses specifically related to cardiovascular responses, and you can review the definitions, etiologies, and signs/symptoms to clarify the most appropriate diagnosis for this patient. Using the taxonomy and terminology in this way supports clinical reasoning, and helps you to navigate a large volume of information/knowledge (235 diagnoses) in an effective and efficient manner. A review of the risk factors or the related factors and defining characteristics of these four diagnoses can (a) provide you with additional data that you need to obtain in order to make an informed decision, and/or (b) enable you to compare your assessment with those diagnostic indicators to diagnose your patient accurately.

Think about a recent patient: Did you struggle to diagnose his human response? Did you find it difficult to know how to identify potential diagnoses? Using the taxonomy can support you in identifying possible diagnoses because of the way the diagnoses are grouped together in classes and domains that represent specific areas of knowledge. Don't forget, however, that *simply looking at the diagnosis label and "picking a diagnosis" is not safe care!* You need to review the definition and diagnostic indicators (defining characteristics and related factors, or the risk factors) for each of the potential diagnoses you identify, which will help you to know what additional data you should collect or if you have enough data to diagnose the patient's human response accurately.

Take a look at the case study on Mrs. Lendo to understand how you might use the taxonomy to help you to identify potential diagnoses.

Case Study: *Mrs. Lendo*

Let's suppose that your patient, Martha Lendo, a 65-year-old married woman, presents with a lower extremity wound, obtained during a minor vehicular accident 15 days ago, that does not show signs of healing. She has 3+ edema in her lower extremities, significantly diminished bilateral peripheral pulses, and a lower extremity capillary refill time of 5 seconds. She is a moderate smoker who is overweight, and she has diabetes mellitus. She describes her life as extremely sedentary, and she states, "Even if I wanted to exercise, I couldn't – my legs hurt so badly when I walk almost any distance at all."

After completing your assessment and reviewing her history, you are confident that Mrs. Lendo has a problem with circulation, but you are new to this area of nursing and so you need some review of potential diagnoses. Since you are considering a circulatory issue, you look at the NANDA-I taxonomy to identify the logical location of these diagnoses. You identify that *Domain 4, Activity/Rest,* deals with production, conservation, expenditure, or balance of energy. Because you know that cardiopulmonary mechanisms support activity/rest, you think this domain will contain diagnoses of relevance to Mrs. Lendo. You then quickly identify *Class 4, Cardiovascular/Pulmonary Responses.* A review of this class leads to the identification of three potential diagnoses: *decreased cardiac output, ineffective peripheral tissue perfusion,* and *risk for ineffective tissue perfusion.*

Questions you should ask yourself include:

- What other human responses should I rule out or consider?
- What other signs/symptoms, or etiologies should I look for to confirm this diagnosis?

Once you review the definitions and diagnostic indicators (related factors, defining characteristics, and risk factors), you diagnose Mrs. Lendo with *ineffective peripheral tissue perfusion* (00204); see Figure 3.7.

Figure 3.7 *Diagnosing Mrs. Lendo*

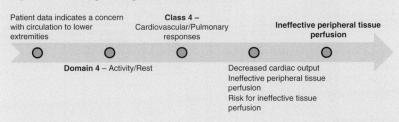

Some final questions should include:

- Am I missing anything?
- Am I diagnosing without sufficient evidence?

If you believe you are correct in your diagnosis, your questions move on to:

- What outcomes can I realistically expect to achieve in Mrs. Lendo?
- What are the evidence-based nursing interventions that I should consider?
- How will I evaluate whether or not they were effective?

The NANDA-I Nursing Diagnosis Taxonomy: A Short History

In 1987, NANDA-I published Taxonomy I, which was structured to reflect nursing theoretical models from North America. In 2002, Taxonomy II was adopted, which was adapted from the Functional Health Patterns assessment framework of Dr. Marjory Gordon. A historical perspective on the NANDA-I taxonomy can be found at our website, at www.nanda. org/nanda-international-history.html.

Table 3.1 demonstrates the domains, classes, and nursing diagnoses and how they are currently located within the NANDA-I Taxonomy II.

Table 3.1   Domains, Classes, and Nursing Diagnoses in the NANDA-I Taxonomy II

DOMAIN 1. HEALTH PROMOTION

The awareness of well-being or normality of function and the strategies used to maintain control of and enhance that well-being or normality of function

Class 1. Health awareness		Recognition of normal function and well-being	
Code	**Diagnosis**	**Code**	**Diagnosis**
00097	Deficient diversional activity	00168	Sedentary lifestyle

Class 2. Health management		Identifying, controlling, performing, and integrating activities to maintain health and well-being	
Code	**Diagnosis**	**Code**	**Diagnosis**
00257	Frail elderly syndrome	00078	Ineffective health management
00231	Risk for frail elderly syndrome	00162	Readiness for enhanced health management
00215	Deficient community health	00080	Ineffective family health management
00188	Risk-prone health behavior	00079	Noncompliance
00099	Ineffective health maintenance	00043	Ineffective protection

DOMAIN 2. Nutrition

The activities of taking in, assimilating, and using nutrients for the purposes of tissue maintenance, tissue repair, and the production of energy

Class 1. Ingestion		Taking food or nutrients into the body	
Code	**Diagnosis**	**Code**	**Diagnosis**
00216	Insufficient breast milk	00163	Readiness for enhanced **nutrition**
00104	Ineffective **breastfeeding**	00232	**Obesity**
00105	Interrupted **breastfeeding**	00233	**Overweight**
00106	Readiness for enhanced **breastfeeding**	00234	Risk for **overweight**
00107	Ineffective infant **feeding pattern**	00103	Impaired **swallowing**
00002	Imbalanced **nutrition**: less than body requirements		

Class 2. Digestion		The physical and chemical activities that convert foodstuffs into substances suitable for absorption and assimilation
None at present time		

Class 3. Absorption		The act of taking up nutrients through body tissues
None at present time		

Class 4. Metabolism		The chemical and physical processes occurring in living organisms and cells for the development and use of protoplasm, the production of waste and energy, with the release of energy for all vital processes
Code	**Diagnosis**	**Code**	**Diagnosis**
00179	Risk for unstable **blood glucose level**	00230	Risk for neonatal **jaundice**
00194	Neonatal **jaundice**	00178	Risk for impaired **liver function**

Class 5. Hydration		The taking in and absorption of **fluids and electrolytes**	
Code	**Diagnosis**	**Code**	**Diagnosis**
00195	Risk for **electrolyte** imbalance	00028	Risk for deficient **fluid volume**
00160	Readiness for enhanced **fluid balance**	00026	Excess **fluid volume**
00027	Deficient **fluid volume**	00025	Risk for imbalanced **fluid volume**

Continued

Table 3.1   Continued

DOMAIN 3. ELIMINATION AND EXCHANGE

Secretion and excretion of waste products from the body

Class 1. Urinary function
The process of secretion, reabsorption, and excretion of urine

Code	Diagnosis	Code	Diagnosis
00016	Impaired urinary elimination	00017	Stress urinary incontinence
00166	Readiness for enhanced urinary elimination	00019	Urge urinary incontinence
00020	Functional urinary incontinence	00022	Risk for urge urinary incontinence
00176	Overflow urinary incontinence	00023	Urinary retention
00018	Reflex urinary incontinence		

Class 2. Gastrointestinal function
The process of absorption and excretion of the end products of digestion

Code	Diagnosis	Code	Diagnosis
00011	Constipation	00013	Diarrhea
00015	Risk for constipation	00196	Dysfunctional gastrointestinal motility
00235	Chronic functional constipation	00197	Risk for dysfunctional gastrointestinal motility
00236	Risk for chronic functional constipation	00014	Bowel incontinence
00012	Perceived constipation		

Class 3. Integumentary function
The process of secretion and excretion through the skin

None at this time

Class 4. Respiratory function
The process of exchange of gases and removal of the end products of metabolism

Code	Diagnosis
00030	Impaired gas exchange

DOMAIN 4. ACTIVITY/REST

The production, conservation, expenditure, or balance of energy resources

Class 1. Sleep/Rest
Slumber, repose, ease, relaxation, or inactivity

Code	Diagnosis	Code	Diagnosis
00095	Insomnia	00165	Readiness for enhanced sleep
00096	**Sleep** deprivation	00198	Disturbed **sleep pattern**

Class 2. Activity/Exercise
Moving parts of the body (mobility), doing work, or performing actions often (but not always) against resistance

Code	Diagnosis	Code	Diagnosis
00040	Risk for **disuse syndrome**	00237	Impaired **sitting**
00091	Impaired **bed mobility**	00238	Impaired **standing**
00085	Impaired physical **mobility**	00090	Impaired **transfer ability**
00089	Impaired **wheelchair mobility**	00088	Impaired **walking**

Class 3. Energy balance
A dynamic state of harmony between intake and expenditure of resources

Code	Diagnosis	Code	Diagnosis
00093	Fatigue	00154	**Wandering**

Class 4. Cardiovascular/pulmonary responses
Cardiopulmonary mechanisms that support activity/rest

Code	Diagnosis	Code	Diagnosis
00092	**Activity** intolerance	00203	Risk for ineffective **renal perfusion**
00094	Risk for **activity intolerance**	00033	Impaired **spontaneous ventilation**
00032	Ineffective **breathing pattern**	00200	Risk for decreased cardiac **tissue perfusion**
00029	Decreased **cardiac output**	00201	Risk for ineffective cerebral **tissue perfusion**
00240	Risk for decreased **cardiac output**	00204	Ineffective peripheral **tissue perfusion**
00239	Risk for impaired **cardiovascular function**	00228	Risk for ineffective peripheral **tissue perfusion**
00202	Risk for ineffective **gastrointestinal perfusion**	00034	Dysfunctional **ventilatory weaning response**

Continued

Table 3.1 Continued

DOMAIN 4. ACTIVITY/REST

The production, conservation, expenditure, or balance of energy resources

Class 5. Self-care | **Ability to perform activities to care for one's body and bodily functions**

Code	Diagnosis	Code	Diagnosis
00098	Impaired **home maintenance**	00110	**Toileting self-care** deficit*
00108	**Bathing self-care** deficit*	00182	Readiness for enhanced **self-care***
00109	**Dressing self-care** deficit*	00193	**Self-neglect**
00102	**Feeding self-care** deficit*		

DOMAIN 5. PERCEPTION/COGNITION

The human information processing system including attention, orientation, sensation, perception, cognition, and communication

Class 1. Attention | **Mental readiness to notice or observe**

Code	Diagnosis	Code	Diagnosis
00123	**Unilateral neglect**		

Class 2. Orientation | **Awareness of time, place, and person**

None at this time

Class 3. Sensation/perception | **Receiving information through the senses of touch, taste, smell, vision, hearing, and kinesthesia, and the comprehension of sensory data resulting in naming, associating, and/or pattern recognition**

None at this time

---

*The editors acknowledge these diagnoses are not in alphabetical order, but a decision was made to maintain all "self-care deficit" diagnoses in sequential order.

Class 4. Cognition		Use of memory, learning, thinking, problem-solving, abstraction, judgment, insight, intellectual capacity, calculation, and language	
Code	Diagnosis	Code	Diagnosis
00128	Acute confusion	00222	Ineffective impulse control
00173	Risk for acute confusion	00126	Deficient knowledge
00129	Chronic confusion	00161	Readiness for enhanced knowledge
00251	Labile emotional control	00131	Impaired memory
Class 5. Communication		Sending and receiving verbal and nonverbal information	
Code	Diagnosis	Code	Diagnosis
00157	Readiness for enhanced communication	00051	Impaired verbal communication

DOMAIN 6. SELF-PERCEPTION

Awareness about the self

Class 1. Self-concept		The perception(s) about the total self	
Code	Diagnosis	Code	Diagnosis
00185	Readiness for enhanced hope	00121	Disturbed personal identity
00124	Hopelessness	00225	Risk for disturbed personal identity
00174	Risk for compromised human dignity	00167	Readiness for enhanced self-concept
Class 2. Self-esteem		Assessment of one's own worth, capability, significance, and success	
Code	Diagnosis	Code	Diagnosis
00119	Chronic low self-esteem	00120	Situational low self-esteem
00224	Risk for chronic low self-esteem	00153	Risk for situational low self-esteem
Class 3. Body image		A mental image of one's own body	
Code	Diagnosis		
00118	Disturbed body image		

Continued

Table 3.1   Continued

DOMAIN 7. ROLE RELATIONSHIPS

The positive and negative connections or associations between people or groups of people and the means by which those connections are demonstrated

Class 1. Caregiving roles		Socially expected behavior patterns by people providing care who are not healthcare professionals	
Code	**Diagnosis**	**Code**	**Diagnosis**
00061	Caregiver role strain	00164	Readiness for enhanced parenting
00062	Risk for caregiver role strain	00057	Risk for impaired parenting
00056	Impaired parenting		
Class 2. Family relationships		Associations of people who are biologically related or related by choice	
Code	**Diagnosis**	**Code**	**Diagnosis**
00058	Risk for impaired attachment	00060	Interrupted family processes
00063	Dysfunctional family processes	00159	Readiness for enhanced family processes
Class 3. Role performance		Quality of functioning in socially expected behavior patterns	
Code	**Diagnosis**	**Code**	**Diagnosis**
00223	Ineffective relationship	00064	Parental role conflict
00207	Readiness for enhanced relationship	00055	Ineffective role performance
00229	Risk for ineffective relationship	00052	Impaired social interaction

DOMAIN 8. SEXUALITY

Sexual identity, sexual function, and reproduction

Class 1. Sexual identity	The state of being a specific person in regard to sexuality and/or gender

None at present time

Class 2. Sexual function	The capacity or ability to participate in sexual activities

Code	Diagnosis
00059	Sexual dysfunction

Class 3. Reproduction	Any process by which human beings are produced

Code	Diagnosis
00221	Ineffective childbearing process
00208	Readiness for enhanced childbearing process

Code	Diagnosis
00065	Ineffective sexuality pattern

Code	Diagnosis
00227	Risk for ineffective childbearing process
00209	Risk for disturbed maternal–fetal dyad

DOMAIN 9. COPING/STRESS TOLERANCE

Contending with life events/life processes

Class 1. Post-trauma responses	Reactions occurring after physical or psychological trauma

Code	Diagnosis
00141	Post-trauma syndrome
00145	Risk for post-trauma syndrome
00142	Rape-trauma syndrome

Code	Diagnosis
00114	Relocation stress syndrome
00149	Risk for relocation stress syndrome

Continued

Table 3.1 Continued

DOMAIN 9. COPING/STRESS TOLERANCE

Table 3.1 Continued

Contending with life events/life processes

Class 2. Coping responses — The process of managing environmental stress

Code	Diagnosis	Code	Diagnosis
00199	Ineffective activity planning	00148	Fear
00226	Risk for ineffective activity planning	00136	Grieving
00146	Anxiety	00135	Complicated grieving
00071	Defensive coping	00172	Risk for complicated grieving
00069	Ineffective coping	00241	Impaired mood regulation
00158	Readiness for enhanced coping	00187	Readiness for enhanced power
00077	Ineffective community coping	00125	Powerlessness
00076	Readiness for enhanced community coping	00152	Risk for powerlessness
00074	Compromised family coping	00210	Impaired resilience
00073	Disabled family coping	00212	Readiness for enhanced resilience
00075	Readiness for enhanced family coping	00211	Risk for impaired resilience
00147	Death anxiety	00137	Chronic sorrow
00072	Ineffective denial	00177	Stress overload

Class 3. Neurobehavioral stress — Behavioral responses reflecting nerve and brain function

Code	Diagnosis	Code	Diagnosis
00049	Decreased intracranial adaptive capacity	00116	Disorganized infant behavior
00009	Autonomic dysreflexia	00117	Readiness for enhanced organized infant behavior
00010	Risk for autonomic dysreflexia	00115	Risk for disorganized infant behavior

DOMAIN 10. LIFE PRINCIPLES

Principles underlying conduct, thought, and behavior about acts, customs, or institutions viewed as being true or having intrinsic worth

Class 1. Values	The identification and ranking of preferred modes of conduct or end states

None at this time

Class 2. Beliefs	Opinions, expectations, or judgments about acts, customs, or institutions viewed as being true or having intrinsic worth

Code	Diagnosis
00068	Readiness for enhanced **spiritual** well-being

Class 3. Value/belief/action congruence	The correspondence or balance achieved among values, beliefs, and actions

Code	Diagnosis	Code	Diagnosis
00184	Readiness for enhanced **decision-making**	00169	Impaired **religiosity**
00083	**Decisional conflict**	00171	Readiness for enhanced **religiosity**
00242	Impaired **emancipated decision-making**	00170	Risk for impaired **religiosity**
00243	Readiness for enhanced **emancipated decision-making**	00066	**Spiritual** distress
00244	Risk for impaired **emancipated decision-making**	00067	Risk for **spiritual** distress
00175	**Moral distress**		

Continued

Table 3.1 Continued

DOMAIN 11. SAFETY/PROTECTION

Freedom from danger, physical injury, or immune system damage; preservation from loss; and protection of safety and security

Class 1. Infection

Code	Diagnosis
00004	Risk for infection

Class 2. Physical injury

Host responses following pathogenic invasion

Bodily harm or hurt

Code	Diagnosis	Code	Diagnosis
00031	Ineffective **airway clearance**	00086	Risk for peripheral neurovascular **dysfunction**
00039	Risk for **aspiration**	00249	Risk for **pressure ulcer**
00206	Risk for **bleeding**	00205	Risk for **shock**
00219	Risk for **dry eye**	00046	Impaired **skin integrity**
00155	Risk for **falls**	00047	Risk for impaired **skin integrity**
00035	Risk for **injury***	00156	Risk for **sudden infant death syndrome**
00245	Risk for **corneal injury***	00036	Risk for **suffocation**
00087	Risk for perioperative **positioning injury***	00100	Delayed **surgical recovery**
00220	Risk for **thermal injury***	00246	Risk for delayed **surgical recovery**
00250	Risk for **urinary tract injury***	00044	Impaired **tissue integrity**
00048	Impaired **dentition**	00248	Risk for impaired **tissue integrity**
00045	Impaired oral **mucous membrane**	00038	Risk for **trauma**
00247	Risk for impaired oral **mucous membrane**	00213	Risk for vascular **trauma**

*The editors acknowledge these diagnoses are not in alphabetical order, but a decision was made to maintain all "Risk for injury" diagnoses in sequential order.

Class 3. Violence	The exertion of excessive force or power so as to cause injury or abuse	
Code	**Diagnosis**	
00138	Risk for other-directed violence	
00140	Risk for self-directed violence	
00151	**Self-mutilation**	

Code	**Diagnosis**	
00139	Risk for self-mutilation	
00150	Risk for suicide	

Class 4. Environmental Hazards	Sources of danger in the surroundings	
Code	**Diagnosis**	
00181	**Contamination**	
00180	Risk for contamination	

Code	**Diagnosis**	
00037	Risk for poisoning	

Class 5. Defensive processes	The processes by which the self protects itself from the nonself	
Code	**Diagnosis**	
00218	Risk for adverse reaction to iodinated contrast media	
00217	Risk for allergy response	

Code	**Diagnosis**	
00041	**Latex allergy response**	
00042	Risk for latex allergy response	

Class 6. Thermoregulation	The physiological process of regulating heat and energy within the body for purposes of protecting the organism	
Code	**Diagnosis**	
00005	Risk for imbalanced body temperature	
00007	**Hyperthermia**	
00006	**Hypothermia**	

Code	**Diagnosis**	
00253	Risk for hypothermia	
00254	Risk for perioperative hypothermia	
00008	Ineffective thermoregulation	

Continued

Table 3.1 Continued

DOMAIN 12. COMFORT

Sense of mental, physical, or social well-being or ease

Class 1. Physical comfort		Sense of well-being or ease and/or freedom from pain	
Code	**Diagnosis**	**Code**	**Diagnosis**
00214	Impaired comfort	00133	Chronic pain
00183	Readiness for enhanced comfort	00256	Labor pain
00134	Nausea	00255	Chronic pain syndrome
00132	Acute pain		

Class 2. Environmental comfort		Sense of well-being or ease in/with one's environment	
Code	**Diagnosis**	**Code**	**Diagnosis**
00214	Impaired comfort	00183	Readiness for enhanced comfort

Class 3. Social comfort		Sense of well-being or ease with one's social situation	
Code	**Diagnosis**	**Code**	**Diagnosis**
00214	Impaired comfort	00054	Risk for loneliness
00183	Readiness for enhanced comfort	00053	**Social isolation**

DOMAIN 13. GROWTH/DEVELOPMENT

Age-appropriate increases in physical dimensions, maturation of organ systems, and/or progression through the developmental milestones

Class 1. Growth		Increases in physical dimensions or maturity of organ systems
Code	**Diagnosis**	
00113	Risk for disproportionate growth	

Class 2. Development		Progress or regression through a sequence of recognized milestones in life
Code	**Diagnosis**	
00112	Risk for delayed development	

As previously noted, taxonomies evolve and change over time. This happens for a variety of reasons. We are always learning more about our professional discipline, and perhaps we discover that what we thought belonged within one domain is really more accurately represented in two distinct domains. New phenomena may be discovered that do not clearly fit within an existing structure. In addition, theoretical perspectives change, which leads professionals to view their knowledge from a different perspective. Recently, NANDA-I was presented with a potential new taxonomy, proposed by Dr. Gunn von Krogh. Work will be occurring over the next few years to test and possibly refine this taxonomy. In 2016, the goal is to bring this taxonomy forward to the membership of NANDA-I to determine if the organization should maintain Taxonomy II, or possibly move to this new view, and adopt a Taxonomy III.

In von Krogh's model (Figure 3.8), seven domains are conceptualized based on significant areas of knowledge in nursing.

Because this is a decision that can have a major impact on the nursing profession, from how we teach, to how computer systems are structured to enable documentation and decision support for nursing diagnoses, we're including here the current structure of the *proposed* Taxonomy III (Figure 3.9). It is important to emphasize that **NANDA-I has not adopted this taxonomic structure**, but that work will be ongoing over the next few years to examine its appropriateness as a taxonomic structure for nursing diagnoses, through worldwide discussion and research. In Table 3.2 we show the difference in how the nursing diagnoses would be slotted in this taxonomy, as compared to our current structure. More information on the testing of this proposed taxonomy will be available as it occurs at our website, at www.nanda.org/ADDLINKHERE.

Figure 3.8 *Seven Domains of the Proposed Taxonomy III*

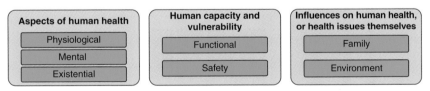

Figure 3.9 *Proposed Taxonomy III Domains and Classes (von Krogh, 2011)*

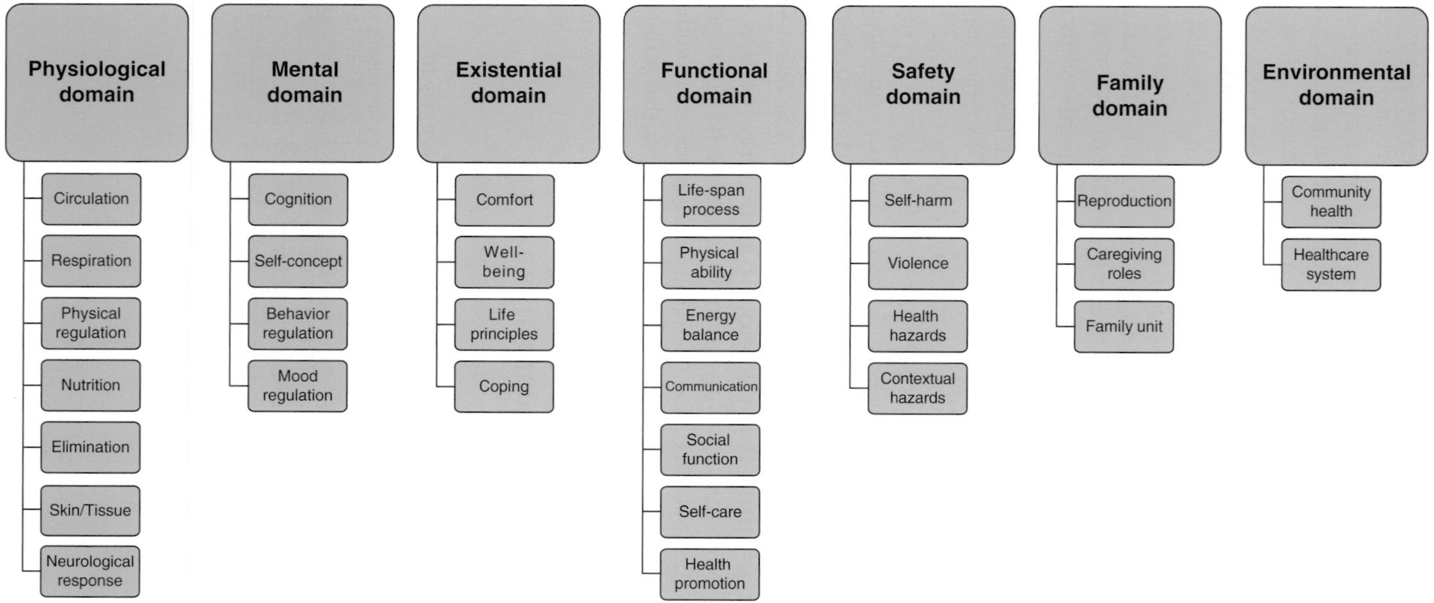

The figure presents the Proposed Taxonomy III with the following domains and their classes:

Physiological domain
- Circulation
- Respiration
- Physical regulation
- Nutrition
- Elimination
- Skin/Tissue
- Neurological response

Mental domain
- Cognition
- Self-concept
- Behavior regulation
- Mood regulation

Existential domain
- Comfort
- Well-being
- Life principles
- Coping

Functional domain
- Life-span process
- Physical ability
- Energy balance
- Communication
- Social function
- Self-care
- Health promotion

Safety domain
- Self-harm
- Violence
- Health hazards
- Contextual hazards

Family domain
- Reproduction
- Caregiving roles
- Family unit

Environmental domain
- Community health
- Healthcare system

Table 3.2   *Proposed Taxonomy III Domains, Classes, and Nursing Diagnoses*

PHYSIOLOGICAL DOMAIN

Anatomical structures and physiological processes essential to human health

Class: Circulation Anatomical structures and physiological processes involved in vital and peripheral circulation	Nursing Diagnosis Code
Decreased cardiac output	00029
Risk for decreased cardiac output	00240
Risk for decreased cardiac tissue perfusion	00200
Risk for impaired cardiovascular function	00239
Risk for ineffective cerebral tissue perfusion	00201
Risk for ineffective gastrointestinal perfusion	00202
Risk for ineffective renal perfusion	00203
Ineffective peripheral tissue perfusion	00204
Risk for ineffective peripheral tissue perfusion	00228
Class: Respiration Anatomical structures and physiological processes involved in ventilation and gas exchange	Nursing Diagnosis Code
Ineffective airway clearance	00031
Ineffective breathing pattern	00032
Impaired gas exchange	00030
Impaired spontaneous ventilation	00033
Dysfunctional ventilatory weaning response	00034
Class: Physical Regulation Anatomical structures and physiological processes involved in hematological, immunological, and metabolic regulatory mechanisms	Nursing Diagnosis Code
Risk for adverse reaction to iodinated contrast media	00218
Risk for allergy response	00217
Risk for unstable blood glucose level	00179
Risk for imbalanced body temperature	00005
Risk for electrolyte imbalance	00195
Readiness for enhanced fluid balance	00160
Deficient fluid volume	00027
Risk for deficient fluid volume	00028
Excess fluid volume	00026
Risk for imbalanced fluid volume	00025

Continued

Table 3.2   *Continued*

Hyperthermia	00007
Risk for hyperthermia	00253
Hypothermia	00006
Risk for hypothermia	00253
Risk for perioperative hypothermia	00254
Neonatal jaundice	00194
Risk for neonatal jaundice	00230
Latex allergy response	00041
Risk for latex allergy response	00042
Risk for impaired liver function	00178
Ineffective thermoregulation	00008
Class: Nutrition Anatomical structures and physiological processes involved in the ingestion, digestion, and absorption of nutrients	Nursing Diagnosis Code
Insufficient breast milk	00216
Ineffective breastfeeding	00104
Interrupted breastfeeding	00105
Readiness for enhanced breastfeeding	00106
Ineffective infant feeding pattern	00107
Imbalanced nutrition: less than body requirements	00002
Readiness for enhanced nutrition	00163
Obesity	00232
Overweight	00233
Risk for overweight	00234
Class: Elimination Anatomical structures and physiological processes involved in discharge of body waste	Nursing Diagnosis Code
Bowel incontinence	00014
Constipation	00011
Risk for constipation	00015
Perceived constipation	00012
Chronic functional constipation	00235
Diarrhea	00013
Dysfunctional gastrointestinal motility	00196
Risk for dysfunctional gastrointestinal motility	00197
Impaired urinary elimination	00016
Readiness for enhanced urinary elimination	00166
Functional urinary incontinence	00020
Overflow urinary incontinence	00176
Reflex urinary incontinence	00018

Table 3.2   *Continued*

Stress urinary incontinence	00017
Urge urinary incontinence	00019
Risk for urge urinary incontinence	00022
Urinary retention	00023
Risk for urinary tract injury	00250
Class: Skin/Tissue Anatomical structures and physiological processes of skin and body tissues involved in structural integrity	Nursing Diagnosis Code
Risk for corneal injury	00245
Impaired dentition	00048
Risk for dry eye	00219
Impaired oral mucous membrane	00045
Risk for impaired oral mucous membrane	00247
Risk for pressure ulcer	00249
Impaired skin integrity	00046
Risk for impaired skin integrity	00047
Risk for thermal injury	00220
Impaired tissue integrity	00044
Risk for impaired tissue integrity	00248
Risk for vascular trauma	00213
Class: Neurological Response Anatomical structures and physiological processes involved in the transmission of nerve impulses	Nursing Diagnosis Code
Decreased intracranial adaptive capacity	00049
Autonomic dysreflexia	00009
Risk for autonomic dysreflexia	00010
Disorganized infant behavior	00116
Readiness for enhanced organized infant behavior	00117
Risk for disorganized infant behavior	00115
Risk for peripheral neurovascular dysfunction	00086
Unilateral neglect	00123
MENTAL DOMAIN	
Mental processes and mental patterns essential to human health	
Class: Cognition Neuropsychological processes involved in orientation, information processing, and memory	Nursing Diagnosis Code
Acute confusion	00128

Continued

Table 3.2   *Continued*

Risk for acute confusion	00173
Chronic confusion	00129
Impaired memory	00131
Class: Self-Concept Psychological patterns involved in self-perception, identity, and self-regulation	Nursing Diagnosis Code
Disturbed body image	00118
Ineffective denial	00072
Labile emotional control	00251
Ineffective impulse control	00222
Chronic low self-esteem	00119
Risk for chronic low self-esteem	00224
Situational low self-esteem	00120
Risk for situational low self-esteem	00153
Disturbed personal identity	00121
Risk for disturbed personal identity	00225
Readiness for enhanced self-concept	00167
Sexual dysfunction	00059
Ineffective sexuality pattern	00065
Class: Mood Regulation Biophysical and emotional interaction processes involved in mood regulation	Nursing Diagnosis Code
Impaired mood regulation	00241
EXISTENTIAL DOMAIN	
Experiences and life perceptions essential to human health	
Class: Comfort Perceptions of symptoms and experience of suffering	Nursing Diagnosis Code
Anxiety	00146
Impaired comfort	00214
Readiness for enhanced comfort	00183
Death anxiety	00147
Fear	00148
Acute pain	00132
Chronic pain	00133
Labor pain	00256
Chronic pain syndrome	00255

Table 3.2   *Continued*

Nausea	00134
Chronic sorrow	00137
Class: Well-Being Perceptions of life qualities and experience of existential needs satisfaction	Nursing Diagnosis Code
Grieving	00136
Complicated grieving	00135
Risk for complicated grieving	00172
Readiness for enhanced hope	00185
Hopelessness	00124
Risk for compromised human dignity	00174
Readiness for enhanced power	00187
Powerlessness	00125
Risk for powerlessness	00152
Spiritual distress	00066
Risk for spiritual distress	00067
Readiness for enhanced spiritual well-being	00068
Class: Life Principles Personal values, beliefs, and religiosity	Nursing Diagnosis Code
Decisional conflict	00083
Moral distress	00175
Noncompliance	00079
Impaired religiosity	00169
Readiness for enhanced religiosity	00171
Risk for impaired religiosity	00170
Class: Coping Perceptions of coping, coping experiences, and coping strategies	Nursing Diagnosis Code
Ineffective activity planning	00199
Risk for ineffective activity planning	00226
Defensive coping	00071
Ineffective coping	00069
Readiness for enhanced coping	00158
Readiness for enhanced decision-making	00184
Impaired emancipated decision-making	00242
Readiness for enhanced emancipated decision-making	00243
Risk for impaired emancipated decision-making	00244
Post-trauma syndrome	00141

Continued

Table 3.2   *Continued*

Risk for post-trauma syndrome	00145
Rape-trauma syndrome	00142
Relocation stress syndrome	00114
Risk for relocation stress syndrome	00149
Impaired resilience	00210
Readiness for enhanced resilience	00212
Risk for impaired resilience	00211
Stress overload	00177

FUNCTIONAL DOMAIN

Life-span processes, basic functions, and skills essential to human health

Class: Lifespan Processes The processes of growth, mental development, physical maturation, and aging	Nursing Diagnosis Code
Risk for delayed development	00112
Risk for disproportionate growth	00113
Class: Physical Ability Audiovisual abilities, sexual function, and mobility	Nursing Diagnosis Code
Impaired bed mobility	00091
Impaired physical mobility	00085
Impaired wheelchair mobility	00089
Impaired sitting	00237
Impaired standing	00238
Impaired transfer ability	00090
Impaired walking	00088
Class: Energy Balance Energy usage and energy regulation pattern	Nursing Diagnosis Code
Activity intolerance	00092
Risk for activity intolerance	00094
Deficient diversional activity	00097
Fatigue	00093
Insomnia	00095
Sedentary lifestyle	00168
Readiness for enhanced sleep	00165
Sleep deprivation	00096
Disturbed sleep pattern	00198
Wandering	00154

Table 3.2   *Continued*

Class: Communication Communication abilities and communication skills	Nursing Diagnosis Code
Readiness for enhanced communication	00157
Impaired verbal communication	00051
Class: Social Function Social network, social roles, social skills, and social interaction	Nursing Diagnosis Code
Risk for loneliness	00054
Readiness for enhanced relationship	00207
Ineffective relationship	00223
Risk for ineffective relationship	00229
Ineffective role performance	00055
Impaired social interaction	00052
Social isolation	00053
Class: Self Care Self-care abilities and home maintenance skills	Nursing Diagnosis Code
Impaired home maintenance	00098
Bathing self-care deficit	00108
Dressing self-care deficit	00109
Feeding self-care deficit	00102
Toileting self-care deficit	00110
Readiness for enhanced self-care	00182
Self-neglect	00193
Class: Health Promotion Health literacy and health maintenance skills	Nursing Diagnosis Code
Ineffective health maintenance	00099
Ineffective health management	00078
Readiness for enhanced health management	00162
Frail elderly syndrome	00230
Risk for frail elderly syndrome	00231
Ineffective protection	00043
Risk-prone health behavior	00188
Deficient knowledge	00126
Readiness for enhanced knowledge	00161

Continued

Table 3.2   *Continued*

SAFETY DOMAIN	
The characteristics of risk behavior, health hazards, and milieu hazards essential to human health	
Class: Self-Harm Self-directed risk behavior and suicidal behavior	Nursing Diagnosis Code
Self-mutilation	00151
Risk for self-mutilation	00139
Risk for self-directed violence	00140
Risk for suicide	00150
Class: Violence Other-directed risk behavior and violent behavior	Nursing Diagnosis Code
Risk for other-directed violence	00138
Class: Health Hazard Health hazards associated with healthcare processes and social processes	Nursing Diagnosis Code
Risk for aspiration	00039
Risk for bleeding	00206
Risk for disuse syndrome	00040
Risk for falls	00155
Risk for infection	00004
Risk for injury	00035
Risk for perioperative positioning injury	00087
Risk for shock	00205
Risk for sudden infant death syndrome	00156
Risk for suffocation	00036
Delayed surgical recovery	00100
Risk for delayed surgical recovery	00246
Impaired swallowing	00103
Risk for trauma	00038
Class: Milieu Hazard Health impacts of economy, housing standard, and working environment	Nursing Diagnosis Code
Contamination	00181
Risk for contamination	00180
Risk for poisoning	00037

Table 3.2   *Continued*

FAMILY	
Reproductive processes, family processes, and family roles essential to human health	
Class: Reproduction Biophysical and psychological processes involved in fertility and conception, and the delivery and postpartum phase of childbirth	Nursing Diagnosis Code
Ineffective childbearing process	00221
Readiness for enhanced childbearing process	00208
Risk for ineffective childbearing process	00227
Risk for disturbed maternal–fetal dyad	00209
Class: Caregiving Roles Caregiving and caregiver functions	Nursing Diagnosis Code
Risk for impaired attachment	00058
Caregiver role strain	00061
Risk for caregiver role strain	00062
Parental role conflict	00064
Impaired parenting	00056
Risk for impaired parenting	00057
Readiness for enhanced parenting	00164
Class: Family Unit Family coping, family functionality, and family integrity	Nursing Diagnosis Code
Compromised family coping	00074
Disabled family coping	00073
Readiness for enhanced family coping	00075
Ineffective family health management	00080
Dysfunctional family processes	00063
Interrupted family processes	00060
Readiness for enhanced family processes	00159

Continued

ENVIRONMENTAL DOMAIN	
Healthcare system and healthcare processes essential to human health	
Class: Community Health Community health needs, risk populations, and healthcare programs	Nursing Diagnosis Code
Deficient community health management	00215
Ineffective community coping	00077
Readiness for enhanced community coping	00076
Class: Healthcare System Healthcare system, healthcare legislations, hospitals treatment, and care processes	Nursing Diagnosis Code
None at present	

References

Abbot, A. (1988) *The Systems of Professions*. Chicago, IL: University of Chicago Press.

Quammen, D. (2007) A passion for order. *National Geographic Magazine*. ngm.national-geographic.com/print/2007/06/Linnaeus-name-giver/david-quammen-text, retrieved November 1, 2013.

Von Krogh, G. (2011) Taxonomy III Proposal. *NANDA International Latin American Symposium*. Sao Paulo, Brazil. May 2011.

Chapter 4

NANDA-I Taxonomy II: Specifications and Definitions

T. Heather Herdman, RN, PhD, FNI

Structure of Taxonomy II

Taxonomy is defined as the "branch of science concerned with classification, especially of organisms; systematics; the classification of something, especially organisms; a scheme of classification" (Oxford Dictionary, 2013). Within a taxonomy, the domains are "a sphere of knowledge, influence, or inquiry"; and the classes are "a group, set, or kind sharing common attributes" (Merriam-Webster, Inc., 2009).

We can adapt the definition for a nursing diagnosis taxonomy; specifically, we are concerned with the orderly classification of diagnostic foci of concern to nursing, according to their presumed natural relationships. Taxonomy II has three levels: domains, classes, and nursing diagnoses. Figure 3.3 (p. 58) depicts the organization of domains and classes in Taxonomy II; Table 3.1 (pp. 66–78) shows Taxonomy II with its 13 domains, 47 classes, and 235 current diagnoses.

The Taxonomy II code structure is a 32-bit integer (or if the user's database uses another notation, the code structure is a five-digit code). This structure provides for the stability, or growth and development, of the taxonomic structure by avoiding the need to change codes when new diagnoses, refinements, and revisions are added. New codes are assigned to newly approved diagnoses. Retired codes are never reused.

Taxonomy II has a code structure that is compliant with recommendations from the National Library of Medicine (NLM) concerning healthcare terminology codes. The NLM recommends that codes do not contain information about the classified concept, as did the Taxonomy I code structure, which included information about the location and the level of the diagnosis.

The NANDA-I terminology is a recognized nursing language that meets the criteria established by the Committee for Nursing Practice

NANDA International, Inc. Nursing Diagnoses: Definitions & Classification 2015–2017, Tenth Edition. Edited by T. Heather Herdman and Shigemi Kamitsuru.
© 2014 NANDA International, Inc. Published 2014 by John Wiley & Sons, Ltd.
Companion website: www.wiley.com/go/nursingdiagnoses

Figure 4.1 *The ISO Reference Terminology Model for a Nursing Diagnosis*

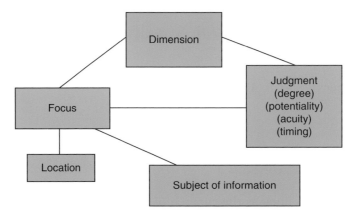

Information Infrastructure (CNPII) of the American Nurses Association (ANA) (Lundberg, Warren, Brokel et al., 2008). The benefit of using a recognized nursing language is the indication that it is accepted as supporting nursing practice by providing clinically useful terminology. The NANDA-I nursing diagnoses also comply with the International Standards Organization (ISO) terminology model for a nursing diagnosis (Figure 4.1). The terminology is also registered with Health Level Seven International (HL7), a healthcare informatics standard, as a terminology to be used in identifying nursing diagnoses in electronic messages among clinical information systems (www.HL7.org).

A Multiaxial System for Constructing Diagnostic Concepts

The NANDA-I diagnoses are concepts constructed by means of a multiaxial system. This system consists of axes out of which components are combined to make the diagnoses substantially equal in form, and in coherence with the ISO model.

An axis, for the purpose of the NANDA-I Taxonomy II, is operationally defined as a dimension of the human response that is considered in the diagnostic process. There are seven axes. The *NANDA-I Model of a Nursing Diagnosis* displays the seven axes and their relationship to each other (Figure 4.2):

- Axis 1: the focus of the diagnosis
- Axis 2: subject of the diagnosis (individual, family, group, caregiver, community, etc.)
- Axis 3: judgment (impaired, ineffective, etc.)
- Axis 4: location (bladder, auditory, cerebral, etc.)

Figure 4.2 *The NANDA-I Model of a Nursing Diagnosis*

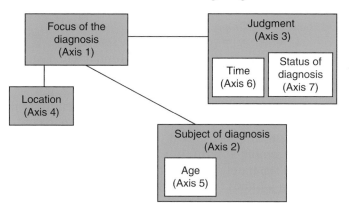

- Axis 5: age (infant, child, adult, etc.)
- Axis 6: time (chronic, acute, intermittent)
- Axis 7: status of the diagnosis (problem-focused, risk, health promotion)

The axes are represented in the labels of the nursing diagnoses through their values. In some cases, they are named explicitly, such as with the diagnoses *Ineffective Community Coping* and *Compromised Family Coping*, in which the subject of the diagnosis (in the first instance "community" and in the second instance "family") is named using the two values "community" and "family" taken from Axis 2 (subject of the diagnosis). "*Ineffective*" and "*compromised*" are two of the values contained in Axis 3 (judgment).

In some cases, the axis is implicit, as is the case with the diagnosis *Activity intolerance*, in which the subject of the diagnosis (Axis 2) is always the patient. In some instances an axis may not be pertinent to a particular diagnosis and therefore is not part of the nursing diagnostic label. For example, the time axis may not be relevant to every diagnosis. In the case of diagnoses without explicit identification of the subject of the diagnosis, it may be helpful to remember that NANDA-I defines patient as "*an individual, family, group or community.*"

Axis 1 (the focus) and Axis 3 (judgment) are essential components of a nursing diagnosis. In some cases, however, the diagnostic focus contains the judgment (for example, *Nausea*); in these cases the judgment is not explicitly separated out in the diagnostic label. Axis 2 (subject of the diagnosis) is also essential, although, as described above, it may be implied and therefore not included in the label. The Diagnosis Development Committee requires these axes for submission; the other axes may be used where relevant for clarity.

Definitions of the Axes

Axis 1 The Focus of the Diagnosis

The focus is the principal element or the fundamental and essential part, the root, of the nursing diagnosis. It describes the "human response" that is the core of the diagnosis.

The focus may consist of one or more nouns. When more than one noun is used (for example, *Activity intolerance*), each one contributes a unique meaning to the focus, as if the two were a single noun; the meaning of the combined term, however, is different from when the nouns are stated separately. Frequently, an adjective (*spiritual*) may be used with a noun (*distress*) to denote the focus, *Spiritual distress* (00066).

In some cases, the focus and the nursing diagnosis are one and the same, as is seen with the diagnosis of *Nausea* (00134). This occurs when the nursing diagnosis is stated at its most clinically useful level and the separation of the focus adds no meaningful level of abstraction. It can be very difficult to determine exactly what should be considered the focus of the diagnosis. For example, using the diagnoses of *bowel incontinence* (00014) and *stress urinary incontinence* (00017), the question becomes: Is the focus *incontinence* alone, or are there two foci, *bowel incontinence* and *urinary incontinence*? In this instance, *incontinence* is the focus, and the location terms (axis 4) of *bowel* and *urinary* provide more clarification about the focus. However, *incontinence* in and of itself is a judgment term that can stand alone, and so it becomes the focus, regardless of location.

In some cases, however, removing the location (axis 4) from the focus would prevent it from providing meaning to nursing practice. For example, if we look at the focus of the diagnosis, *risk for imbalanced body temperature* (00005), is it *body temperature* or simply *temperature*? Or if you look at the diagnosis, *disturbed personal identity* (00121), is the focus *identity* or *personal identity*? Decisions about what constitutes the essence of the focus of the diagnosis, then, are made on the basis of what helps to identify the nursing practice implication, and whether or not the term indicates a human response. *Temperature* could mean environmental temperature, which is not a human response, so it is important to identify *body temperature* as the nursing diagnosis. Similarly, *identity* could mean nothing more than one's gender, eye color, height, or age – again, these are characteristics but not human responses; *personal identity*, however, indicates one's self-perception and is a human response. In some cases the focus may seem similar, but is in fact quite distinct: *other-directed violence* and *self-directed violence* are two different human responses, and therefore must be identified separately in terms of foci within Taxonomy II. The foci of the NANDA-I nursing diagnoses are shown in Table 4.1.

Table 4.1   Foci of the NANDA-I Nursing Diagnoses

Activity planning	**D**eath anxiety	**G**as exchange	**M**aternal–fetal dyad	**R**ape-trauma syndrome	**T**hermal injury
Activity tolerance	Decisional conflict	Gastrointestinal motility	Memory	Reaction to iodinated contrast media	Thermoregulation
Adaptive capacity	Decision-making	Gastrointestinal perfusion	Mobility	Relationship	Tissue integrity
Airway clearance	Denial	Grieving	Mood regulation	Religiosity	Tissue perfusion
Allergy response	Dentition	Growth	Moral distress	Relocation stress syndrome	Toileting self-care
Anxiety	Development		Mucous membrane		Transfer ability
Aspiration	Diarrhea	**H**ealth		Renal perfusion	Trauma
Attachment	Disorganized behavior	Health behavior	**N**ausea	Resilience	
Autonomic dysreflexia	Disuse syndrome	Health maintenance	Nutrition	Role conflict	**U**nilateral neglect
	Diversional activity	Health management		Role performance	Urinary retention
	Dressing self-care	Home maintenance		Role strain	
	Dry eye	Hope			**V**entilatory weaning response
	Dysfunction	Human dignity			Verbal communication
		Hyperthermia			
Bathing self-care	**E**lectrolyte balance	Hypothermia	**O**besity	**S**elf-care	**W**alking
Bleeding	Elimination		Organized behavior	Self-concept	Wandering
Blood glucose level	Emancipated decision-making	**I**mpulse control	Other-directed violence	Self-directed violence	
Body image	Emotional control	Incontinence	Overweight	Self-esteem	
Body temperature		Infection		Self-mutilation	
Breastfeeding		Injury		Self-neglect	
Breast milk		Insomnia		Sexual dysfunction	
Breathing pattern				Sexuality pattern	
				Shock	

(Continued)

Table 4.1 (Continued)

Cardiac output	Falls	Jaundice	Pain	Sitting
Cardiovascular function	Family processes	Knowledge	Pain syndrome	Skin integrity
Childbearing process	Fatigue	Latex allergy response	Parenting	Sleep
Comfort	Fear	Lifestyle	Personal identity	Sleep pattern
Communication	Feeding pattern	Liver function	Poisoning	Social interaction
Compliance	Feeding self-care	Loneliness	Positioning injury	Social isolation
Confusion	Fluid balance		Post-trauma syndrome	Sorrow
Constipation	Fluid volume		Power	Spiritual distress
Contamination	Frail elderly syndrome		Pressure ulcer	Spiritual well-being
Coping			Protection	Spontaneous ventilation
				Standing
				Stress
				Sudden infant death syndrome
				Suffocation
				Suicide
				Surgical recovery
				Swallowing

The subject of the diagnosis is defined as the person(s) for whom a nursing diagnosis is determined. The values in Axis 2 are individual, caregiver, family, group, and community, representing the NANDA-I definition of "patient":

- *Individual:* a single human being distinct from others, a person
- *Caregiver:* a family member or helper who regularly looks after a child or a sick, elderly, or disabled person
- *Family:* two or more people having continuous or sustained relationships, perceiving reciprocal obligations, sensing common meaning, and sharing certain obligations toward others; related by blood and/or choice
- *Group:* a number of people with shared characteristics
- *Community:* a group of people living in the same locale under the same governance. Examples include neighborhoods and cities

When the subject of the diagnosis is not explicitly stated, it becomes the individual by default. However, it is perfectly appropriate to consider such diagnoses for the other subjects of the diagnosis as well. The diagnosis *Grieving* could be applied to an individual or family who has lost a loved one. It could also be appropriate for a community that has experienced a mass casualty, suffered the loss of an important community leader, devastation due to natural disasters, or even the loss of a symbolic structure within the community (a school, religious structure, historic building, etc.).

Axis 3 Judgment

A judgment is a descriptor or modifier that limits or specifies the meaning of the diagnostic focus. The diagnostic focus, together with the nurse's judgment about it, forms the diagnosis. All of the definitions used are found in the Oxford Dictionary On-Line (2013). The values in Axis 3 are found in Table 4.2.

Axis 4 Location

Location describes the parts/regions of the body and/or their related functions – all tissues, organs, anatomical sites, or structures. The values in Axis 4 are shown in Table 4.3.

Table 4.2 Definitions of Judgment Terms for Axis 3, NANDA-I Taxonomy II, adapted from the Oxford Dictionary On-Line (2013).

Judgment	Definition	Judgment	Definition
Complicated	Consisting of many interconnecting parts or elements; involving many different and confusing aspects	Frail	Weak and delicate
Compromised	Made vulnerable, or to function less effectively	Functional	Affecting the operation, rather than the structure, of an organ
Decreased	Smaller or fewer in size, amount, intensity, or degree	Imbalanced	Lack of proportion or relation between corresponding things
Defensive	Used or intended to defend or protect	Impaired	Weakened or damaged (something, especially a faculty or function)
Deficient/Deficit	Not having enough of a specified quality or ingredient; a deficiency or failing, especially in a neurological or psychological function	Ineffective	Not producing any significant or desired effect
Delayed	A period of time by which something is late, slow, or postponed	Insufficient	Not enough, inadequate; incapable, incompetent
Disabled	Limited in movements, senses, or activities	Interrupted	A stop in continuous progress of (an activity or process); to break the continuity of something
Disorganized	Not properly arranged or controlled; scattered or inefficient	Labile	Of or characterized by emotions that are easily aroused, freely expressed, and tend to alter quickly and spontaneously
Disproportionate	Too large or too small in comparison with something else (norm)	Low	Below average in amount, extent, or intensity; small

Disturbed	Having had its normal pattern or function disrupted
Dysfunctional	Not operating normally or properly; deviating from the norms of social behavior in a way regarded as bad
Emancipated	Free from legal, social, or political restrictions; liberated
Effective	Successful in producing a desired or intended result
Enhanced	Intensified, increased, or further improved the quality, value, or extent of something
Excess	An amount of something that is more than necessary, permitted, or desirable
Failure	The action or state of not functioning
Organized	Properly arranged or controlled; efficient
Perceived	Became aware of (something) by the use of one of the senses, especially that of sight; interpreted or looked upon (someone or something) in a particular way; regarded as; became aware or conscious of (something); realized or understood
Readiness	Willingness to do something; state of being fully prepared for something
Risk	Situation involving exposure to danger; possibility or vulnerability that something unpleasant or unwelcome will happen
Risk-prone	Likely to or liable to suffer from, do, or experience something, typically something regrettable or unwelcome/dangerous
Unstable	Prone to change, fail, or give way; not stable

Table 4.3   *Locations in Axis 4, NANDA-I Taxonomy II*

Bed	Cerebral	Neurovascular	Urinary tract
Bladder	Corneal	Peripheral	Vascular
Bowel	Gastrointestinal	Renal	Wheelchair
Cardiac	Intracranial	Urinary	

Axis 5 Age

Age refers to the age of the person who is the subject of the diagnosis (Axis 2). The values in Axis 5 are noted below, with all definitions *except* that of older adult being drawn from the World Health Organization (2013):

- **Fetus**: an unborn human more than eight weeks after conception, until birth
- **Neonate**: a child <28 days of age
- **Infant**: a child ≥28 days and <1 year of age
- **Child**: person aged 1 to 9 years, inclusive
- **Adolescent**: person aged 10 to 19 years, inclusive
- **Adult**: a person older than 19 years of age unless national law defines a person as being an adult at an earlier age
- **Older adult**: a person ≥65 years of age

Axis 6 Time

Time describes the duration of the nursing diagnosis (Axis 1). The values in Axis 6 are:

- *Acute:* lasting <3 months
- *Chronic:* lasting ≥3 months
- *Continuous:* uninterrupted, going on without stop
- *Intermittent:* stopping or starting again at intervals, periodic, cyclic
- *Perioperative:* occurring or performed at or around the time of an operation
- *Situational:* Related to a set of circumstances in which one finds oneself

Axis 7 Status of the Diagnosis

The status of the diagnosis refers to the actuality or potentiality of the problem/syndrome or to the categorization of the diagnosis as a health promotion diagnosis. The values in Axis 7 are:

- *Problem-focused:* an undesirable human response to health conditions/life processes that exists in the current moment (includes problem-focused syndrome diagnoses)
- *Health promotion:* motivation and desire to increase well-being and to actualize human health potential that exists in the current moment (Pender, Murduagh, & Parsons, 2006)
- *Risk:* vulnerability for developing in the future an undesirable human response to health conditions/life processes (includes risk syndrome diagnoses)

Developing and Submitting a Nursing Diagnosis

A nursing diagnosis is constructed by combining the values from Axis 1 (the diagnostic focus), Axis 2 (subject of the diagnosis), and Axis 3 (judgment) where needed, and adding values from the other axes for relevant clarity. Thus you start with the diagnostic focus (Axis 1) and add the judgment (Axis 3) about it. Remember that these two axes are sometimes combined to form a nursing diagnosis label in which judgment is implicit, as can be seen with *Fatigue* (00093). Next, you specify the subject of the diagnosis (Axis 2). If the subject is an "individual," you need not make it explicit (Figure 4.3). You can then use the remaining axes, if they are appropriate, to add more detail. Figures 4.4 and 4.5 illustrate other examples, using a risk diagnosis and health promotion diagnosis, respectively.

NANDA-I does not support the **random construction** of nursing diagnoses that would occur by simply matching terms from one axis to another to create a diagnosis label to represent judgments based on a

Figure 4.3 *A NANDA-I Nursing Diagnosis Model: (Individual) Impaired Standing*

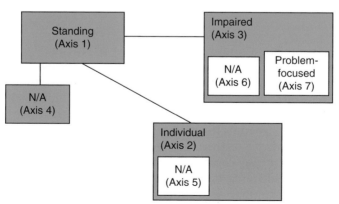

Figure 4.4 *A NANDA-I Nursing Diagnosis Model: Risk for Disorganized Infant Behavior*

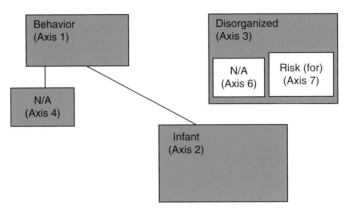

Figure 4.5 *A NANDA-I Nursing Diagnosis Model: Readiness for Enhanced Family Coping*

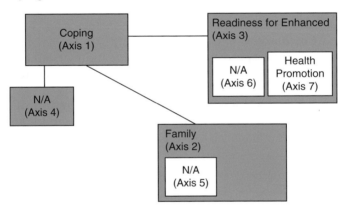

patient assessment. Clinical problems/areas of nursing foci that are identified and that do not have a NANDA-I label should be carefully described in documentation to ensure the accuracy of other nurses'/healthcare professionals' interpretation of the clinical judgment.

Creating a diagnosis to be used in clinical practice and/or documentation by matching terms from different axes, without development of the definition and other component parts of a diagnosis (defining characteristics, related factors, or risk factors) in an evidence-based manner, negates the purpose of a standardized language as a method to truly represent, inform, and direct clinical judgment and practice.

This is a serious concern with regard to patient safety, because the lack of the knowledge inherent within the component diagnostic parts makes it impossible to ensure diagnostic accuracy. Nursing terms arbitrarily created at the point of care could result in misinterpretation of the clinical problem/area of focus, and subsequently lead to inappropriate outcome-setting and intervention choice. It also makes it impossible to accurately research the incidence of nursing diagnoses, or to conduct outcome or intervention studies related to diagnoses, since, without clear component diagnostic parts (definitions, defining characteristics, related or risk factors) it is impossible to know if human response that are given the same label truly represent the same phenomena.

Therefore, when discussing the construction of nursing diagnoses in this chapter, the intent is to inform nurses about how nursing diagnoses are developed, and to provide clarity for individuals who are developing diagnoses for submission into the NANDA-I Taxonomy; it *should not* be interpreted to suggest that NANDA-I supports the creation of diagnoses by nurses at the point of patient care.

Further Development

A taxonomy and a multiaxial framework for developing nursing diagnoses allow clinicians to see where the nursing discipline lacks diagnoses, and provides the opportunity to develop clinically useful new diagnoses. If you develop a new diagnosis that is useful to your practice, please submit it to NANDA-I so that others can share in the discovery. Submission forms and information can be found on the NANDA-I website (www.nanda.org). The Diagnosis Development Committee (DDC) will be glad to support you as you prepare your submission.

References

Lundberg, C., Warren, J., Brokel, J., Bulechek, G., Butcher, H., Dochterman, J., Johnson, M., Maas, M., Martin, K., Moorhead, S., Spisla, C., Swanson, E., & S. Giarrizzo-Wilson (2008). Selecting a standardized terminology for the electronic health record that reveals the impact of nursing on patient care. *Online Journal of Nursing Informatics, 12*(2). Available at http://ojni.org/12_2/lundberg.pdf

Merriam-Webster, Inc. (2009). *Merriam-Webster's Collegiate Dictionary* (11th ed.) Springfield, MA: Merriam-Webster, Inc.

Oxford Dictionary On-Line, British and World Version. (2013). Oxford University Press. Available at http://www.oxforddictionaries.com/

Pender, N. J., Murdaugh, C. L., & Parsons, M. A. (2006). *Health promotion in nursing practice* (5th ed.). Upper Saddle River, NJ: Pearson Prentice-Hall.

World Health Organization (2013). Health topics: Infant, newborn. Available at: http://www.who.int/topics/infant_newborn/en/

World Health Organization (2013). Definition of key terms. Available at: http://www.who.int/hiv/pub/guidelines/arv2013/intro/keyterms/en/

Other Recommended Reading

Matos, F. G. O. A., & Cruz, D. A. L. M. (2009). Development of an instrument to evaluate diagnosis accuracy. *Revista da Escola de Enfermagem USP 43*(Spe): 1087–1095.

Paans, W., Nieweg, R. M. B, Van der Schans, C. P, & Sermeus, W. (2011). What factors influence the prevalence and accuracy of nursing diagnoses documentation in clinical practice? A systematic literature review. *Journal of Clinical Nursing, 20*, 2386–2403.

Chapter 5

Frequently Asked Questions

T. Heather Herdman, RN, PhD, FNI and Shigemi Kamitsuru,
RN, PhD, FNI

We routinely receive questions via our website, email, and when members of the NANDA-I Board of Directors or the CEO/Executive Director travel and present at a variety of conferences. We have decided to include some of the most common questions here, along with their answers, with the hope that it will help others who may have the same questions.

Basic Questions about Standardized Nursing Languages

What is standardized nursing language?

Standardized nursing language (SNL) is a commonly understood set of terms used to describe the clinical judgments involved in assessments (nursing diagnoses), along with the interventions and outcomes related to the documentation of nursing care.

How many standardized nursing languages are there?

The American Nurses Association recognizes 12 SNLs for nursing.

What are the differences among standardized nursing languages?

Many nursing languages claim to be standardized; some are simply a list of terms, others provide definitions of those terms. NANDA-I maintains that a standardized language that represents any profession should provide, at a minimum, an evidence-based definition, list of defining

NANDA International, Inc. Nursing Diagnoses: Definitions & Classification 2015–2017,
Tenth Edition. Edited by T. Heather Herdman and Shigemi Kamitsuru.
© 2014 NANDA International, Inc. Published 2014 by John Wiley & Sons, Ltd.
Companion website: www.wiley.com/go/nursingdiagnoses

characteristics (signs/symptoms), and related factors (etiologic factors); risk diagnoses should include an evidence-based definition, and a list of risk factors. Without these, anyone can define any term in his/her own way, which obviously violates the purpose of standardization.

I see people use terms such as "select a diagnosis," "choose a diagnosis," "pick a diagnosis" – this sounds like there is an easy way to know what diagnosis to use. Is that correct?

When we speak about diagnosing, we really are not talking about something as simplistic as picking a term from a list, or choosing something that "sounds right" for our patient. We are speaking about the diagnostic decision-making process, in which nurses diagnose. So, rather than using these simplistic terms (selecting, choosing, picking), we should really describe the process of diagnosing. Rather than saying "choose a diagnosis," we should be saying "diagnose the patient/family"; rather than saying "picking a diagnosis," we could use "ensure accuracy in your diagnosis," or again, simply "diagnose the patient/family." Words are powerful – so when we say things such as choose, pick, or select, it *does* sound simple, like reading through a list of terms and picking one. Using diagnostic reasoning, however, is much more than that – and *diagnosing* is what we are doing, which is far more than just "picking" something.

Basic Questions about NANDA-I

What is NANDA International?

Implementation of nursing diagnosis enhances every aspect of nursing practice, from garnering professional respect to assuring consistent documentation representing nurses' professional clinical judgment, and accurate documentation to enable reimbursement. NANDA-I exists to develop, refine, and promote terminology that accurately reflects nurses' clinical judgments.

What is taxonomy?

Taxonomy is the practice and science of categorization and classification. The NANDA-I taxonomy currently includes 235 nursing diagnoses that are grouped (classified) within 13 domains (categories) of nursing practice: Health Promotion; Nutrition; Elimination and Exchange; Activity/Rest; Perception/Cognition; Self-Perception; Role Relationships; Sexuality; Coping/Stress Tolerance; Life Principles; Safety/Protection; Comfort; Growth/Development.

In any field, development and maintenance of a research-based body of work require an investment of time and expertise, and dissemination of that work is an additional expense. As a volunteer organization, we sponsor committee meetings for the review of submitted diagnoses, to ensure they meet the level of evidence criteria. We also provide educational courses and offerings in English, Spanish, and Portuguese due to the high demand for this content. We have committee members from all over the world, and video conferencing and the occasional face-to-face meeting are expenses – as are our conferences and educational events. Our fees support this work on a break-even basis, and are quite modest in comparison to fees charged for a license to ICD-10 medical diagnoses.

If we buy a book, and type the contents into software ourselves, do we still have to pay?

NANDA International, Inc. depends on the funds received from the sale of our textbooks and electronic licensing to maintain and improve the state of the science within our terminology. The NANDA-I terminology is a copyrighted terminology, therefore **no part of the NANDA-I publication,** *NANDA International Nursing Diagnoses: Definitions and Classification,* **can be reproduced, stored in a retrieval system, or transmitted by any means, electronic, mechanical, photocopying, recording, or otherwise, without the prior permission of the publisher. This includes publication in online blogs, websites, etc.**

This is true regardless of the language in which you intend to use the work. For usage other than reading or consulting the book, a license is required from Blackwell Publishing, Ltd (a company of John Wiley & Sons Inc.) or the approved publisher of the book in any other language. The official translation rights holders for our work in languages other than English can be found at http://www.nanda.org/nanda-interntional-taxonomy-translation-licensees.html. Use of this content requires that you apply for and receive permission from the publisher to reproduce our work in any format. Further information is available on our website (www.nanda.org) or you can contact Wiley-Blackwell at wiley@nanda.org or visit their website at www.wiley.com/wiley-blackwell.

Should the structure of Taxonomy II be used as a nursing assessment framework?

The purpose of the taxonomy is to provide organization to the terms (diagnoses) within NANDA-I. It was never intended to serve as an assessment framework. Please see our Position Statement on the use of the NANDA-I taxonomy as a nursing assessment framework, on p. 459.

"PES" is an acronym that stands for **P**roblem, **E**tiology (related factors), and **S**igns/Symptoms (defining characteristics). The PES format was first published by Dr. Marjory Gordon, a founder and former President of NANDA-I. The component parts of NANDA-I diagnoses are now referred to as *related factors* and *defining characteristics*, and therefore the wording "PES format" is not used in current NANDA-I books. It is still used in several countries and in many publications. Formulating accurate diagnoses relies on assessing and documenting related factors and defining characteristics, and the PES format supports this, which is critical for accuracy in nursing diagnoses, a focus that NANDA-I strongly supports.

However, NANDA-I does not require the PES format, or any other particular format, to document nursing diagnoses. We are aware of the wide variety of electronic documentation systems in use and in development around the world, and it seems that there are as many ways of providing nursing documentation as there are systems. Many computer systems do not allow the use of the "related to…as evidenced by" model. However, it is important that nurses are able to communicate the assessment data that support the diagnosis they make, so that others caring for the patient know why a diagnosis was selected. Please see the NANDA-I Position Statement on the structure of the nursing diagnosis statement when included in a care plan (p. 459).

The PES format remains a strong method for teaching clinical reasoning and for supporting students and nurses as they learn the skill of diagnosis. Because patients usually have more than one related factor and/or defining characteristic, many sites replace the wording "as manifested/as evidenced by" and "related to" with a list of the defining characteristics and related factors following the diagnostic statement. This list is based on the individual patient situation and can use the standardized NANDA-I terms. Informatics codes are now available for all diagnostic indicators within the NANDA-I terminology, on our website.

Regardless of the requirements for documentation, it is important to remember that for safe patient care in clinical areas, it is crucial to survey or assess defining characteristics (manifestations of diagnoses) and related factors (or causes) of nursing diagnoses. Choosing effective interventions is based on related factors and defining characteristics.

Documentation systems differ by organization, so in some cases you may write (or select from a computerized list) the diagnostic label that corresponds to the human response you have diagnosed. Assessment data may be found in a different section (or "screen") of the computer system, and you would select your related factors and defining characteristics, or your risk factors, in that location. Here are some examples of PES charting.

Problem-Focused Diagnosis

To use the PES format, start with the diagnosis itself, followed by the etiological factors (related factors in a problem-focused diagnosis). Finally, identify the major signs/symptoms (defining characteristics).

- *Anxiety* **related to** situational crises and stress (related factors) **as evidenced by** restlessness, insomnia, anguish and anorexia (defining characteristics)

Risk Diagnosis

For risk diagnoses, there are no related factors (etiological factors), since you are identifying a *vulnerability* in a patient for a potential problem; the problem is not yet present. Different experts recommend different phrasing (some use "related to," others use "as evidenced by" for risk diagnoses). Because the term "related to" is used to suggest an etiology, in the case of a problem-focused diagnosis, and because there is only a vulnerability to a problem when a risk diagnosis is used, NANDA-I has decided to recommend the use of the phrase "as evidenced by" to refer to the evidence of risk that exists, if the PES format is used.

- *Risk for infection* **as evidenced by** inadequate vaccination and immunosuppression (risk factors)

Health Promotion Diagnosis

Because health promotion diagnoses do not require a related factor, there is no "related to" in the writing of this diagnosis. Instead, the defining characteristic(s) are provided as evidence of the desire on the part of the patient to improve his/her current health state.

- *Readiness for enhanced self-care* **as evidenced by** expressed desire to enhance self-care

Does NANDA-I provide a list of its diagnoses?

There is no real use for simply providing a list of terms – to do so defeats the purpose of a SNL. Unless the definition, defining characteristics, related and/or risk factors are known, the label itself is meaningless. Therefore, we do not believe it is in the interest of patient safety to produce simple lists of terms that could be misunderstood or used inappropriately in a clinical context.

It is essential to have the definition of the diagnosis and, more importantly, the diagnostic indicators (assessment data/patient history data) required to make the diagnosis: for example, the signs/symptoms that you collect through your assessment ("defining characteristics") and the cause of the diagnosis ("related factors") or those things that place a patient at significant risk for a diagnosis ("risk factors"). As you assess the patient, you will rely on both your clinical knowledge and "book knowledge" to see patterns in the data, diagnostic indicators that cluster together that may relate to a diagnosis. Questions to ask to identify and validate the correct diagnosis include:

1. Are the majority of the defining characteristics/risk factors present in the patient?
2. Are there etiological factors ("related factors") for the diagnosis evident in your patient?
3. Have you validated the diagnosis with the patient/family or with another nurse peer (when possible)?

Basic Questions about Nursing Diagnoses

Can nursing diagnosis be used safely other than in an inpatient unit, such as in the operating room and outpatient clinics?

Absolutely! Nursing diagnoses are used in operating rooms, ambulatory clinics, psychiatric facilities, home health, and hospice organizations, as well as in public health, school nursing, occupational health – and, of course, in hospitals. As diverse as nursing practice is, there are core diagnoses that seem to cross them all – *acute pain* (00132), *anxiety* (00146), *deficient knowledge* (00126), *readiness for enhanced health management* (00162), for example, can probably be found anywhere a nurse might practice. That said, we know that there is a need for the development of diagnoses to further expand the terms we use to describe nursing knowledge across all of these areas of nursing. Work is underway in some areas, such as pediatrics and mental health, and across a great number of countries, and we are eagerly awaiting the results!

Should nurses in a critical care unit use nursing diagnosis?
We are busy taking care of medical conditions.

What an interesting question! Should nurses practice nursing? Yes, of course! There is no question that critical care nurses have a high focus on interventions as a result of medical conditions, and often intervene with patients using "standing protocols" (standing medical orders) that require critical thinking to implement correctly. But let's be honest: nurses in critical care units need to practice nursing. Patients in critical condition are at risk for many complications that can be prevented by nurses: ventilator-related pneumonias (*risk for infection*, 00004), pressure ulcers (*risk for pressure ulcer*, 00249), corneal injury (*risk for corneal injury*, 00245). They are often scared (*fear*, 00148), and families are stressed but need to know how to care for their loved one when he comes home: *deficient knowledge* (00126), *stress overload* (00177), *risk for caregiver role strain* (00162). If nurses only attend to the obvious medical condition, then, as the old adage says, they may win the battle, but still lose the war. These patients may develop sequelae that could have been avoided, length of stay may be prolonged, or discharge home could result in untoward events and increased readmission rates. Attend to the medical conditions? Certainly! *And* focus on the human responses? Absolutely!

What are the types of nursing diagnoses in the NANDA-I classification?

NANDA-I identifies three categories of nursing diagnosis: problem-focused, health promotion, and risk diagnoses. Within these categories, you can also find the use of syndromes. Definitions for each of these categories, and syndromes, can be found in the Glossary of Terms, on p. 464.

What are nursing diagnoses, and why should I use them?

A nursing diagnosis is a clinical judgment concerning a human response to health conditions/life processes, or a vulnerability for that response, by an individual, family, group, or community. It requires a nursing assessment to diagnose your patient correctly – you cannot safely standardize nursing diagnoses by using a medical diagnosis. Although it is true that there are common nursing diagnoses that frequently occur in patients with various medical diagnoses, the fact is that you will not know if the nursing diagnosis is accurate unless you assess for defining characteristics and establish that key related factors exist.

A nursing diagnosis provides the basis for selection of nursing interventions to achieve outcomes for which the nurse has accountability. This means that nursing diagnoses are used to determine the appropriate plan of care for the patient, driving patient outcomes and interventions. You cannot standardize a nursing diagnosis, but it is possible to standardize nursing interventions, once you have selected the appropriate outcome for the nursing diagnosis, as interventions should be evidence-based whenever possible.

Nursing diagnoses also provide a standard language for use in the Electronic Health Record, enabling clear communication among care team members and the collection of data for continuous improvement in patient care.

What is the difference between a medical diagnosis and a nursing diagnosis?

A medical diagnosis deals with a disease, illness or injury. A nursing diagnosis deals with actual or potential human responses to health problems and life processes. For example, a medical diagnosis of *cerebrovascular attack* (CVA or stroke) provides information about the patient's pathology. The nursing diagnoses of *impaired verbal communication, risk for falls, interrupted family processes, chronic pain,* and *powerlessness* provide a more holistic understanding of the impact of that stroke on this particular patient and his/her family – they also direct nursing interventions to obtain patient-specific outcomes. If nurses only focus on the stroke, they might miss the *chronic pain* the patient suffers, his sense of *powerlessness,* and even the *interrupted family processes.* All of these issues will have an impact on his potential discharge home, his ability to manage his new therapeutic regimen, and his overall quality of life. It is also important to remember that, while a medical diagnosis belongs only to the patient, **nursing treats the patient *and* his family**, so diagnoses regarding the family are critical because they have the potential to influence – positively or negatively – the outcomes you are trying to achieve with the patient.

What are the component parts of a diagnosis, and what do they mean for nurses in practice?

There are several parts of a nursing diagnosis: the *diagnostic label, definition,* and the assessment criteria used to diagnose, the *defining characteristics* and *related factors* or *risk factors.* As we noted in Chapter 4, NANDA-I has strong concerns about the safety of using terms (diagnosis labels) that have no standardized meaning, and/or no assessment criteria. Picking a diagnosis from a list, or making up a term at a patient's bedside, is a dangerous practice for a couple of very important reasons. First, communication between healthcare team members must be clear, concise, and consistent. If every person defines a "diagnosis" in a different way, there is no clarity. Secondly, how can we assess the validity of a diagnosis, or the diagnostic ability of a nurse, if we have no data to support the diagnosis?

Let's look at the example of Myra Johansen. This case study shows the problem with "picking" a diagnosis from a list of terms, without knowledge of the definition or the assessment data needed to diagnose the response.

Case Study: *Myra Johansen*

Myra Johansen is a 57-year-old obese patient with a 30-year history of smoking (she quit 6 years ago), who was admitted due to severe respiratory complications of her chronic obstructive pulmonary disease (COPD). Her condition is starting to stabilize, and you are assuming her care at the beginning of your shift. You notice in the chart that the nurse caring for her previously documented three nursing diagnoses: *ineffective breathing pattern* (00032), *anxiety* (00146), and *deficient knowledge* (00126). Based on that communication, you form a picture in your mind of this patient and how you will want to approach her. The *anxiety* alerts you that you will want to be calming and reassuring in your approach, while the *ineffective breathing pattern* tells you that Ms. Johansen is still having difficulty with ventilation. The diagnosis of *deficient knowledge* concerns you because you have a lot of teaching to do with the patient about her new medications, as well as nutritional changes to support her in losing weight, which can help to improve her breathing.

A little while later, you complete your assessment and find that you have identified some differences from the previous nurse. The diagnosis of *ineffective breathing pattern* is clearly accurate – she has orthopnea, tachypnea, dyspnea, an increased anterior-posterior diameter; nasal flaring is evident, as is pursed-lip breathing, and she is using her intercostal muscles to breathe. She is also sitting in the classic "three-point position" to attempt to ease her breathing. Her related factors include fatigue, obesity, and respiratory muscle fatigue. The *anxiety*, too, is obvious. She states that she is an anxious person, she is "always worried about something," and now she is preoccupied by many issues, such as having to miss work, who is taking care of her teenage son, and what the hospitalization is going to mean in terms of her finances. She says that she lost her full-time job three months ago, and has only been able to find part-time, temporary work. She is barely able to pay her mortgage and buy groceries, and has no health insurance. She tells you that she has not been able to afford her medications for her COPD for the past 6–7 weeks, and she canceled her routine appointment with her pulmonologist because she could not afford to pay for the visit. She is knowledgeable about her disease, and clearly aware of the consequences of not taking the medication, but was unable to afford to continue with treatment. It is clear that the financial concern is affecting her anxiety, which in turn increases her breathing difficulties. Your assessment did not confirm any of the defining characteristics of *deficient knowledge*, nor did you identify any related factors. Rather, you identify *noncompliance* (00079), which is evident in the development of complications and exacerbations of her symptoms, and her statements that she could not continue her treatment regimen. The related factor is the cost of treatment, and her inability to afford medication and physician follow-up.

When you mention your difference in assessment to your colleague the next day, she responds, "I picked *deficient knowledge* because it's a standard diagnosis for every patient: everyone has a knowledge deficit of some kind!" Clearly, this is faulty thinking, and had your colleague validated the diagnosis by reviewing the definition, defining characteristics, and related factors – and by speaking with the patient – it would have been obvious that this was not a relevant nursing diagnosis. Indeed, many patients with chronic disease often know as much or more about their health condition, their responses to it, and what improves or worsens their symptoms than the health professional.

Focusing on *deficient knowledge* in Ms. Johansen's case would not be appropriate, as she clearly understands her disease and the implications of not following her regimen – focusing on the *noncompliance*, however, can direct appropriate intervention. Recognizing the financial barriers, the nurse can begin to work with the patient and the interdisciplinary team to identify potential sources of financial support for obtaining her medications, attending her follow-up visits, and possibly even sources to support her hospitalization and follow-up care costs. Focusing on the "standard" diagnosis of *deficient knowledge*, for which there was no assessment support noted, wastes the nurse's time and leads to provision of unnecessary care, while at the same time limiting time spent on care that could influence the patient's outcomes.

Which nursing diagnosis is most applicable to a patient with cerebral vascular accident? How do I write a care plan including a nursing diagnosis for patients with a specific medical condition/diagnosis, e.g., hip fracture?

Nursing diagnoses are individual (family, group, or community) responses to health problems or life processes. This means that one cannot standardize nursing diagnoses based on medical diagnoses or procedures. Although many patients with a hip fracture, for example, may suffer from *acute pain, risk for falls,* and/or *self-care deficits* (bathing and hygiene), others might respond with *anxiety, disturbed sleep pattern,* or *noncompliance*. Without a nursing assessment, it is simply impossible to determine the correct diagnosis – and it is does not contribute to safe, quality patient care.

The care plan for each individual patient is based on assessment data. The assessment data and patient preferences guide the nurse in prioritizing nursing diagnoses and interventions – the medical diagnosis is only one piece of assessment data, and therefore cannot be used as the only determining factor for selection of a nursing diagnosis. A thinking tool used by our colleagues in medicine can be useful as you determine your diagnoses: it uses the acronym SEA TOW (Rencic, 2011; refer to Figure 2.5, pp. 48).

It is always a good idea to ask a colleague, or an expert, for a second opinion if you are unsure of the diagnosis. Is the diagnosis you are considering the result of a "Eureka" moment? Did you recognize a pattern in the data from your assessment and patient interview? Can you confirm this pattern by reviewing the diagnostic indicators? Did you collect data that seem to oppose this diagnosis? Can you justify the diagnosis even with this data, or do this data suggest you need to look deeper? Think about your thinking – was it logical, reasoned, built on your knowledge of nursing science and the human response that you are diagnosing? Do you need additional information about the response before you are ready to confirm it? Are you overconfident? This can happen when you are accustomed to patients presenting with particular diagnoses, and so you "jump" to a diagnosis, rather than truly applying clinical reasoning skills. Finally, what other data might you need to collect or review in order to validate, confirm, or rule out a potential nursing diagnosis? Use of the SEA TOW acronym can help you validate your clinical reasoning process and increase the likelihood of accurate diagnosis.

How many diagnoses should my patient have?

Students are often encouraged to identify every diagnosis that a patient has – this is a learning method to improve clinical reasoning and mastery of nursing science. However, in practice it is important to prioritize nursing diagnoses, as these should form the basis for nursing interventions. You should consider which diagnoses are the most critical – from the patient's perspective as well as from a nursing perspective – and the resources and time available for treatment. Other diagnoses may require referral to other healthcare providers or settings, such as home healthcare, a different hospital unit, skilled nursing facility, etc. In a practical sense, having one diagnosis per NANDA-I domain, or a minimum of 5 or 10 diagnoses, does not reflect reality. Although it is important to identify all diagnoses (problem-focused, risk, and health promotion), nurses must focus on high-priority, high-risk diagnoses first; other diagnoses may be added later (moved up on the priority list) to replace those that are resolved, or for which interventions are clearly being effective. Also, if the patient's condition deteriorates or additional data is identified that leads to a more urgent diagnosis, prioritization of the diagnoses must be readdressed. Planning care for patients is not a "one-time thing" – as with all facets of the nursing process, it needs to be continually reevaluated and adjusted to meet the needs of the patient and his/her family.

Can I change a nursing diagnosis after it has been documented in a patient record?

Absolutely! As you continue to assess your patient and collect additional data, you may find that your initial diagnosis wasn't the most critical – or your patient's condition may have resolved, or new data become available that refocuses the priority. It is very important to continually evaluate your patient to determine if the diagnosis is still the most accurate for the patient at any particular point in time.

Can I document nursing diagnoses of a patient's family members in the patient chart?

Documentation rules vary by organization and by particular state and country requirements. However, the concept of family-based care is becoming quite standard, and certainly diagnoses that have an impact on the patient, and can contribute to patient outcomes, should be considered by nurses. For example, if a patient is admitted for exacerbation of a chronic condition, and the nurse recognizes that the spouse is exhibiting signs/symptoms of *caregiver role strain* (00061), it is critical that the nurse confirms or refutes this diagnosis. Taking advantage of the patient's hospitalization, the nurse can work with the spouse to mobilize resources for caregiving at home, such as identifying sources of support for stress management, respite, financial concerns, etc. A review of the therapeutic regimen, along with recommendations to simplify or organize care, may be very helpful. Diagnosis and treatment of the spouse's *caregiver role strain* will not only affect the caregiver, but will have a significant impact on the patient's outcomes when s/he returns home.

Can all nursing diagnoses be used safely and legally in every country?

The NANDA-I classification represents international nursing practice, therefore all diagnoses will not be appropriate for every nurse in the world. Please see *International Considerations on the Use of the NANDA-I Nursing Diagnoses*, pp. 133–135.

Questions about Defining Characteristics

What are defining characteristics?

Defining characteristics are observable cues/inferences that cluster as manifestations of a problem-focused or health promotion diagnosis or syndrome. This does not only imply those things that the nurse can see, but things that are seen, heard (e.g., the patient/family tells us), touched, or smelled.

Defining characteristics in the book are not always observable data; some are judgments (e.g., complicated grieving or deficient knowledge). How can we use them in assessment?

Given the current definition of defining characteristics, nursing diagnoses (inferences) are considered to be acceptable defining characteristics for diagnoses. Although this is logical for syndromes, which are defined as a cluster of two or more nursing diagnoses, it can be confusing for other types of diagnoses. If you have a nursing diagnosis as a defining characteristic, it means you have already made a judgment. Yet, some degree of inference, such as that made through comparison of data to standardized norms, is appropriate for driving diagnosis (e.g., inferring that the heart rate of 174 in an elderly male is above normal). The definition of defining characteristic is currently under review to clarify the intent.

Are the defining characteristics in the book arranged in order of importance?

No. The defining characteristics (and related/risk factors) are listed in alphabetical order, based on the original English-language version. Ultimately, the goal is to validate critical defining characteristics through research – those that must be present for the diagnosis to be made. As that occurs, we will reorganize the diagnostic indicators by order of importance.

How many defining characteristics do I need to identify to diagnose a patient with a particular nursing diagnosis?

That is a difficult question, and it really depends on the diagnosis. For some diagnoses, one defining characteristic is all that is necessary; for example, with the health promotion diagnoses, a patient's expressed desire to enhance a particular facet of a human response is all that is required. Other diagnoses require a cluster of symptoms, probably three or four, to have accuracy in diagnosis. In the future, we would like to be able to limit the number of diagnostic indicators provided within NANDA-I, because long lists of signs/symptoms are not necessarily that clinically useful. As more research is conducted on nursing concepts, this work will be facilitated.

Questions about Related Factors

What are related factors?

Related factors can be considered etiological factors, or those data that appear to show some type of patterned relationship with the nursing diagnosis. Such factors may be described as antecedent to, associated with, related to, contributing to, or abetting. Only problem-focused nursing diagnoses and syndromes must have related factors; health promotion diagnoses may have related factors, if they help to clarify the diagnosis.

How many related factors do I need to identify to diagnose a patient with a particular nursing diagnosis?

As with the defining characteristics, this really depends on the diagnosis. One factor is probably not adequate, and this is especially true if you are using a medical diagnosis alone as a related factor. This can lead to the practice in which every patient admitted for a mastectomy gets "labeled" with *disturbed body image* (00118), or every patient with a surgical procedure gets "labeled" with *acute pain* (00132). This practice is not a diagnostic practice, it truly is labeling a patient, based on an assumption that one person's response will be exactly the same as another's. This is an erroneous assumption at best, and can risk misdiagnosis and lead to nurses spending time on unnecessary interventions. In the worst-case scenario, it can lead to an error of omission in which a significant diagnosis goes unnoticed, and results in significant problems with patient care and quality outcomes.

Related factors within NANDA-I diagnoses are not always factors that a nurse can eliminate or decrease. Should I include them in a diagnosis statement?

Currently, many of our related factors are nonmodifiable factors, such as age or gender. Although these are important factors to know when assessing and diagnosing, it may be that these are more accurately characteristics of "at-risk groups" (e.g., adolescents, elderly, females, etc.). These are factors that help in our diagnosis, but we cannot intervene on age or gender, for example, so it is possible that they should be considered separately from the related factors. This issue is under consideration at this time. In the meantime, although it is technically acceptable to use these related factors in a PES statement, the better practice would be to identify those related factors on which you could intervene, and for which intervention could lead to a decrease in or cessation of the unfavorable human response you have diagnosed.

Questions about Risk Factors

What are risk factors?

These are environmental factors and physiological, psychological, genetic, or chemical elements that increase the vulnerability of an individual, family, group, or community to an unhealthy event. Only risk diagnoses have risk factors.

How many risk factors do I need to identify to diagnose
a patient with a particular risk nursing diagnosis?

As with the defining characteristics and related factors, this really depends on the diagnosis. For example, in the new diagnosis *risk for pressure ulcer* (00249), having a Braden Q score of < 16 in a child, or a Braden Scale score of <18 in an adult, or a low score on the Risk Assessment Pressure Sore (RAPS) Scale might be all that is needed to diagnose this risk. That is because these standardized tools have been clinically validated as predictors of risk for pressure ulcer. For other diagnoses that do not yet have this level of diagnostic indicator validation, a clustering of risk factors is needed.

Risk factors in the book are not always factors that a nurse can
eliminate or decrease. Should I include them in a diagnosis statement?

See the answer regarding related factors.

Is there a relationship between related factors and risk factors,
such as with diagnoses that have a problem-based and/or health
promotion diagnosis, and a risk diagnosis?

Yes. You should notice strong similarities between the related factors for a problem-focused diagnosis and the risk factors of a risk diagnosis related to the same concept. Indeed, the lists of factors could be identical. The same condition that puts you at risk for an undesirable response would most often be an etiology of that response if it were to occur. For example, in the diagnosis *risk for disorganized infant behavior* (00115), environmental overstimulation is noted as a risk factor. In the problem-focused diagnosis *disorganized infant behavior* (00116), environmental sensory overstimulation is noted as a related factor. In both cases, this is something for which many nursing interventions are available that can decrease the unfavorable response, or modify its risk of occurrence.

Differentiating between Similar Nursing Diagnoses

How can I decide between diagnoses that are very similar – how do
I know which one is the most accurate diagnosis?

Accuracy in diagnosis is critical. Avoid reaching a conclusion too quickly, and use some easy tools to reflect on your decision-making process. A diagnostic aid that is used in medicine for differentiation between diagnoses can be easily adapted for nursing: SNAPPS (Rencic, 2011); see Figure 5.1. Using this tool, you summarize the data you collected in your

Figure 5.1   *The SNAPPS diagnostic aid*

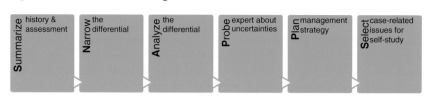

interview and assessment, as well as any other relevant data from the patient record. You then seek to narrow the differential between the diagnoses: eliminate the data that fits for both diagnoses, so you are left with only that data that differ. Analyze this data – is a pattern more evident now that you are looking at a narrower cluster of data? Probe a colleague, professor, or expert when you have doubts or unanswered questions – don't ask for the answer, ask them to walk through their thinking with you to help you determine the more appropriate diagnosis. Plan a management strategy, which should include frequent reassessment, especially at the beginning of the plan, to ensure that your diagnosis truly was accurate. Finally, select case-related issues for further investigation and study. Find an article, a case study in a journal, or information from a recent text that can deepen your understanding of the human response you have just diagnosed.

Can I add "risk for" to a problem-focused diagnosis to make it a risk diagnosis? Or remove "risk for" from a risk diagnosis to make it a problem-focused diagnosis?

Simply put, the answer to this question is "no." In fact, to randomly "make up" a label is meaningless, and we believe could be dangerous. Why? Ask yourself these questions: How is the diagnosis defined? What are the risk factors (for risk diagnoses) or the defining characteristics/related factors (for problem-focused diagnoses) that should be identified during your nursing assessment? How do other people know what you mean if the diagnosis is not clearly defined and provided in a resource format (text, computer system) to review and to enable validation of the diagnosis?

If you identify a patient whom you feel might be at risk for something for which there is not a nursing diagnosis, it is better to document very clearly what it is that you are seeing in your patient or why you feel he is at risk, so that others can easily follow your clinical reasoning. This is critical for patient safety.

When considering whether or not a risk diagnosis should be modified to create an actual diagnosis, the question should be asked: "Is this already identified as a medical diagnosis?" If so, there is no reason to rename it as a nursing diagnosis, unless there is a distinctive view that nursing would bring to it phenomena different from those of medicine. For example, "anxiety" is a nursing/medical/psychiatric diagnosis, and all disciplines may approach it differently from their disciplinary perspectives. On the other hand, when considering a diagnosis such as "pneumonia" (infection), what viewpoint would the nurse bring that would differ from that of medicine? To date, we have not identified that there would be a difference in treatment among disciplines, so it is a medical diagnosis for which nurses utilize nursing interventions. That's perfectly acceptable.

Finally, if you have identified a human response that you believe should be identified as a nursing diagnosis, check out our information on diagnosis development, review the literature or work with experts to develop it, and submit it to NANDA-I. It is generally nurses in practice who identify diagnoses that we need, which allows the terminology to grow or to be refined, and to better reflect the reality of practice.

Questions Regarding the Development of a Treatment Plan

Does every nursing intervention require a nursing diagnosis? Is all nursing practice related to patient care driven by nursing diagnoses?

Not all nursing interventions or actions are based on nursing diagnoses. Nurses intervene on conditions described by medical diagnoses as well as nursing diagnoses; they also provide interventions that result from organizational protocols versus patient-specific needs. We do not rename medical diagnoses or terms to create nursing diagnoses, nor do we need a nursing diagnosis for every nursing intervention. Kamitsuru's *Tripartite Model of Nursing Practice* (2008) may be helpful as you consider the interventions that nurses perform, and what the underlying rationale or support is for those interventions (Figure 5.2).

Figure 5.2   *Tripartite Model of Nursing Practice (Kamitsuru, 2008)*

Foundation for what nurses do	Medical diagnoses	Nursing diagnoses	Organizational protocols
What nurses do	Treatment, surveillance, collaboration	Nursing interventions	Basic care
Standards	Standards of medical care	Standards of nursing care	Standards of organizational care

As you can see, there are three foundational "pillars" of this model, each of which represents different theoretical positions/standards that provide rationale/knowledge for nursing interventions (the bottom level of the model): medical standards of care, nursing standards of care, and organizational standards. At the top of the model the focus of the interventions is indicated: medical diagnosis, nursing diagnosis, and organizational protocol. All of these drive nursing intervention or activities, some of which are dependent, some are interdependent, and others are independent.

How do I find interventions to be used with nursing diagnoses?

Interventions should be directed at the related or etiological factors whenever possible. Sometimes, however, that is not possible and so interventions are chosen to control symptoms (defining characteristics). Take a look at two different situations using the same diagnosis:

- *Acute pain* (related factors: inappropriate lifting technique and body posture; defining characteristics: report of sharp back pain, guarding behavior and positioning to avoid pain)
- *Acute pain* (related factors: surgical procedures; defining characteristics: verbal report of sharp incisional pain, guarding behavior, and positioning to avoid pain)

In the first example, the nurse can aim interventions at the symptoms (providing pain relief interventions) but also at the etiology (providing education on proper lifting techniques, proper body mechanics, and exercises to strengthen the core muscles and back muscles).

In the second example, the nurse cannot intervene to remove the causative factor (the surgical procedure), so the interventions are all aimed at symptom control (providing pain relief interventions).

Choosing interventions for a specific patient is also influenced by the severity and duration of the nursing diagnosis, effectiveness of interventions, patient preferences, organizational guidelines, and ability to perform the intervention (e.g., whether the intervention is realistic).

When does a nursing care plan need revision?

There is not a clear-cut standard for the frequency for revision: it depends on the patient's condition, the severity and complexity of care, as well as organizational standards. In general, a minimum guideline would be once every 24 hours, but in intensive care environments or with complex patient conditions it is often done one or more times per shift.

What does it mean to "revise" the care plan? This requires a reassessment of the patient's current conditions, to identify current human responses that require nursing intervention, and that means reviewing those that were previously identified to determine:

1. Are the previously identified nursing diagnoses still present?
2. Are they still high priority?
3. Are they improving, staying the same, worsening?
4. Are the current interventions effective? Has the desired outcome been achieved/partially achieved?
5. Perhaps most importantly, did you identify the correct response to treat (did you diagnose accurately)?

All of these questions require ongoing reassessment of the patient. When intervention is not being successful in reaching determined patient outcomes, continuing the same intervention may not be the best policy. Is it possible that there is something else going on that wasn't noted previously? What other data might you need to collect to identify other issues? Is the patient in agreement with you about prioritization of care? Are there other interventions that might be more effective? All of this is involved in reviewing and revising the plan of care.

Remember that the nursing care plan is a computerized (or written) representation of your clinical judgment. It isn't something you do and then forget about – it should drive every single thing you are doing with that patient. Every question you ask, every diagnostic test result, every piece of physical assessment data adds more information to consider when looking at patient responses. Thus, assessment and evaluation should be occurring every time you look at, talk with, or touch a patient, and every time you interact with his/her family and with data in his/her patient record.

Clinical reasoning, diagnosis, and appropriate treatment planning require mindful, reflective practice. Planning of patient care isn't a task to check off so you can move on to something else – it is the key component of professional nursing practice.

Questions about Teaching/Learning Nursing Diagnoses

I never learned about nursing diagnosis while I was in school. What is the best way to study nursing diagnosis? I am not comfortable teaching nursing diagnoses because I never learned about them while I was in school. Any recommendations?

You are getting a good start by using this book! But first, we really recommend that you spend some time learning/reviewing the concepts that support the diagnoses. Think about how much you know about ventilation, coping, activity tolerance, mobility, feeding patterns, sleep patterns, tissue perfusion, etc. You really need to start with a solid understanding of these "neutral" phenomena: What is *normal*? What would you expect to see in a healthy patient? What physiological/ psychological/sociological factors influence these normal patterns? Once you really understand the concepts, then you can move into deviations from the norm: How would you assess for these? What other areas of the person's health might be affected if a deviation occurred? What kinds of things would put someone at risk for developing an undesired response? What are the strengths that people might draw on to improve this area of their health? What are nurses saying about these phenomena – what research is being done? Are there clinical guidelines for practice? All of these areas of knowledge will contribute to your understanding of nursing diagnosis – after all, nursing diagnoses name the knowledge of the discipline.

It simply isn't enough to pick up this book, or any other, and start writing down diagnoses that "sound like" they fit your patient, or that have been linked to a medical diagnosis in some standardized way. Once you truly understand the concepts, you will start to see the patterns in your assessment data that will point you to risk states, problem states, and strengths – then you can begin to sharpen your understanding of the diagnoses by reviewing the definitions and diagnostic indicators for the diagnoses that seem to represent the majority of patient responses that you see in your practice. There are core diagnoses in every area of practice, and those are the ones on which you will want to focus so that you build expertise in them first.

Should I choose one diagnosis from each of the 13 domains and combine those diagnoses at the end of the assessment?

Although we know that some professors teach this way, it is not really a method that we support. Arbitrarily assigning a set number of diagnoses to consider is neither practical nor necessarily reflective of the patient's reality. Also, as noted previously, the domains are not an assessment format. You should complete a nursing assessment, and as you are conducting your assessment you will begin to hypothesize about potential diagnoses. That in turn should lead you to more focused assessment either to rule out or confirm those hypotheses. Assessment is a fluid process – one piece of data may lead you back to previously obtained data, or it may require further in-depth assessment to collect additional information. We recommend the use of an assessment based on a nursing model, such as Gordon's Functional Health Patterns. Although the taxonomy is currently adapted from these patterns, the assessment framework provides support for nurses in conducting an interview and patient assessment, allowing (and encouraging!) a fluid consideration of how data and information obtained from other patterns interact while assessment is occurring.

My professors do not allow us to use risk diagnoses, because they say we have to focus on the "real" diagnoses. Aren't patient risks "real"?

Absolutely! Risk diagnoses can actually be the highest-priority diagnosis that a patient may have – a patient with a significant vulnerability to infection, falls, a pressure ulcer, or bleeding may have no more critical diagnosis that this risk. The prior use of the term "actual" diagnosis may have led to this confusion – some people interpreted this to mean that the actual (problem-focused) diagnosis was more "real" than the risk. Think about the young woman who has just given birth to a healthy newborn baby, but who developed disseminated intravascular coagulation during this pregnancy and has a history of postpartum hemorrhage. She most likely has no higher-priority nursing diagnosis than *risk for bleeding* (00206). She may have *acute pain* (00132) from her episiotomy, she may have *anxiety* (00146), and she may have *readiness for enhanced breastfeeding* (00106) – but any perinatal nurse will tell you that the number one focus will be the *risk for bleeding*.

Our basic nursing curriculum is already full. When and who should teach nursing diagnoses?

Nursing, as with other disciplines, is struggling to move from a content-laden educational system to a learner-based, reasoning-focused educational process. For at least the last several decades, the pattern within nursing education has been to try to include more and more information in lectures, readings, and assignments, leading to a pattern of memorization and regurgitation of knowledge (often followed by forgetting most of what was "learned" shortly thereafter) – it simply does not work! The speed of knowledge development has increased exponentially – we cannot continue to teach every piece of information necessary. Instead, we need to teach core concepts, teach students how to reason, how to discover knowledge and know if it is trustworthy, and how to apply it. We have to give them the tools that lead to life-long learning, and clinical reasoning is probably the most critical of these. But critical reasoning requires a field of knowledge – nursing, in this case – and that requires mastery of our disciplinary knowledge, which is represented by nursing diagnoses.

Every nursing professor needs to teach nursing diagnoses – in every course, and as the focus of the course. By being taught the concepts, students will learn about related disciplines, their diagnoses and standard treatments; they will also learn about human responses and how they differ under a variety of situations or by age, gender, culture, etc. Restructuring curricula to truly focus on nursing may sound radical, but it is the only way to solidly provide nursing content to the nurses of our future. Teach the core diagnoses that cross all areas of practice first, then as students gain knowledge, teach the core specialty diagnoses. The remainder – those that don't occur often or only occur in very specialized conditions – they will learn as they practice and as they encounter patients who exhibit these responses.

Questions about Using NANDA-I in Electronic Health Records

Is there any regulatory mandate that patient problems, interventions, and outcomes included in an electronic health record should be stated using NANDA-I terminology? Why should we use NANDA-I nursing diagnoses with an electronic health system?

There is no regulatory mandate. However, NANDA International nursing diagnoses are strongly suggested by standards organizations for inclusion in the EHR. Several international expert papers and studies promote inclusion of the NANDA-I taxonomy in the EHR based on several reasons:

- The safety of patients requires accurate documentation of health problems (e.g. risk states, actual diagnoses, health promotion diagnoses) and NANDA-I is the single classification having a broad literature base (with some diagnoses evidence-based, including a level of evidence (LOE) format). Most importantly, NANDA-I diagnoses are comprehensive concepts have been defined and include related factors and defining characteristics. This is a major difference from other nursing terminologies
- NANDA-I, NIC, and NOC (NNN) not only are the most frequently used classifications internationally, studies have shown them to be the most evidence-based and comprehensive classifications (Tastan, Linch, Keenan, Stifter, McKinney, Fahey... & Wilkie, 2013).
- NANDA-I diagnoses are under continual refinement and development. The classification is not a single-author product, it is based on the work of professional nurses around the world, members and nonmembers of NANDA International (Anderson, Keenan, & Jones, 2009; Bernhard-Just, Hillewerth, Holzer-Pruss, et al., 2009; Keenan, Tschannen, & Wesley, 2008; Lunney, 2006; Lunney, Delaney, Duffy, et al., 2005; Müller-Staub, 2007, 2009; Müller-Staub, Lavin, Needham, et al., 2007)

Questions about Diagnosis Development and Review

Who develops and revises NANDA-I diagnoses?

New and revised diagnoses are submitted to the NANDA-I Diagnosis Development Committee (DDC) by nurses from around the world. Primarily these nurses come from the areas of practice and education, although we have researchers and theorists who occasionally submit diagnoses, too. The DDC formulates and conducts review processes of proposed diagnoses. The duties of the committee include but are not limited to: the review of proposed new or revised diagnoses, or proposed deletions of current nursing diagnoses; soliciting and disseminating feedback from experts; implementing processes for review by the membership; and voting by the general assembly/membership on diagnosis development matters.

I understand that nurses can submit new nursing diagnoses as well as revise the current nursing diagnoses. How does NANDA-I help us? Is there a service fee charged for this support?

NANDA-I's Diagnosis Development Committee (DDC) provides a mentor for you during the submission process. When you contact us with a diagnosis submission or revision, that individual is assigned and becomes your primary contact to the committee. He or she will work with you to understand any questions that may arise from the DDC members, or to clarify your submission to make sure that it meets the requirements identified in the submission process. No fee is charged for this support.

Why are certain diagnoses revised?

Knowledge is continually evolving within nursing practice, and as research clarifies and refines that knowledge, it is important that the NANDA-I terminology reflects those changes. Nurses in practice, as well as educators and researchers, submit revisions based on their own work or a review of research literature. The purpose is to refine the diagnoses, providing information that enables accuracy in diagnosis.

Questions about the *NANDA-I Definitions and Classification* Text

How do I know which diagnoses are new?

All of the new and revised diagnoses are highlighted in the section of this book entitled ***What's New in the 2015–2017 Edition of* Diagnoses and Classification?** (pp. 4–15).

When I reviewed the informatics codes provided in the book, I noticed that there were some codes missing – does that mean that there are missing diagnoses?

No, the missing codes represent codes that were not assigned, or diagnoses that have been retired, or removed, from the taxonomy over time. Codes are not reused, but rather are retired along with the diagnosis. Likewise, unassigned codes are never assigned later, out of sequence, but simply remain permanently unassigned.

When a diagnosis is revised, how do we know what was changed? I noticed changes to some diagnoses, but they are not listed as revisions – why?

The section **What's New in the 2015–2017 Edition of Diagnoses and Classification?** (pp. 4–15) provides detailed information on changes made in this edition. However, the best way to see each individual change is to compare the current edition with the previous one. We did not list all of the edits made as we standardized terms for the diagnostic indicators; nor were these changes considered as revisions but rather as editorial changes. There was an emphasis during this cycle to continue the previous work of refining and standardizing terms of the defining characteristics, related factors, and risk factors. This work enabled the coding of these terms to facilitate the development of an assessment structure within an electronic health record. This is a work in progress, as there are currently >5,600 diagnostic indicators within the terminology (defining characteristics, related factors, and risk factors), and this requires slow and meticulous work to ensure that changes do not have an impact on the intended meaning of the terms. The 2015–2017 edition provides the first full standardization and coding of these terms (coding is available on the NANDA-I website).

Why don't all of the diagnoses show a level of evidence (LOE)?

NANDA International did not begin using LOE criteria until 2002, therefore diagnoses that were entered into the taxonomy prior to that time do not show an LOE criteria because none was identified when the diagnoses were submitted. All diagnoses that existed in the taxonomy in 2002 were "grandfathered" into the taxonomy, with those clearly not meeting criteria (e.g., no identified related factors, multiple diagnostic foci in the label, etc.) targeted for revision or removal over the next few editions. The last of these diagnoses is being removed in this edition. We strongly encourage work on the older diagnoses to bring them up to a level of evidence consistent with a minimum LOE of 2.1 for maintenance in the terminology, and slotting within the taxonomic structure.

What happened to the references? Why doesn't NANDA-I print all of the references used for all of the diagnoses?

NANDA-I began publishing references by asking submitters to identify their three most important references. In the 2009–2011 edition, we began to publish the full list of references, due to the large number of requests received from individuals regarding the literature reviewed for different diagnoses. We have now heard from many individuals that they would prefer to have access to the references online, rather than in the book. There have also been concerns raised about the environmental impact of a larger book, and recommendations to publish information specific to researchers and informaticists on our website, for those who want to access this information. After discussion, we determined that this course of action would be the best one for the purposes of this text. Therefore, all references that we have for all diagnoses will be placed in the knowledge base of the NANDA-I website (www.nanda.org), as well as on the companion website for this text, to enable ease of searching for and retrieving this information.

Student Resources

References

Anderson, C. A., Keenan, G., & Jones, J. (2009). Using bibliometrics to support your selection of a nursing terminology set. *CIN: Computers, Informatics, Nursing,* 27(2), 82–90.

Bernhard-Just, A., Hillewerth, K., Holzer-Pruss, C., Paprotny, M., & Zimmermann Heinrich, H. (2009). Die elektronische Anwendung der NANDA-, NOC- und NIC - Klassifikationen und Folgerungen für die Pflegepraxis. *Pflege,* 22(6), 443–454.

Kamitsuru, S. (2008). *Kango shindan seminar shiryou* [Nursing diagnosis seminar handout]. Kango Laboratory (Japanese).

Keenan, G., Tschannen, D., & Wesley, M. L. (2008). Standardized nursing teminologies can transform practice. *Journal of Nursing Administration,* 38(3), 103–106.

Lunney, M. (2006). NANDA diagnoses, NIC interventions, and NOC outcomes used in an electronic health record with elementary school children. *Journal of School Nursing,* 22(2), 94–101.

Lunney, M. (2008). Critical need to address accuracy of nurses' diagnoses. *OJIN: The Online Journal of Issues in Nursing,* 13(1).

Lunney, M., Delaney, C., Duffy, M., Moorhead, S., & Welton, J. (2005). Advocating for standardized nursing languages in electronic health records. *Journal of Nursing Administration,* 35(1), 1–3.

Müller-Staub, M. (2007). *Evaluation of the implementation of nursing diagnostics: A study on the use of nursing diagnoses, interventions and outcomes in nursing documentation.* Wageningen: Ponsen & Looijen.

Müller-Staub, M. (2009). Preparing nurses to use standardized nursing language in the electronic health record. Studies in health technology and informatics. *Connecting Health and Humans,* 146, 337–341.

Müller-Staub, M., Lavin, M. A., Needham, I., & van Achterberg, T. (2007). Meeting the criteria of a nursing diagnosis classification: Evaluation of ICNP®, ICF, NANDA and ZEFP. *International Journal of Nursing Studies*, 44(5), 702–713.

Rencic, J. (2011). Twelve tips for teaching expertise in clinical reasoning. *Medical Teacher*, 33(11), 887–892.

Tastan, S., Linch, G. C., Keenan, G. M., Stifter, J., McKinney, D., Fahey, L., ... & Wilkie, D. J. (2013). Evidence for the existing American Nurses Association-recognized standardized nursing terminologies: A systematic review. *International journal of nursing studies*.

Part 3
The NANDA International Nursing Diagnoses

International Considerations on the use of the
NANDA-I Nursing Diagnoses   **133**

Domain 1: Health Promotion   **137**

Domain 2: Nutrition   **153**

Domain 3: Elimination and Exchange   **181**

Domain 4: Activity/Rest   **205**

Domain 5: Perception/Cognition   **249**

Domain 6: Self-Perception   **263**

Domain 7: Role Relationships   **277**

Domain 8: Sexuality   **303**

Domain 9: Coping/Stress Tolerance   **313**

Domain 10: Life Principles   **359**

Domain 11: Safety/Protection   **375**

Domain 12: Comfort   **435**

Domain 13: Growth/Development   **449**

**Nursing Diagnoses Accepted for Development
and Clinical Validation 2015–2017**   **455**

NANDA International, Inc. Nursing Diagnoses: Definitions & Classification 2015–2017,
Tenth Edition. Edited by T. Heather Herdman and Shigemi Kamitsuru.
© 2014 NANDA International, Inc. Published 2014 by John Wiley & Sons, Ltd.
Companion website: www.wiley.com/go/nursingdiagnoses

International Considerations on the Use of the *NANDA-I Nursing Diagnoses*

T. Heather Herdman, RN, PhD, FNI

As we noted previously, NANDA International, Inc. began as a North American organization and therefore the earliest nursing diagnoses were primarily developed by nurses from the United States and Canada. However, over the past 20 years there has been increasing involvement from nurses around the world, and membership in NANDA International includes nurses from nearly 40 countries, with nearly two-thirds of its members coming from countries outside North America. Work is occurring across all continents using NANDA-I nursing diagnoses in curricula, clinical practice, research, and informatics applications. Development and refinement of diagnoses are ongoing across multiple countries.

As a reflection of this increased international activity, contribution, and utilization, the North American Nursing Diagnosis Association changed its scope to an international organization in 2002, changing its name to **NANDA International, Inc.** So, please, we ask that you **do not refer to the organization as the North American Nursing Diagnosis Association (or as the North American Nursing Diagnosis Association International)**, unless referring to something that happened prior to 2002 – it simply doesn't reflect our international scope, and it is not the legal name of the organization. We retained "NANDA" within our name because of its status in the nursing profession, so think of it more as a trademark or brand name than as an acronym, since it no longer stands for the original name.

As NANDA-I experiences increased worldwide adoption, issues related to differences in the scope of nursing practice, diversity of nurse practice models, divergent laws and regulations, nurse competence, and educational differences must be addressed. At the 2009 Think Tank Meeting, which included 86 individuals representing 16 countries, significant discussions occurred as to how best to handle these and other issues. Nurses in some countries are not able to utilize nursing diagnoses of a more physiological nature because they are in conflict with their current scope of nursing practice. Nurses in other

NANDA International, Inc. Nursing Diagnoses: Definitions & Classification 2015–2017,
Tenth Edition. Edited by T. Heather Herdman and Shigemi Kamitsuru.
© 2014 NANDA International, Inc. Published 2014 by John Wiley & Sons, Ltd.
Companion website: www.wiley.com/go/nursingdiagnoses

nations are facing regulations to ensure that everything done within nursing practice can be demonstrated to be evidence-based, and therefore face difficulties with some of the older nursing diagnoses and/or linked interventions that are not supported by a strong level of research literature. Discussions were therefore held with international leaders in nursing diagnosis use and research, looking for direction that would meet the needs of the worldwide community.

These discussions resulted in a unanimous decision to maintain the taxonomy as an intact body of knowledge in all languages, in order to enable nurses around the world to view, discuss, and consider diagnostic concepts being used by nurses within and outside of their countries and to engage in discussions, research, and debate regarding the appropriateness of all of the diagnoses. The full minutes of the Think Tank Summit can be found on our website (www.nanda.org). However, a critical statement agreed upon in that Summit is noted here prior to introducing the nursing diagnoses themselves:

Not every nursing diagnosis within the NANDA-I taxonomy is appropriate for every nurse in practice – nor has it ever been. Some of the diagnoses are specialty-specific, and would not necessarily be used by all nurses in clinical practice … There are diagnoses within the taxonomy that may be outside the scope or standards of nursing practice governing a particular geographic area in which a nurse practices.

Those diagnoses would, in these instances, not be appropriate for practice, and should not be used if they lie outside the scope or standards of nursing practice for a particular geographic region. However, it is appropriate for these diagnoses to remain visible in the taxonomy because the taxonomy represents clinical judgments made by nurses around the world, not just those made in a particular region or country. Every nurse should be aware of, and work within, the standards and scope of practice and any laws or regulations within which he or she is licensed to practice. However, it is also important for all nurses to be aware of the areas of nursing practice that exist globally, as this informs discussion and may over time support the broadening of nursing practice across other countries. Conversely, these individuals may be able to provide evidence that would support the removal of diagnoses from the current taxonomy, which, if they were not shown in their translations, would be unlikely to occur.

Ultimately, nurses must identify those diagnoses that are appropriate for their area of practice, that fit within their scope of practice or legal regulations, and for which they have competence. Nurse educators, clinical experts, and nurse administrators are critical to ensuring that nurses are aware of diagnoses that are truly outside the scope of nursing practice in a particular geographic region. Multiple textbooks in many languages are available that include the entire NANDA-I taxonomy, so for the NANDA-I text to remove diagnoses from country to country would no doubt lead to a great level of confusion worldwide. Publication of the taxonomy in no way requires that a nurse utilize every diagnosis within it, nor does it justify practicing outside the scope of an individual's nursing license or regulations to practice.

Domain 1
Health Promotion

DOMAIN 1. HEALTH PROMOTION		
The awareness of well-being or normality of function and the strategies used to maintain control of and enhance that well-being or normality of function		

Class 1. Health awareness
Recognition of normal function and well-being

Code	Diagnosis	Page
00097	Deficient **diversional activity**	139
00168	Sedentary **lifestyle**	140

Class 2. Health management
Identifying, controlling, performing, and integrating activities to maintain health and well-being

Code	Diagnosis	Page
00257	**Frail elderly syndrome**	141
00231	Risk for **frail elderly syndrome**	142
00215	Deficient community **health**	144
00188	Risk-prone **health behavior**	145
00099	Ineffective **health maintenance**	146
00078	Ineffective **health management**	147

NANDA International, Inc. Nursing Diagnoses: Definitions & Classification 2015–2017,
Tenth Edition. Edited by T. Heather Herdman and Shigemi Kamitsuru.
© 2014 NANDA International, Inc. Published 2014 by John Wiley & Sons, Ltd.
Companion website: www.wiley.com/go/nursingdiagnoses

Class 2. Health management (continued)		
Code	**Diagnosis**	**Page**
00162	Readiness for enhanced **health management**	148
00080	Ineffective family **health management**	149
00079	Non**compliance**	150
00043	Ineffective **protection**	152

00097

Deficient **diversional activity**
(1980)

Definition
Decreased stimulation from (or interest or engagement in) recreational or leisure activities.

Defining Characteristics

- Boredom
- Current setting does not allow engagement in activity

Related Factors

- Insufficient diversional activity
- Extremes of age
- Prolonged hospitalization
- Prolonged institutionalization

00168

Sedentary lifestyle
(2004; LOE 2.1)

Definition
Reports a habit of life that is characterized by a low physical activity level.

Defining Characteristics

- Average daily physical activity is less than recommended for gender and age
- Physical deconditioning
- Preference for activity low in physical activity

Related Factors

- Insufficient interest in physical activity
- Insufficient knowledge of health benefits associated with physical exercise
- Insufficient motivation for physical activity
- Insufficient resources for physical activity
- Insufficient training for physical exercise

Original literature support available at www.nanda.org

00257

Frail elderly syndrome
(2013; LOE 2.1)

Definition
Dynamic state of unstable equilibrium that affects the older individual experiencing deterioration in one or more domain of health (physical, functional, psychological, or social) and leads to increased susceptibility to adverse health effects, in particular disability.

Defining Characteristics

- Activity intolerance (00092)
- Bathing self-care deficit (00108)
- Decreased cardiac output (00029)
- Dressing self-care deficit (00109)
- Fatigue (00093)
- Feeding self-care deficit (00102)
- Hopelessness (00124)
- Imbalanced nutrition: less than body requirements (00002)
- Impaired memory (00131)
- Impaired physical mobility (00085)
- Impaired walking (00088)
- Social isolation (00053)
- Toileting self-care deficit (00110)

Related Factors

- Alteration in cognitive functioning
- Chronic illness
- History of falls
- Living alone
- Malnutrition
- Prolonged hospitalization
- Psychiatric disorder
- Sarcopenia
- Sarcopenic obesity
- Sedentary lifestyle

Original literature support available at **www.nanda.org**

00231

Risk for **frail elderly syndrome**
(2013; LOE 2.1)

1. Health Promotion

Definition
Vulnerable to a dynamic state of unstable equilibrium that affects the older individual experiencing deterioration in one or more domain of health (physical, functional, psychological, or social) and leads to increased susceptibility to adverse health effects, in particular disability.

Risk Factors

- Activity intolerance
- Age > 70 years
- Alteration in cognitive functioning
- Altered clotting process (e.g., Factor VII, D-dimers)
- Anorexia
- Anxiety
- Average daily physical activity is less than recommended for gender and age
- Chronic illness
- Constricted life space
- Decrease in energy
- Decrease in muscle strength
- Decrease in serum 25-hydroxyvitamin D concentration
- Depression
- Economically disadvantaged
- Endocrine regulatory dysfunction (e.g., glucose intolerance, increase in IGF-1, androgen, DHEA, and cortisol)
- Ethnicity other than Caucasian
- Exhaustion
- Fear of falling
- Female gender
- History of falls
- Immobility
- Impaired balance
- Impaired mobility
- Insufficient social support
- Living alone
- Low educational level
- Malnutrition
- Muscle weakness
- Obesity
- Prolonged hospitalization
- Sadness
- Sarcopenia
- Sarcopenic obesity
- Sedentary lifestyle
- Sensory deficit (e.g., visual, hearing)
- Social isolation
- Social vulnerability (e.g., disempowerment, decreased life control)

- Suppressed inflammatory response (e.g., IL-6, CRP)
- Unintentional loss of 25% of body weight over one year
- Unintentional weight loss >10 pounds (>4.5 kg) in one year
- Walking 15 feet requires >6 seconds (4 meter >5 seconds)

Original literature support available at www.nanda.org

00215

Deficient community **health**
(2010; LOE 2.1)

Definition
Presence of one or more health problems or factors that deter wellness or increase the risk of health problems experienced by an aggregate.

Defining Characteristics

- Health problem experienced by aggregates or populations
- Program unavailable to eliminate health problem(s) of an aggregate or population
- Program unavailable to enhance wellness of an aggregate or population
- Program unavailable to prevent health problem(s) of an aggregate or population
- Program unavailable to reduce health problem(s) of an aggregate or population
- Risk of hospitalization experienced by aggregates or population
- Risk of physiological states experienced by aggregates or populations
- Risk of psychological states experienced by aggregates or population

Related Factors

- Inadequate consumer satisfaction with program
- Inadequate program budget
- Inadequate program evaluation plan
- Inadequate program outcome data
- Inadequate social support for program
- Insufficient access to healthcare provider
- Insufficient community experts
- Insufficient resources (e.g., financial, social, knowledge)
- Program incompletely addresses health problem

Original literature support available at www.nanda.org

00188

Risk-prone **health behavior**
(1986, 1998, 2006, 2008; LOE 2.1)

Definition
Impaired ability to modify lifestyle/behaviors in a manner that improves health status.

Defining Characteristics

- Failure to achieve optimal sense of control
- Failure to take action that prevents health problem
- Minimizes health status change
- Nonacceptance of health status change

Related Factors

- Economically disadvantaged
- Inadequate comprehension
- Insufficient social support
- Low self-efficacy
- Negative attitude toward healthcare
- Smoking
- Stressors
- Substance abuse

Original literature support available at **www.nanda.org**

00099

Ineffective **health maintenance**
(1982)

Definition
Inability to identify, manage, and/or seek out help to maintain health.

Defining Characteristics

- Absence of adaptive behaviors to environmental changes
- Absence of interest in improving health behaviors
- Inability to take responsibility for meeting basic health practices
- Insufficient knowledge about basic health practices
- Insufficient social support
- Pattern of lack of health-seeking behavior

Related Factors

- Alteration in cognitive functioning
- Complicated grieving
- Decrease in fine motor skills
- Decrease in gross motor skills
- Impaired decision-making
- Ineffective communication skills
- Ineffective coping strategies
- Insufficient resources (e.g., financial, social, knowledge)
- Perceptual impairment
- Spiritual distress
- Unachieved developmental tasks

00078

Ineffective **health management**
(1994, 2008; LOE 2.1)

Definition
Pattern of regulating and integrating into daily living a therapeutic regimen for the treatment of illness and its sequelae that is unsatisfactory for meeting specific health goals.

Defining Characteristics

- Difficulty with prescribed regimen
- Failure to include treatment regimen in daily living
- Failure to take action to reduce risk factor
- Ineffective choices in daily living for meeting health goal

Related Factors

- Complex treatment regimen
- Complexity of healthcare system
- Decisional conflict
- Economically disadvantaged
- Excessive demands
- Family conflict
- Family pattern of healthcare
- Inadequate number of cues to action
- Insufficient knowledge of therapeutic regimen
- Insufficient social support
- Perceived barrier
- Perceived benefit
- Perceived seriousness of condition
- Perceived susceptibility
- Powerlessness

Original literature support available at www.nanda.org

00162

Readiness for enhanced **health management**
(2002, 2010, 2013; LOE 2.1)

Definition
A pattern of regulating and integrating into daily living a therapeutic regimen for the treatment of illness and its sequelae, which can be strengthened.

Defining Characteristics

- Expresses desire to enhance choices of daily living for meeting goals
- Expresses desire to enhance management of illness
- Expresses desire to enhance management of prescribed regimens
- Expresses desire to enhance management of risk factors
- Expresses desire to enhance management of symptoms
- Expresses desire to enhance immunization/vaccination status

Original literature support available at **www.nanda.org**

00080

Ineffective family **health management**
(1992)

Definition
A pattern of regulating and integrating into family processes a program for the treatment of illness and its sequelae that is unsatisfactory for meeting specific health goals.

Defining Characteristics

- Acceleration of illness symptoms of a family member
- Decrease in attention to illness
- Difficulty with prescribed regimen
- Failure to take action to reduce risk factor
- Inappropriate family activities for meeting health goal

Related Factors

- Complex treatment regimen
- Complexity of healthcare system
- Decisional conflict
- Economically disadvantaged
- Family conflict

00079

Non**compliance**
(1973, 1996, 1998)

Definition
Behavior of person and/or caregiver that fails to coincide with a health-promoting or therapeutic plan agreed on by the person (and/or family and/or community) and healthcare professional. In the presence of an agreed-upon, health-promoting, or therapeutic plan, the person's or caregiver's behavior is fully or partly nonadherent and may lead to clinically ineffective or partially effective outcomes.

Defining Characteristics

- Development-related complication
- Exacerbation of symptoms
- Failure to meet outcomes
- Missing of appointments
- Nonadherence behavior

Related Factors

Health System
- Difficulty in client–provider relationship
- Inadequate access to care
- Inconvenience of care
- Ineffective communication skills of the provider
- Insufficient follow-up with provider
- Insufficient health insurance coverage
- Insufficient provider reimbursement
- Insufficient teaching skill of the provider
- Low satisfaction with care
- Perceived low credibility of provider
- Provider discontinuity

Healthcare plan
- Complex treatment regimen
- Financial barriers
- High-cost regimen
- Intensity of regimen
- Lengthy duration of regimen

Individual

- Cultural incongruence
- Expectations incongruent with developmental phase
- Health beliefs incongruent with plan
- Insufficient knowledge about the regimen
- Insufficient motivation
- Insufficient skills to perform regimen
- Insufficient social support
- Spiritual values incongruent with plan
- Values incongruent with plan

Network

- Insufficient involvement of members in plan
- Low social value attributed to plan
- Perception that beliefs of significant other differ from plan

00043

Ineffective **protection**
(1990)

Definition
Decrease in the ability to guard self from internal or external threats such as illness or injury.

Defining Characteristics

- Alteration in clotting
- Alteration in perspiration
- Anorexia
- Chilling
- Coughing
- Deficient immunity
- Disorientation
- Dyspnea
- Fatigue
- Immobility
- Insomnia
- Itching
- Maladaptive stress response
- Neurosensory impairment
- Pressure ulcer
- Restlessness
- Weakness

Related Factors

- Abnormal blood profile
- Cancer
- Extremes of age
- Immune disorder (e.g., HIV-associated neuropathy, varicella-zoster virus)
- Inadequate nutrition
- Pharmaceutical agent
- Substance abuse
- Treatment regimen

DOMAIN 2. NUTRITION

The activities of taking in, assimilating, and using nutrients for the purposes of tissue maintenance, tissue repair, and the production of energy

Class 1. Ingestion
Taking food or nutrients into the body

Code	Diagnosis	Page
00216	Insufficient **breast milk**	155
00104	Ineffective **breastfeeding**	156
00105	Interrupted **breastfeeding**	158
00106	Readiness for enhanced **breastfeeding**	159
00107	Ineffective infant **feeding pattern**	160
00002	Imbalanced **nutrition**: less than body requirements	161
00163	Readiness for enhanced **nutrition**	162
00232	**Obesity**	163
00233	**Overweight**	165
00234	Risk for **overweight**	167
00103	Impaired **swallowing**	169

NANDA International, Inc. Nursing Diagnoses: Definitions & Classification 2015–2017, Tenth Edition. Edited by T. Heather Herdman and Shigemi Kamitsuru.
© 2014 NANDA International, Inc. Published 2014 by John Wiley & Sons, Ltd.
Companion website: www.wiley.com/go/nursingdiagnoses

| **Class 2. Digestion** | |
| *The physical and chemical activities that convert foodstuffs into* | |
substances suitable for absorption and assimilation	
None at present time	

| **Class 3. Absorption** | |
The act of taking up nutrients through body tissues	
None at present time	

Class 4. Metabolism
The chemical and physical processes occurring in living organisms
and cells for the development and use of protoplasm, the production
of waste and energy, with the release of energy for all vital
processes

Code	**Diagnosis**	**Page**
00179	Risk for unstable **blood glucose level**	171
00194	Neonatal **jaundice**	172
00230	Risk for neonatal **jaundice**	173
00178	Risk for impaired **liver function**	174

Class 5. Hydration
The taking in and absorption of fluids and electrolytes

Code	**Diagnosis**	**Page**
00195	Risk for **electrolyte** imbalance	175
00160	Readiness for enhanced **fluid balance**	176
00027	Deficient **fluid volume**	177
00028	Risk for deficient **fluid volume**	178
00026	Excess **fluid volume**	179
00025	Risk for imbalanced **fluid volume**	180

Insufficient **breast milk**
(2010; LOE 2.1)

Definition
Low production of maternal breast milk.

Defining Characteristics

Infant
- Constipation
- Frequent crying
- Frequently seeks to suckle at breast
- Prolonged breastfeeding time
- Refuses to suckle at breast
- Suckling time at breast appears unsatisfactory
- Voids small amounts of concentrated urine
- Weight gain <500 g in a month

Mother
- Absence of milk production with nipple stimulation
- Delay in milk production
- Expresses breast milk less than prescribed volume

Related Factors

Infant
- Ineffective latching on to breast
- Ineffective sucking reflex
- Insufficient opportunity for suckling at the breast
- Insufficient suckling time at breast
- Rejection of breast

Mother
- Alcohol consumption
- Insufficient fluid volume
- Malnutrition
- Pregnancy
- Smoking
- Treatment regimen

Original literature support available at **www.nanda.org**

2. Nutrition

00104

Ineffective **breastfeeding**
(1988, 2010, 2013; LOE 2.2)

Definition
Difficulty providing milk to an infant or young child directly from the breasts, which may compromise nutritional status of the infant/child.

Defining Characteristics

- Inadequate infant stooling
- Infant arching at breast
- Infant crying at the breast
- Infant crying within the first hour after breastfeeding
- Infant fussing within one hour of breastfeeding
- Infant inability to latch on to maternal breast correctly
- Infant resisting latching on to breast
- Infant unresponsive to other comfort measures
- Insufficient emptying of each breast per feeding
- Insufficient infant weight gain
- Insufficient signs of oxytocin release
- Perceived inadequate milk supply
- Sore nipples persisting beyond first week
- Sustained infant weight loss
- Unsustained suckling at the breast

Related Factors

- Delayed lactogenesis II
- Inadequate milk supply
- Insufficient family support
- Insufficient opportunity for suckling at the breast
- Insufficient parental knowledge regarding breastfeeding techniques
- Insufficient parental knowledge regarding importance of breastfeeding
- Interrupted breastfeeding
- Maternal ambivalence
- Maternal anxiety
- Maternal breast anomaly
- Maternal fatigue
- Maternal obesity
- Maternal pain
- Oropharyngeal defect
- Pacifier use
- Poor infant sucking reflex
- Prematurity

- Previous breast surgery
- Previous history of breastfeeding failure
- Short maternity leave
- Supplemental feedings with artificial nipple

Original literature support available at www.nanda.org

2. Nutrition

00105

Interrupted **breastfeeding**
(1992, 2013; LOE 2.2)

Definition
Break in the continuity of providing milk to an infant or young child directly from the breasts, which may compromise breastfeeding success and/or nutritional status of the infant/child.

Defining Characteristics

- Nonexclusive breastfeeding

Related Factors

- Contraindications to breastfeeding (e.g., pharmaceutical agents)
- Hospitalization of child
- Infant illness
- Maternal employment
- Maternal illness
- Maternal–infant separation
- Need to abruptly wean infant
- Prematurity

Original literature support available at www.nanda.org

00106

Readiness for enhanced **breastfeeding**
(1990, 2010, 2013; LOE 2.2)

Definition
A pattern of providing milk to an infant or young child directly from the breasts, which may be strengthened.

Defining Characteristics

- Mother expresses desire to enhance ability to provide breast milk for child's nutritional needs

- Mother expresses desire to enhance ability to exclusively breastfeed

Original literature support available at www.nanda.org

00107

Ineffective infant **feeding pattern**
(1992, 2006; LOE 2.1)

Definition
Impaired ability of an infant to suck or coordinate the suck/swallow response resulting in inadequate oral nutrition for metabolic needs.

Defining Characteristics

- Inability to coordinate sucking, swallowing, and breathing
- Inability to initiate an effective suck
- Inability to sustain an effective suck

Related Factors

- Neurological delay
- Neurological impairment (e.g., positive EEG, head trauma, seizure disorders)
- Oral hypersensitivity
- Oropharyngeal defect
- Prematurity
- Prolonged nil per os (NPO) status

Original literature support available at www.nanda.org

00002

Imbalanced **nutrition**: less than body requirements
(1975, 2000)

> ### Definition
> Intake of nutrients insufficient to meet metabolic needs.

Defining Characteristics

- Abdominal cramping
- Abdominal pain
- Alteration in taste sensation
- Body weight 20% or more below ideal weight range
- Capillary fragility
- Diarrhea
- Excessive hair loss
- Food aversion
- Food intake less than recommended daily allowance (RDA)
- Hyperactive bowel sounds
- Insufficient information
- Insufficient interest in food
- Insufficient muscle tone
- Misinformation
- Misperception
- Pale mucous membranes
- Perceived inability to ingest food
- Satiety immediately upon ingesting food
- Sore buccal cavity
- Weakness of muscles required for mastication
- Weakness of muscles required for swallowing
- Weight loss with adequate food intake

Related Factors

- Biological factors
- Economically disadvantaged
- Inability to absorb nutrients
- Inability to digest food
- Inability to ingest food
- Insufficient dietary intake
- Psychological disorder

00163

Readiness for enhanced **nutrition**
(2002, 2013; LOE 2.1)

> **Definition**
> A pattern of nutrient intake, which can be strengthened.

Defining Characteristics

- Expresses desire to enhance nutrition

00232

Obesity
(2013; LOE 2.2)

Definition
A condition in which an individual accumulates abnormal or excessive fat for age and gender that exceeds overweight.

Defining Characteristics

- ADULT: BMI of >30 kg/m²
- CHILD <2 years: Term not used with children at this age
- CHILD 2–18 years: BMI of >30 kg/m² or >95th percentile for age and gender

Related Factors

- Average daily physical activity is less than recommended for gender and age
- Consumption of sugar-sweetened beverages
- Disordered eating behaviors
- Disordered eating perceptions
- Economically disadvantaged
- Energy expenditure below energy intake based on standard assessment (e.g., WAVE assessment*)
- Excessive alcohol consumption
- Fear regarding lack of food supply
- Formula- or mixed-fed infants
- Frequent snacking
- Genetic disorder
- Heritability of interrelated factors (e.g., adipose tissue distribution, energy expenditure, lipoprotein lipase activity, lipid synthesis, lipolysis)
- High disinhibition and restraint eating behavior score
- High frequency of restaurant or fried food
- Low dietary calcium intake in children
- Maternal diabetes mellitus
- Maternal smoking
- Overweight in infancy
- Parental obesity
- Portion sizes larger than recommended

*WAVE assessment = Weight, activity, variety in diet, excess.

- Premature pubarche
- Rapid weight gain during childhood
- Rapid weight gain during infancy, including the first week, first 4 months, and first year
- Sedentary behavior occurring for >2 hours/day
- Shortened sleep time
- Sleep disorder
- Solid foods as major food source at <5 months of age

Original literature support available at www.nanda.org

00233

Overweight
(2013; LOE 2.2)

Definition
A condition in which an individual accumulates abnormal or excessive fat for age and gender.

Defining Characteristics

- ADULT: BMI > 25 kg/m²
- CHILD < 2 years: Weight-for-length > 95th percentile
- CHILD 2–18 years: BMI > 85th but < 95th percentile, or 25 kg/m² (whichever is smaller)

Related Factors

- Average daily physical activity is less than recommended for gender and age
- Consumption of sugar-sweetened beverages
- Disordered eating behaviors (e.g., binge eating, extreme weight control)
- Disordered eating perceptions
- Economically disadvantaged
- Energy expenditure below energy intake based on standard assessment (e.g., WAVE assessment*)
- Excessive alcohol consumption
- Fear regarding lack of food supply
- Formula- or mixed-fed infants
- Frequent snacking
- Genetic disorder
- Heritability of interrelated factors (e.g., adipose tissue distribution, energy expenditure, lipoprotein lipase activity, lipid synthesis, lipolysis)
- High disinhibition and restraint eating behavior score
- High frequency of restaurant or fried food
- Low dietary calcium intake in children
- Maternal diabetes mellitus
- Maternal smoking
- Obesity in childhood
- Parental obesity
- Portion sizes larger than recommended
- Premature pubarche
- Rapid weight gain during childhood

*WAVE assessment = Weight, activity, variety in diet, excess.

2. Nutrition

- Rapid weight gain during infancy, including the first week, first 4 months, and first year
- Sedentary behavior occurring for >2 hours/day
- Shortened sleep time
- Sleep disorder
- Solid foods as major food source at <5 months of age

Original literature support available at www.nanda.org

Risk for **overweight**
(2013; LOE 2.2)

Definition
Vulnerable to abnormal or excessive fat accumulation for age and gender, which may compromise health.

Risk Factors

- ADULT: BMI approaching 25 kg/m^2
- Average daily physical activity is less than recommended for gender and age
- CHILD < 2 years: Weight-for-length approaching 95th percentile
- CHILD 2–18 years: BMI approaching 85th percentile, or 25 kg/m^2 (whichever is smaller)
- Children who are crossing BMI percentiles upward
- Children with high BMI percentiles
- Consumption of sugar-sweetened beverages
- Disordered eating behaviors (e.g., binge eating, extreme weight control)
- Disordered eating perceptions
- Eating in response to external cues (e.g., time of day, social situations)
- Eating in response to internal cues other than hunger (e.g., anxiety)
- Economically disadvantaged
- Energy expenditure below energy intake based on standard assessment (e.g., WAVE assessment*)
- Excessive alcohol consumption
- Fear regarding lack of food supply
- Formula- or mixed-fed infants
- Frequent snacking
- Genetic disorder
- Heritability of interrelated factors (e.g., adipose tissue distribution, energy expenditure, lipoprotein lipase activity, lipid synthesis, lipolysis)
- High disinhibition and restraint eating behavior score
- High frequency of restaurant or fried food
- Higher baseline weight at beginning of each pregnancy
- Low dietary calcium intake in children
- Maternal diabetes mellitus
- Maternal smoking

*WAVE assessment = Weight, activity, variety in diet, excess.

- Obesity in childhood
- Parental obesity
- Portion sizes larger than recommended
- Premature pubarche
- Rapid weight gain during childhood
- Rapid weight gain during infancy, including the first week, first 4 months, and first year
- Sedentary behavior occurring for >2 hours/day
- Shortened sleep time
- Sleep disorder
- Solid foods as major food source at <5 months of age

Original literature support available at www.nanda.org

00103

Impaired **swallowing**
(1986, 1998)

> ## Definition
> Abnormal functioning of the swallowing mechanism associated with deficits in oral, pharyngeal, or esophageal structure or function.

Defining Characteristics

First Stage: Oral

- Abnormal oral phase of swallow study
- Choking prior to swallowing
- Coughing prior to swallowing
- Drooling
- Food falls from mouth
- Food pushed out of mouth
- Gagging prior to swallowing
- Inability to clear oral cavity
- Incomplete lip closure
- Inefficient nippling
- Inefficient suck
- Insufficient chewing
- Nasal reflux
- Piecemeal deglutition
- Pooling of bolus in lateral sulci
- Premature entry of bolus
- Prolonged bolus formation
- Prolonged meal time with insufficient consumption
- Tongue action ineffective in forming bolus

Second Stage: Pharyngeal

- Abnormal pharyngeal phase of swallow study
- Alteration in head position
- Choking
- Coughing
- Delayed swallowing
- Fevers of unknown etiology
- Food refusal
- Gagging sensation
- Gurgly voice quality
- Inadequate laryngeal elevation
- Nasal reflux
- Recurrent pulmonary infection
- Repetitive swallowing

Third Stage: Esophageal

- Abnormal esophageal phase of swallow study
- Acidic-smelling breath
- Bruxism
- Difficulty swallowing
- Epigastric pain
- Food refusal
- Heartburn
- Hematemesis
- Hyperextension of head
- Nighttime awakening
- Nighttime coughing
- Odynophagia
- Regurgitation
- Repetitive swallowing
- Reports "something stuck"
- Unexplained irritability surrounding mealtimes
- Volume limiting
- Vomiting
- Vomitus on pillow

Related Factors

Congenital Deficits

- Behavioral feeding problem
- Conditions with significant hypotonia
- Congenital heart disease
- Failure to thrive
- History of enteral feeding
- Mechanical obstruction
- Neuromuscular impairment
- Protein-energy malnutrition
- Respiratory condition
- Self-injurious behavior
- Upper airway abnormality

Neurological Problems

- Achalasia
- Acquired anatomic defects
- Brain injury (e.g., cerebrovascular impairment, neurological illness, trauma, tumor)
- Cerebral palsy
- Cranial nerve involvement
- Developmental delay
- Esophageal reflux disease
- Laryngeal abnormality
- Laryngeal defect
- Nasal defect
- Nasopharyngeal cavity defect
- Neurological problems
- Oropharynx abnormality
- Prematurity
- Tracheal defect
- Trauma
- Upper airway anomaly

00179

Risk for unstable **blood glucose level**
(2006, 2013; LOE 2.1)

Definition
Vulnerable to variation in blood glucose/sugar levels from the normal range, which may compromise health.

Risk Factors

- Alteration in mental status
- Average daily physical activity is less than recommended for gender and age
- Compromised physical health status
- Delay in cognitive development
- Does not accept diagnosis
- Excessive stress
- Excessive weight gain
- Excessive weight loss
- Inadequate blood glucose monitoring
- Ineffective medication management
- Insufficient diabetes management
- Insufficient dietary intake
- Insufficient knowledge of disease management
- Nonadherence to diabetes management plan
- Pregnancy
- Rapid growth period

Original literature support available at www.nanda.org

00194

Neonatal **jaundice**
(2008, 2010; LOE 2.1)

Definition
The yellow-orange tint of the neonate's skin and mucous membranes that occurs after 24 hours of life as a result of unconjugated bilirubin in the circulation.

Defining Characteristics

- Abnormal blood profile
- Bruised skin
- Yellow mucous membranes
- Yellow sclera
- Yellow-orange skin color

Related Factors

- Age < 7 days
- Deficient feeding pattern
- Delay in meconium passage
- Infant experiences difficulty making the transition to extra-uterine life
- Unintentional weight loss

Original literature support available at www.nanda.org

00230

Risk for neonatal **jaundice**
(2010, 2013; LOE 2.1)

2. Nutrition

Definition
Vulnerable to the yellow-orange tint of the neonate's skin and mucous membranes that occur after 24 hours of life as a result of unconjugated bilirubin in the circulation, which may compromise health.

Risk Factors

- Abnormal weight loss (>7–8% in breastfeeding newborn, 15% in nonbreast-feeding newborn)
- Age < 7 days
- Delay in meconium passage
- Feeding pattern not well established
- Infant experiences difficulty making the transition to extra-uterine life
- Prematurity

Original literature support available at www.nanda.org

00178

Risk for impaired **liver function**
(2006, 2008, 2013; LOE 2.1)

Definition
Vulnerable to a decrease in liver function, which may compromise health.

Risk Factors

- HIV coinfection
- Pharmaceutical agent
- Substance abuse
- Viral infection

Original literature support available at www.nanda.org

00195

Risk for **electrolyte imbalance**
(2008, 2013; LOE 2.1)

> **Definition**
> Vulnerable to changes in serum electrolyte levels, which may compromise health.

Risk Factors

- Compromised regulatory mechanism
- Diarrhea
- Endocrine regulatory dysfunction (e.g., glucose intolerance, increase in IGF-1, androgen, DHEA, and cortisol)
- Excessive fluid volume
- Insufficient fluid volume
- Renal dysfunction
- Treatment regimen
- Vomiting

Original literature support available at www.nanda.org

00160
Readiness for enhanced **fluid balance**
(2002, 2013; LOE 2.1)

Definition
A pattern of equilibrium between the fluid volume and chemical composition of body fluids, which can be strengthened.

Defining Characteristics

- Expresses desire to enhance fluid balance

00027

Deficient **fluid volume**
(1978, 1996)

> ### Definition
> Decreased intravascular, interstitial, and/or intracellular fluid. This refers to dehydration, water loss alone without change in sodium.

Defining Characteristics

- Alteration in mental status
- Alteration in skin turgor
- Decrease in blood pressure
- Decrease in pulse pressure
- Decrease in pulse volume
- Decrease in tongue turgor
- Decrease in urine output
- Decrease in venous filling
- Dry mucous membranes
- Dry skin
- Increase in body temperature
- Increase in heart rate
- Increase in hematocrit
- Increase in urine concentration
- Sudden weight loss
- Thirst
- Weakness

Related Factors

- Active fluid volume loss
- Compromised regulatory mechanism

00028

Risk for deficient **fluid volume**
(1978, 2010, 2013)

Definition
Vulnerable to experiencing decreased intravascular, interstitial, and/or intracellular fluid volumes, which may compromise health.

Risk Factors

- Active fluid volume loss
- Barrier to accessing fluid
- Compromised regulatory mechanism
- Deviations affecting fluid absorption
- Deviations affecting fluid intake
- Excessive fluid loss through normal route
- Extremes of age
- Extremes of weight
- Factors influencing fluid needs
- Fluid loss through abnormal route
- Insufficient knowledge about fluid needs
- Pharmaceutical agent

00026

Excess **fluid volume**
(1982, 1996, 2013)

Definition
Increased isotonic fluid retention.

Defining Characteristics

- Adventitious breath sounds
- Alteration in blood pressure
- Alteration in mental status
- Alteration in pulmonary artery pressure (PAP)
- Alteration in respiratory pattern
- Alteration in urine specific gravity
- Anasarca
- Anxiety
- Azotemia
- Decrease in hematocrit
- Decrease in hemoglobin
- Dyspnea
- Edema
- Electrolyte imbalance
- Hepatomegaly
- Increase in central venous pressure (CVP)
- Intake exceeds output
- Jugular vein distension
- Oliguria
- Orthopnea
- Paroxysmal nocturnal dyspnea
- Pleural effusion
- Positive hepatojugular reflex
- Pulmonary congestion
- Restlessness
- Presence of S3 heart sound
- Weight gain over short period of time

Related Factors

- Compromised regulatory mechanism
- Excessive fluid intake
- Excessive sodium intake

00025

Risk for imbalanced **fluid volume**
(1998, 2008, 2013; LOE 2.1)

> ### Definition
> Vulnerable to a decrease, increase, or rapid shift from one to the other of intravascular, interstitial, and/or intracellular fluid, which may compromise health. This refers to body fluid loss, gain, or both.

Risk Factors

- Apheresis
- Ascites
- Burns
- Intestinal obstruction
- Pancreatitis
- Sepsis
- Trauma
- Treatment regimen

Original literature support available at www.nanda.org

Domain 3
Elimination and Exchange

DOMAIN 3. ELIMINATION AND EXCHANGE		
Secretion and excretion of waste products from the body		

Class 1. Urinary function
The process of secretion, reabsorption, and excretion of urine

Code	Diagnosis	Page
00016	Impaired urinary **elimination**	183
00166	Readiness for enhanced urinary **elimination**	184
00020	Functional urinary **incontinence**	185
00176	Overflow urinary **incontinence**	186
00018	Reflex urinary **incontinence**	187
00017	Stress urinary **incontinence**	188
00019	Urge urinary **incontinence**	189
00022	Risk for urge urinary **incontinence**	190
00023	**Urinary retention**	191

Class 2. Gastrointestinal function
The process of absorption and excretion of the end products of digestion

Code	Diagnosis	Page
00011	**Constipation**	192
00015	Risk for **constipation**	194

NANDA International, Inc. Nursing Diagnoses: Definitions & Classification 2015–2017, Tenth Edition. Edited by T. Heather Herdman and Shigemi Kamitsuru.
© 2014 NANDA International, Inc. Published 2014 by John Wiley & Sons, Ltd.
Companion website: www.wiley.com/go/nursingdiagnoses

Class 2. Gastrointestinal function (continued)		
Code	**Diagnosis**	**Page**
00235	Chronic functional **constipation**	196
00236	Risk for chronic functional **constipation**	198
00012	Perceived **constipation**	199
00013	**Diarrhea**	200
00196	Dysfunctional **gastrointestinal motility**	201
00197	Risk for dysfunctional **gastrointestinal motility**	202
00014	Bowel **incontinence**	203

Class 3. Integumentary function
The process of secretion and excretion through the skin

None at this time	

Class 4. Respiratory function
The process of exchange of gases and removal of the end products of metabolism

Code	**Diagnosis**	**Page**
00030	Impaired **gas exchange**	204

00016

Impaired urinary **elimination**
(1973, 2006; LOE 2.1)

> **Definition**
> Dysfunction in urine elimination.

Defining Characteristics

- Dysuria
- Frequent voiding
- Hesitancy
- Nocturia
- Urinary incontinence

- Urinary retention
- Urinary urgency

Related Factors

- Anatomic obstruction
- Multiple causality

- Sensory motor impairment
- Urinary tract infection

Original literature support available at www.nanda.org

00166

Readiness for enhanced urinary **elimination**
(2002, 2013; LOE 2.1)

Definition
A pattern of urinary functions for meeting eliminatory needs, which can be strengthened.

Defining Characteristics

- Expresses desire to enhance urinary elimination

00020

Functional urinary **incontinence**
(1986, 1998)

3. Elimination and Exchange

> ### Definition
> Inability of a usually continent person to reach the toilet in time to avoid unintentional loss of urine.

Defining Characteristics

- Completely empties bladder
- Early morning urinary incontinence
- Sensation of need to void
- Time between sensation of urge and ability to reach toilet is too short
- Voiding prior to reaching toilet

Related Factors

- Alteration in cognitive functioning
- Alteration in environmental factor
- Impaired vision
- Neuromuscular impairment
- Psychological disorder
- Weakened supporting pelvic structure

00176

Overflow urinary **incontinence**
(2006; LOE 2.1)

Definition
Involuntary loss of urine associated with overdistention of the bladder.

Defining Characteristics

- Bladder distention
- High post-void residual volume
- Involuntary leakage of small volume of urine
- Nocturia

Related Factors

- Bladder outlet obstruction
- Detrusor external sphincter dyssynergia
- Detrusor hypocontractility
- Fecal impaction
- Severe pelvic prolapse
- Treatment regimen
- Urethral obstruction

Original literature support available at www.nanda.org

00018

Reflex urinary **incontinence**
(1986, 1998)

Definition
Involuntary loss of urine at somewhat predictable intervals when a specific bladder volume is reached.

Defining Characteristics

- Absence of sensation of bladder fullness
- Absence of urge to void
- Absence of voiding sensation
- Inability to voluntarily inhibit voiding
- Inability to voluntarily initiate voiding
- Incomplete emptying of bladder with lesion above pontine micturition center
- Predictable pattern of voiding
- Sensation of bladder fullness
- Sensation of urgency to void without voluntary inhibition of bladder contraction

Related Factors

- Neurological impairment above level of pontine micturition center
- Neurological impairment above level of sacral micturition center
- Tissue damage

00017

Stress urinary **incontinence**
(1986, 2006; LOE 2.1)

Definition
Sudden leakage of urine with activities that increase intra-abdominal pressure.

Defining Characteristics

- Involuntary leakage of small volume of urine (e.g., with coughing, laughing, sneezing, on exertion)

- Involuntary leakage of small volume of urine in the absence of detrusor contraction
- Involuntary leakage of small volume of urine in the absence of overdistended bladder

Related Factors

- Degenerative changes in pelvic muscles
- Increase in intra-abdominal pressure

- Intrinsic urethral sphincter deficiency
- Weak pelvic muscles

Original literature support available at www.nanda.org

00019

Urge urinary **incontinence**
(1986, 2006; LOE 2.1)

Definition
Involuntary passage of urine occurring soon after a strong sense of urgency to void.

Defining Characteristics

- Inability to reach toilet in time to avoid urine loss
- Involuntary loss of urine with bladder contractions
- Involuntary loss of urine with bladder spasms
- Urinary urgency

Related Factors

- Alcohol consumption
- Atrophic urethritis
- Atrophic vaginitis
- Bladder infection
- Caffeine intake
- Decrease in bladder capacity
- Detrusor hyperactivity with impaired bladder contractility
- Fecal impaction
- Treatment regimen

Original literature support available at www.nanda.org

00022

Risk for urge urinary **incontinence**
(1998, 2008, 2013; LOE 2.1)

> ### Definition
> Vulnerable to involuntary passage of urine occurring soon after a strong sensation or urgency to void, which may compromise health.

Risk Factors

- Alcohol consumption
- Atrophic urethritis
- Atrophic vaginitis
- Detrusor hyperactivity with impaired bladder contractility
- Fecal impaction
- Impaired bladder contractility
- Ineffective toileting habits
- Involuntary sphincter relaxation
- Small bladder capacity
- Treatment regimen

Original literature support available at www.nanda.org

00023

Urinary retention
(1986)

Definition
Incomplete emptying of the bladder.

Defining Characteristics

- Absent urinary output
- Bladder distention
- Dribbling of urine
- Dysuria
- Frequent voiding
- Overflow incontinence
- Residual urine
- Sensation of bladder fullness
- Small voiding

Related Factors

- Blockage in urinary tract
- High urethral pressure
- Reflex arc inhibition
- Strong sphincter

00011

Constipation
(1975, 1998)

Definition
Decrease in normal frequency of defecation accompanied by difficult or incomplete passage of stool and/or passage of excessively hard, dry stool.

Defining Characteristics

- Abdominal pain
- Abdominal tenderness with palpable muscle resistance
- Abdominal tenderness without palpable muscle resistance
- Anorexia
- Atypical presentations in older adults (e.g., changes in mental status, urinary incontinence, unexplained falls, elevated body temperature)
- Borborygmi
- Bright red blood with stool
- Change in bowel pattern
- Decrease in stool frequency
- Decrease in stool volume
- Distended abdomen
- Fatigue
- Hard, formed stool
- Headache
- Hyperactive bowel sounds
- Hypoactive bowel sounds
- Inability to defecate
- Increase in intra-abdominal pressure
- Indigestion
- Liquid stool
- Pain with defecation
- Palpable abdominal mass
- Palpable rectal mass
- Percussed abdominal dullness
- Rectal fullness
- Rectal pressure
- Severe flatus
- Soft, paste-like stool in rectum
- Straining with defecation
- Vomiting

Related Factors

Functional
- Abdominal muscle weakness
- Average daily physical activity is less than recommended for gender and age
- Habitually ignores urge to defecate
- Inadequate toileting habits
- Irregular defecation habits
- Recent environmental change

Mechanical
- Electrolyte imbalance
- Hemorrhoids
- Hirschprung's disease
- Neurological impairment (e.g., positive EEG, head trauma, seizure disorders)
- Obesity
- Postsurgical bowel obstruction
- Pregnancy
- Prostate enlargement
- Rectal abscess
- Rectal anal fissure
- Rectal anal stricture
- Rectal prolapse
- Rectal ulcer
- Rectocele
- Tumor

Pharmacological
- Laxative abuse
- Pharmaceutical agent

Physiological
- Decrease in gastrointestinal motility
- Dehydration
- Eating habit change (e.g., foods, eating times)
- Inadequate dentition
- Inadequate oral hygiene
- Insufficient dietary habits
- Insufficient fiber intake
- Insufficient fluid intake

Psychological
- Confusion
- Depression
- Emotional disturbance

00015

Risk for **constipation**
(1998, 2013)

> **Definition**
> Vulnerable to a decrease in normal frequency of defecation accompanied by difficult or incomplete passage of stool, which may compromise health.

Risk Factors

Functional
- Abdominal muscle weakness
- Average daily physical activity is less than recommended for gender and age
- Habitually ignores urge to defecate
- Inadequate toileting habits
- Irregular defecation habits
- Recent environmental change

Mechanical
- Electrolyte imbalance
- Hemorrhoids
- Hirschprung's disease
- Neurological impairment (e.g., positive EEG, head trauma, seizure disorders)
- Obesity
- Postsurgical bowel obstruction
- Pregnancy
- Prostate enlargement
- Rectal abscess
- Rectal anal fissure
- Rectal anal stricture
- Rectal prolapse
- Rectal ulcer
- Rectocele
- Tumor

Pharmacological
- Iron salts
- Laxative abuse
- Pharmaceutical agent

Physiological
- Decrease in gastrointestinal motility
- Dehydration
- Eating habit change (e.g., foods, eating times)

- Inadequate dentition
- Inadequate oral hygiene
- Insufficient dietary habits
- Insufficient fiber intake
- Insufficient fluid intake

Psychological
- Confusion
- Depression

- Emotional disturbance

3. Elimination and Exchange

3. Elimination and Exchange

00235

Chronic functional **constipation**
(2013; LOE 2.2)

Definition

Infrequent or difficult evacuation of feces, which has been present for at least three of the prior 12 months.

Defining Characteristics

- Abdominal distention
- ADULT: Presence of ≥2 of the following symptoms on Rome III classification system: * Lumpy or hard stools in ≥25% defecations; * Straining during ≥25% of defecations; * Sensation of incomplete evacuation for ≥25% of defecations; * Sensation of anorectal obstruction/blockage for ≥25% of defecations; * Manual manuevers to facilitate ≥25% of defecations (digital manipulation, pelvic floor support); * ≤3 evacuations per week
- CHILD ≤4 years: Presence of ≥2 criteria on Roman III Pediatric classification system for ≥1 month: * ≤2 defecations per week; * ≥1 episode of fecal incontinence per week; * Stool retentive posturing; * Painful or hard bowel movements; * Presence of large fecal mass in the rectum; * Large-diameter stools that may obstruct the toilet
- CHILD ≥4 years: Presence of ≥2 criteria on Roman III Pediatric classification system for ≥2 months: * ≤2 defecations per week; * ≥1 episode of fecal incontinence per week; * Stool retentive posturing; * Painful or hard bowel movements; * Presence of large fecal mass in the rectum; * Large diameter stools that may obstruct the toilet
- Fecal impaction
- Fecal incontinence (in children)
- Leakage of stool with digital stimulation
- Pain with defecation
- Palpable abdominal mass
- Positive fecal occult blood test
- Prolonged straining
- Type 1 or 2 on Bristol Stool Chart

Related Factors

- Amyloidosis
- Anal fissure
- Anal stricture
- Autonomic neuropathy
- Cerebral vascular accident
- Chronic intestinal pseudo-obstruction
- Chronic renal insufficiency
- Colorectal cancer
- Dehydration
- Dementia
- Depression
- Dermatomyositis
- Diabetes mellitus
- Diet disproportionally high in protein and fat
- Extra intestinal mass
- Failure to thrive
- Habitually ignores urge to defecate
- Hemorrhoids
- Hirschprung's disease
- Hypercalcemia
- Hypothyroidism
- Impaired mobility
- Inflammatory bowel disease
- Insufficient dietary intake
- Insufficient fluid intake
- Ischemic stenosis
- Low caloric intake
- Low fiber diet
- Multiple sclerosis
- Myotonic dystrophy
- Panhypopituitarism
- Paraplegia
- Parkinson's disease
- Pelvic floor dysfunction
- Perineal damage
- Pharmaceutical agent
- Polypharmacy
- Porphyria
- Postinflammatory stenosis
- Pregnancy
- Proctitis
- Scleroderma
- Sedentary lifestyle
- Slow colon transit time
- Spinal cord injury
- Surgical stenosis

Original literature support available at www.nanda.org

3. Elimination and Exchange

00236

Risk for chronic functional **constipation**
(2013; LOE 2.2)

> ### Definition
> Vulnerable to infrequent or difficult evacuation of feces, which has been present nearly 3 of the prior 12 months, which may compromise health.

Risk Factors

- Aluminum-containing antacids
- Anti-epileptics
- Antihypertensives
- Anti-Parkinsonian agents (anticholinergic or dopaminergic)
- Calcium-channel antagonists
- Chronic intestinal pseudo-obstruction
- Decreased food intake
- Dehydration
- Depression
- Diet proportionally high in protein and fat
- Diuretics
- Failure to thrive
- Habitual ignoring of urge to defecate
- Impaired mobility
- Low-fiber diet
- Insufficient fluid intake
- Inactive lifestyle
- Iron preparations
- Low caloric intake
- Non-steroidal anti-inflammatories (NSAIDs)
- Opioids
- Polypharmacy
- Slow colon transit time
- Tricyclic antidepressants

Original literature support available at www.nanda.org

00012

Perceived **constipation**
(1988)

Definition
Self-diagnosis of constipation combined with abuse of laxatives, enemas, and/or suppositories to ensure a daily bowel movement.

Defining Characteristics

- Enema abuse
- Expects daily bowel movement
- Expects daily bowel movement at same time every day
- Laxative abuse
- Suppository abuse

Related Factors

- Cultural health beliefs
- Family health beliefs
- Impaired thought process

00013

Diarrhea
(1975, 1998)

> ## Definition
> Passage of loose, unformed stools.

Defining Characteristics

- Abdominal pain
- Bowel urgency
- Cramping
- Hyperactive bowel sounds
- Loose liquid stools > 3 in 24 hours

Related Factors

Physiological
- Gastrointestinal inflammation
- Gastrointestinal irritation
- Infection
- Malabsorption
- Parasite

Psychological
- Anxiety
- Increase in stress level

Situational
- Enteral feedings
- Exposure to contaminant
- Exposure to toxin
- Laxative abuse
- Substance abuse
- Travel
- Treatment regimen

00196

Dysfunctional **gastrointestinal motility**
(2008; LOE 2.1)

Definition
Increased, decreased, ineffective, or lack of peristaltic activity within the gastrointestinal system.

Defining Characteristics

- Abdominal cramping
- Abdominal distention
- Abdominal pain
- Absence of flatus
- Acceleration of gastric emptying
- Bile-colored gastric residual
- Change in bowel sounds

- Diarrhea
- Difficulty with defecation
- Hard, formed stool
- Increase in gastric residual
- Nausea
- Regurgitation
- Vomiting

Related Factors

- Aging
- Anxiety
- Enteral feedings
- Food intolerance
- Immobility

- Ingestion of contaminated material (e.g., radioactive, food, water)
- Malnutrition
- Prematurity
- Sedentary lifestyle
- Treatment regimen

Original literature support available at www.nanda.org

00197

Risk for dysfunctional **gastrointestinal motility**
(2008, 2013; LOE 2.1)

Definition
Vulnerable to a decrease in normal frequency of defecation accompanied by difficult or incomplete passage of stool, which may compromise health.

Risk Factors

- Aging
- Anxiety
- Change in water source
- Decrease in gastrointestinal circulation
- Diabetes mellitus
- Eating habit change (e.g., foods, eating times)
- Food intolerance
- Gastroesophageal reflux disease
- Immobility
- Infection
- Pharmaceutical agent
- Prematurity
- Sedentary lifestyle
- Stressors
- Unsanitary food preparation

Original literature support available at www.nanda.org

00014

Bowel incontinence
(1975, 1998)

Definition
Change in normal bowel habits characterized by involuntary passage of stool.

Defining Characteristics

- Bowel urgency
- Constant passage of soft stool
- Does not recognize urge to defecate
- Fecal odor
- Fecal staining of bedding
- Fecal staining of clothing
- Inability to delay defecation
- Inability to expel formed stool despite recognition of rectal fullness
- Inability to recognize rectal fullness
- Inattentive to urge to defecate
- Reddened perianal skin

Related Factors

- Abnormal increase in abdominal pressure
- Abnormal increase in intestinal pressure
- Alteration in cognitive functioning
- Chronic diarrhea
- Colorectal lesion
- Deficient dietary habits
- Difficulty with toileting self-care
- Dysfunctional rectal sphincter
- Environmental factor (e.g., inaccessible bathroom)
- Generalized decline in muscle tone
- Immobility
- Impaction
- Impaired reservoir capacity
- Incomplete emptying of bowel
- Laxative abuse
- Lower motor nerve damage
- Pharmaceutical agent
- Rectal sphincter abnormality
- Stressors
- Upper motor nerve damage

00030

Impaired **gas exchange**
(1980, 1996, 1998)

Definition
Excess or deficit in oxygenation and/or carbon dioxide elimination at the alveolar-capillary membrane.

Defining Characteristics

- Abnormal arterial blood gases
- Abnormal arterial pH
- Abnormal breathing pattern (e.g., rate, rhythm, depth)
- Abnormal skin color (e.g., pale, dusky, cyanosis)
- Confusion
- Cyanosis
- Decrease in carbon dioxide (CO_2) level
- Diaphoresis
- Dyspnea
- Headache upon awakening
- Hypercapnia
- Hypoxemia
- Hypoxia
- Irritability
- Nasal flaring
- Restlessness
- Somnolence
- Tachycardia
- Visual disturbance

Related Factors

- Alveolar-capillary membrane changes
- Ventilation-perfusion imbalance

Domain 4
Activity/Rest

DOMAIN 4. ACTIVITY/REST		
The production, conservation, expenditure, or balance of energy resources		

Class 1. Sleep/Rest
Slumber, repose, ease, relaxation, or inactivity

Code	Diagnosis	Page
00095	**Insomnia**	209
00096	**Sleep** deprivation	210
00165	Readiness for enhanced **sleep**	212
00198	Disturbed **sleep pattern**	213

Class 2. Activity/Exercise
Moving parts of the body (mobility), doing work, or performing actions often (but not always) against resistance

Code	Diagnosis	Page
00040	Risk for **disuse syndrome**	214
00091	Impaired bed **mobility**	215
00085	Impaired physical **mobility**	216
00089	Impaired wheelchair **mobility**	218
00237	Impaired **sitting**	219
00238	Impaired **standing**	220

NANDA International, Inc. Nursing Diagnoses: Definitions & Classification 2015–2017, Tenth Edition. Edited by T. Heather Herdman and Shigemi Kamitsuru.
© 2014 NANDA International, Inc. Published 2014 by John Wiley & Sons, Ltd.
Companion website: www.wiley.com/go/nursingdiagnoses

Class 2. Activity/Exercise (continued)		
Code	**Diagnosis**	**Page**
00090	Impaired **transfer ability**	221
00088	Impaired **walking**	222

Class 3. Energy balance
A dynamic state of harmony between intake and expenditure of resources

Code	**Diagnosis**	**Page**
00093	**Fatigue**	223
00154	**Wandering**	224

Class 4. Cardiovascular/pulmonary responses
Cardiopulmonary mechanisms that support activity/rest

Code	**Diagnosis**	**Page**
00092	**Activity** intolerance	225
00094	Risk for **activity** intolerance	226
00032	Ineffective **breathing pattern**	227
00029	Decreased **cardiac output**	228
00240	Risk for decreased **cardiac output**	230
00239	Risk for impaired **cardiovascular function**	231
00202	Risk for ineffective **gastrointestinal perfusion**	232
00203	Risk for ineffective **renal perfusion**	233
00033	Impaired **spontaneous ventilation**	234
00200	Risk for decreased cardiac **tissue perfusion**	235
00201	Risk for ineffective cerebral **tissue perfusion**	236
00204	Ineffective peripheral **tissue perfusion**	237
00228	Risk for ineffective peripheral **tissue perfusion**	238
00034	Dysfunctional **ventilatory weaning response**	239

Class 5. Self-care
Ability to perform activities to care for one's body and bodily functions

Code	**Diagnosis**	**Page**
00098	Impaired **home maintenance**	241
00108	**Bathing self-care** deficit*	242
00109	**Dressing self-care** deficit*	243

Class 5. Self-care (continued)		
Code	Diagnosis	Page
00102	**Feeding self-care** deficit*	244
00110	**Toileting self-care** deficit*	245
00182	Readiness for enhanced **self-care**＊	246
00193	**Self-neglect**	247

* The editors acknowledge these concepts are not in alphabetical order, but the decision was made to maintain all "self-care deficit" diagnoses in sequential order.

00095

Insomnia
(2006; LOE 2.1)

Definition
A disruption in amount and quality of sleep that impairs functioning.

Defining Characteristics

- Alteration in affect
- Alteration in concentration
- Alteration in mood
- Alteration in sleep pattern
- Compromised health status
- Decrease in quality of life
- Difficulty initiating sleep
- Difficulty maintaining sleep
- Dissatisfaction with sleep
- Early awakening
- Increase in absenteeism
- Increase in accidents
- Insufficient energy
- Nonrestorative sleep pattern (i.e., due to caregiver responsibilities, parenting practices, sleep partner)
- Sleep disturbance producing next-day consequences

Related Factors

- Alcohol consumption
- Anxiety
- Average daily physical activity is less than recommended for gender and age
- Depression
- Environmental barrier (e.g., ambient noise, daylight/ darkness exposure, ambient temperature/humidity, unfamiliar setting)
- Fear
- Frequent naps
- Grieving
- Hormonal change
- Inadequate sleep hygiene
- Pharmaceutical agent
- Physical discomfort
- Stressors

Original literature support available at www.nanda.org

4. Activity/Rest

00096

Sleep deprivation
(1998)

Definition
Prolonged periods of time without sleep (sustained natural, periodic suspension of relative consciousness).

Defining Characteristics

- Agitation
- Alteration in concentration
- Anxiety
- Apathy
- Combativeness
- Confusion
- Decrease in functional ability
- Decrease in reaction time
- Drowsiness
- Fatigue
- Fleeting nystagmus
- Hallucinations
- Hand tremors
- Heightened sensitivity to pain
- Irritability
- Lethargy
- Listlessness
- Malaise
- Perceptual disorders
- Restlessness
- Transient paranoia

Related Factors

- Age-related sleep stage shifts
- Average daily physical activity is less than recommended for gender and age
- Conditions with periodic limb movement (e.g., restless leg syndrome, nocturnal myoclonus)
- Dementia
- Environmental barrier
- Familial sleep paralysis
- Idiopathic central nervous system hypersomnolence
- Narcolepsy
- Nightmares
- Nonrestorative sleep pattern (i.e., due to caregiver responsibilities, parenting practices, sleep partner)
- Overstimulating environment
- Prolonged discomfort (e.g., physical, psychological)

- Sleep apnea
- Sleep terror
- Sleep walking
- Sleep-related enuresis
- Sleep-related painful erections

- Sundowner's syndrome
- Sustained circadian asynchrony
- Sustained inadequate sleep hygiene
- Treatment regimen

000165

Readiness for enhanced **sleep**
(2002, 2013; LOE 2.1)

Definition
A pattern of natural, periodic suspension of relative consciousness to provide rest and sustain a desired lifestyle, which can be strengthened.

Defining Characteristics

- Expresses desire to enhance sleep

000198

Disturbed **sleep pattern**
(1980, 1998, 2006; LOE 2.1)

Definition
Time-limited interruptions of sleep amount and quality due to external factors.

Defining Characteristics

- Alteration in sleep pattern
- Difficulty in daily functioning
- Difficulty initiating sleep
- Dissatisfaction with sleep
- Feeling unrested
- Unintentional awakening

Related Factors

- Disruption caused by sleep partner
- Environmental barrier (e.g., ambient noise, daylight/darkness exposure, ambient temperature/humidity, unfamiliar setting)
- Immobilization
- Insufficient privacy
- Nonrestorative sleep pattern (i.e., due to caregiver responsibilities, parenting practices, sleep partner)

00040

Risk for **disuse syndrome**
(1988, 2013)

Definition
Vulnerable to deterioration of body systems as the result of prescribed or unavoidable musculoskeletal inactivity, which may compromise health.

Risk Factors

- Alteration in level of consciousness
- Mechanical immobility

- Pain
- Paralysis
- Prescribed immobility

00091

Impaired bed **mobility**
(1998, 2006; LOE 2.1)

Definition
Limitation of independent movement from one bed position to another.

Defining Characteristics

- Impaired ability to move between long sitting and supine positions
- Impaired ability to move between prone and supine positions

- Impaired ability to move between sitting and supine positions
- Impaired ability to reposition self in bed
- Impaired ability to turn from side to side

Related Factors

- Alteration in cognitive functioning
- Environmental barrier (e.g., bed size, bed type, equipment, restraints)
- Insufficient knowledge of mobility strategies

- Insufficient muscle strength
- Musculoskeletal impairment
- Neuromuscular impairment
- Obesity
- Pain
- Pharmaceutical agent
- Physical deconditioning

Original literature support available at www.nanda.org

4. Activity/Rest

00085

Impaired physical **mobility**
(1973, 1998, 2013; LOE 2.1)

> ### Definition
> Limitation in independent, purposeful physical movement of the body or of one or more extremities

Defining Characteristics

- Alteration in gait
- Decrease in fine motor skills
- Decrease in gross motor skills
- Decrease in range of motion
- Decrease in reaction time
- Difficulty turning
- Discomfort
- Engages in substitutions for movement (e.g., attention to other's activity, controlling behavior, focus on pre-illness activity)
- Exertional dyspnea
- Movement-induced tremor
- Postural instability
- Slowed movement
- Spastic movement
- Uncoordinated movement

Related Factors

- Activity intolerance
- Alteration in bone structure integrity
- Alteration in cognitive functioning
- Alteration in metabolism
- Anxiety
- Body mass index >75th age-appropriate percentile
- Contractures
- Cultural belief regarding appropriate activity
- Decrease in endurance
- Decrease in muscle control
- Decrease in muscle mass
- Decrease in muscle strength
- Depression
- Developmental delay
- Disuse
- Insufficient environmental support (e.g., physical, social)
- Insufficient knowledge of value of physical activity
- Joint stiffness
- Malnutrition
- Musculoskeletal impairment

- Neuromuscular impairment
- Pain
- Pharmaceutical agent
- Physical deconditioning
- Prescribed movement restrictions
- Reluctance to initiate movement
- Sedentary lifestyle
- Sensoriperceptual impairment

Original literature support available at www.nanda.org

00089

Impaired wheelchair **mobility**
(1998, 2006; LOE 2.1)

Definition
Limitation of independent operation of wheelchair within environment.

Defining Characteristics

- Impaired ability to operate power wheelchair on a decline
- Impaired ability to operate power wheelchair on an incline
- Impaired ability to operate power wheelchair on curbs
- Impaired ability to operate power wheelchair on even surface
- Impaired ability to operate power wheelchair on uneven surface
- Impaired ability to operate wheelchair on a decline
- Impaired ability to operate wheelchair on an incline
- Impaired ability to operate wheelchair on curbs
- Impaired ability to operate wheelchair on even surface
- Impaired ability to operate wheelchair on uneven surface

Related Factors

- Alteration in cognitive functioning
- Alteration in mood
- Decrease in endurance
- Environmental barrier (e.g., stairs, inclines, uneven surfaces, obstacles, distance)
- Impaired vision
- Insufficient knowledge of wheelchair use
- Insufficient muscle strength
- Musculoskeletal impairment
- Neuromuscular impairment
- Obesity
- Pain
- Physical deconditioning

Original literature support available at **www.nanda.org**

000237

Impaired **sitting**
(2013; LOE 2.1)

Definition
Limitation of ability to independently and purposefully attain and/or maintain a rest position that is supported by the buttocks and thighs, in which the torso is upright.

Defining Characteristics

- Impaired ability to adjust position of one or both lower limbs on uneven surface
- Impaired ability to attain a balanced position of the torso
- Impaired ability to flex or move both hips
- Impaired ability to flex or move both knees
- Impaired ability to maintain the torso in balanced position
- Impaired ability to stress torso with body weight
- Insufficient muscle strength

Related Factors

- Alteration in cognitive functioning
- Impaired metabolic functioning
- Insufficient endurance
- Insufficient energy
- Malnutrition
- Neurological disorder
- Orthopedic surgery
- Pain
- Prescribed posture
- Psychological disorder
- Sarcopenia
- Self-imposed relief posture

Original literature support available at www.nanda.org

4. Activity/Rest

000238

Impaired **standing**
(2013; LOE 2.1)

Definition
Limitation of ability to independently and purposefully attain and/or maintain the body in an upright position from feet to head.

Defining Characteristics

- Impaired ability to adjust position of one or both lower limbs on uneven surface
- Impaired ability to attain a balanced position of the torso
- Impaired ability to extend one or both hips
- Impaired ability to extend one or both knees
- Impaired ability to flex one or both hips
- Impaired ability to flex one or both knees
- Impaired ability to maintain the torso in balanced position
- Impaired ability to stress torso with body weight
- Insufficient muscle strength

Related Factors

- Circulatory perfusion disorder
- Emotional disturbance
- Impaired metabolic functioning
- Injury to lower extremity
- Insufficient endurance
- Insufficient energy
- Malnutrition
- Neurological disorder
- Obesity
- Pain
- Prescribed posture
- Sarcopenia
- Self-imposed relief posture
- Surgical procedure

Original literature support available at www.nanda.org

00090

Impaired **transfer ability**
(1998, 2006; LOE 2.1)

Definition
Limitation of independent movement between two nearby surfaces.

Defining Characteristics

- Impaired ability to transfer between bed and chair
- Impaired ability to transfer between bed and standing position
- Impaired ability to transfer between car and chair
- Impaired ability to transfer between chair and floor
- Impaired ability to transfer between chair and standing position
- Impaired ability to transfer between floor and standing position
- Impaired ability to transfer between uneven levels
- Impaired ability to transfer in or out of bath tub
- Impaired ability to transfer in or out of shower
- Impaired ability to transfer on or off a commode
- Impaired ability to transfer on or off a toilet

Related Factors

- Alteration in cognitive functioning
- Environmental barrier (e.g., bed height, inadequate space, wheelchair type, treatment equipment, restraints)
- Impaired balance
- Impaired vision
- Insufficient knowledge of transfer techniques
- Insufficient muscle strength
- Musculoskeletal impairment
- Neuromuscular impairment
- Obesity
- Pain
- Physical deconditioning

Original literature support available at www.nanda.org

00088

Impaired **walking**
(1998, 2006; LOE 2.1)

Definition
Limitation of independent movement within the environment on foot.

Defining Characteristics

- Impaired ability to climb stairs
- Impaired ability to navigate curbs
- Impaired ability to walk on decline
- Impaired ability to walk on incline
- Impaired ability to walk on uneven surface
- Impaired ability to walk required distance

Related Factors

- Alteration in cognitive functioning
- Alteration in mood
- Decrease in endurance
- Environmental barrier (e.g., stairs, inclines, uneven surfaces, obstacles, distance, lack of assistive device)
- Fear of falling
- Impaired balance
- Impaired vision
- Insufficient knowledge of mobility strategies
- Insufficient muscle strength
- Musculoskeletal impairment
- Neuromuscular impairment
- Obesity
- Pain
- Physical deconditioning

Original literature support available at www.nanda.org

00093

Fatigue
(1988, 1998)

Definition
An overwhelming sustained sense of exhaustion and decreased capacity for physical and mental work at the usual level.

Defining Characteristics

- Alteration in concentration
- Alteration in libido
- Disinterest in surroundings
- Drowsiness
- Guilt about difficulty maintaining responsibilities
- Impaired ability to maintain usual physical activity
- Impaired ability to maintain usual routines
- Increase in physical symptoms
- Increase in rest requirement
- Ineffective role performance
- Insufficient energy
- Introspection
- Lethargy
- Listlessness
- Nonrestorative sleep pattern (i.e., due to caregiver responsibilities, parenting practices, sleep partner)
- Tiredness

Related Factors

- Anxiety
- Depression
- Environmental barrier (e.g., ambient noise, daylight/darkness exposure, ambient temperature/humidity, unfamiliar setting)
- Increase in physical exertion
- Malnutrition
- Negative life event
- Nonstimulating lifestyle
- Occupational demands (e.g., shift work, high level of activity, stress)
- Physical deconditioning
- Physiological condition (e.g., anemia, pregnancy, disease)
- Sleep deprivation
- Stressors

000154

Wandering
(2000)

Definition
Meandering, aimless, or repetitive locomotion that exposes the individual to harm; frequently incongruent with boundaries, limits, or obstacles.

Defining Characteristics

- Continuous movement from place to place
- Eloping behavior
- Frequent movement from place to place
- Fretful locomotion
- Haphazard locomotion
- Hyperactivity
- Impaired ability to locate landmarks in a familiar setting
- Locomotion into unauthorized spaces
- Locomotion resulting in getting lost
- Locomotion that cannot be easily dissuaded
- Long periods of locomotion without an apparent destination
- Pacing
- Periods of locomotion interspersed with periods of nonlocomotion (e.g., sitting, standing, sleeping)
- Persistent locomotion in search of something
- Scanning behavior
- Searching behavior
- Shadowing a caregiver's locomotion
- Trespassing

Related Factors

- Alteration in cognitive functioning
- Cortical atrophy
- Overstimulating environment
- Physiological state (e.g., hunger, thirst, pain, need to urinate)
- Premorbid behavior (e.g., outgoing, sociable personality)
- Psychological disorder
- Sedation
- Separation from familiar environment
- Time of day

00092

Activity intolerance
(1982)

Definition
Insufficient physiological or psychological energy to endure or complete required or desired daily activities.

Defining Characteristics

- Abnormal blood pressure response to activity
- Abnormal heart rate response to activity
- ECG change (e.g., arrhythmia, conduction abnormality, ischemia)
- Exertional discomfort
- Exertional dyspnea
- Fatigue
- Generalized weakness

Related Factors

- Bed rest
- Generalized weakness
- Imbalance between oxygen supply/demand
- Immobility
- Sedentary lifestyle

00094

Risk for **activity intolerance**
(1982, 2013)

Definition
Vulnerable to experiencing insufficient physiological or psychological energy to endure or complete required or desired daily activities, which may compromise health.

Risk Factors

- Circulatory problem
- History of previous intolerance
- Inexperience with an activity
- Physical deconditioning
- Respiratory condition

00032

Ineffective **breathing pattern**
(1980, 1996, 1998, 2010; LOE 2.1)

Definition
Inspiration and/or expiration that does not provide adequate ventilation.

Defining Characteristics

- Abnormal breathing pattern (e.g., rate, rhythm, depth)
- Altered chest excursion
- Bradypnea
- Decrease in expiratory pressure
- Decrease in inspiratory pressure
- Decrease in minute ventilation
- Decrease in vital capacity
- Dyspnea
- Increase in anterior-posterior chest diameter
- Nasal flaring
- Orthopnea
- Prolonged expiration phase
- Pursed-lip breathing
- Tachypnea
- Use of accessory muscles to breathe
- Use of three-point position

Related Factors

- Anxiety
- Body position that inhibits lung expansion
- Bony deformity
- Chest wall deformity
- Fatigue
- Hyperventilation
- Hypoventilation syndrome
- Musculoskeletal impairment
- Neurological immaturity
- Neurological impairment (e.g., positive EEG, head trauma, seizure disorders)
- Neuromuscular impairment
- Obesity
- Pain
- Respiratory muscle fatigue
- Spinal cord injury

Original literature support available at www.nanda.org

4. Activity/Rest

00029

Decreased cardiac output
(1975, 1996, 2000)

Definition
Inadequate blood pumped by the heart to meet the metabolic demands of the body.

Defining Characteristics

Altered Heart Rate/Rhythm
- Bradycardia
- ECG change (e.g., arrhythmia, conduction abnormality, ischemia)
- Heart palpitations
- Tachycardia

Altered Preload
- Decreased central venous pressure (CVP)
- Decrease in pulmonary artery wedge pressure (PAWP)
- Edema
- Fatigue
- Heart murmur
- Increase in central venous pressure (CVP)
- Increase in pulmonary artery wedge pressure (PAWP)
- Jugular vein distension
- Weight gain

Altered Afterload
- Abnormal skin color (e.g., pale, dusky, cyanosis)
- Alteration in blood pressure
- Clammy skin
- Decrease in peripheral pulses
- Decrease in pulmonary vascular resistance (PVR)
- Decrease in systemic vascular resistance (SVR)
- Dyspnea
- Increase in pulmonary vascular resistance (PVR)
- Increase in systemic vascular resistance (SVR)
- Oliguria
- Prolonged capillary refill

Altered Contractility
- Adventitious breath sounds
- Coughing
- Decreased cardiac index
- Decrease in ejection fraction
- Decrease in left ventricular stroke work index (LVSWI)
- Decrease in stroke volume index (SVI)
- Orthopnea
- Paroxysmal nocturnal dyspnea
- Presence of S3 heart sound
- Presence of S4 heart sound

Behavioral/Emotional
- Anxiety
- Restlessness

Related Factors

- Alteration in heart rate
- Alteration in heart rhythm
- Altered afterload
- Altered contractility
- Altered preload
- Altered stroke volume

00240

Risk for decreased **cardiac output**
(2013; LOE 2.1)

Definition
Vulnerable to inadequate blood pumped by the heart to meet metabolic demands of the body, which may compromise health.

Risk Factors

- Alteration in heart rate
- Alteration in heart rhythm
- Altered afterload
- Altered contractility
- Altered preload
- Altered stroke volume

Original literature support available at www.nanda.org

00239

Risk for impaired **cardiovascular function**
(2013; LOE 2.1)

Definition
Vulnerable to internal or external causes that can damage one or more vital organs and the circulatory system itself.

Risk Factors

- Age ≥ 65 years
- Diabetes mellitus
- Dyslipidemia
- Family history of cardiovascular disease
- History of cardiovascular disease
- Hypertension
- Insufficient knowledge of modifiable risk factors
- Obesity
- Pharmaceutical agent
- Sedentary lifestyle
- Smoking

Original literature support available at www.nanda.org

00202

Risk for ineffective **gastrointestinal perfusion**
(2008, 2013; LOE 2.1)

Definition
Vulnerable to decrease in gastrointestinal circulation, which may compromise health.

Risk Factors

- Abdominal aortic aneurysm
- Abdominal compartment syndrome
- Abnormal partial thromboplastin time (PTT)
- Abnormal prothrombin time (PT)
- Acute gastrointestinal hemorrhage
- Age > 60 years
- Anemia
- Cerebral vascular accident
- Coagulopathy (e.g., sickle cell anemia)
- Decrease in left ventricular performance
- Diabetes mellitus
- Disseminated intravascular coagulopathy
- Female gender
- Gastroesophageal varicies
- Gastrointestinal condition (e.g., ulcer, ischemic colitis, ischemic pancreatitis)
- Hemodynamic instability
- Impaired liver function (e.g., cirrhosis, hepatitis)
- Myocardial infarction
- Renal disease (e.g., polycystic kidney, renal artery stenosis, failure)
- Smoking
- Trauma
- Treatment regimen
- Vascular disease

Original literature support available at www.nanda.org

00203

Risk for ineffective **renal perfusion**
(2008, 2013; LOE 2.1)

Definition
Vulnerable to a decrease in blood circulation to the kidney, which may compromise health.

Risk Factors

- Abdominal compartment syndrome
- Alteration in metabolism
- Bilateral cortical necrosis
- Burns
- Cardiac surgery
- Cardiopulmonary bypass
- Diabetes mellitus
- Exposure to nephrotoxin
- Extremes of age
- Female gender
- Glomerulonephritis
- Hypertension
- Hypovolemia
- Hypoxemia
- Hypoxia
- Infection
- Interstitial nephritis
- Malignancy
- Malignant hypertension
- Polynephritis
- Renal disease (e.g., polycystic kidney, renal artery stenosis, failure)
- Smoking
- Substance abuse
- Systemic inflammatory response syndrome (SIRS)
- Trauma
- Treatment regimen
- Vascular embolism
- Vasculitis

Original literature support available at www.nanda.org

00033

Impaired **spontaneous ventilation**
(1992)

Definition
Decreased energy reserves resulting in an inability to maintain independent breathing that is adequate to support life.

Defining Characteristics

- Alteration in metabolism
- Apprehensiveness
- Decrease in arterial oxygen saturation (SaO_2)
- Decrease in cooperation
- Decrease in partial pressure of oxygen (PO_2)
- Decrease in tidal volume
- Dyspnea
- Increase in accessory muscle use
- Increase in heart rate
- Increase in partial pressure of carbon dioxide (PCO_2)
- Restlessness

Related Factors

- Alteration in metabolism
- Respiratory muscle fatigue

00200

Risk for decreased cardiac **tissue perfusion**
(2008, 2013; LOE 2.1)

Definition
Vulnerable to a decrease in cardiac (coronary) circulation, which may compromise health.

Risk Factors

- Cardiac tamponade
- Cardiovascular surgery
- Coronary artery spasm
- Diabetes mellitus
- Family history of cardivascular disease
- Hyperlipidemia
- Hypertension
- Hypovolemia
- Hypoxemia
- Hypoxia
- Increase in C-reactive protein
- Insufficient knowledge about modifiable risk factors (e.g., smoking, sedentary lifestyle, obesity)
- Pharmaceutical agent
- Substance abuse

Original literature support available at www.nanda.org

00201

Risk for ineffective cerebral **tissue perfusion**
(2008, 2013; LOE 2.1)

Definition
Vulnerable to a decrease in cerebral tissue circulation, which may compromise health.

Risk Factors

- Abnormal partial thromboplastin time (PTT)
- Abnormal prothrombin time (PT)
- Akinetic left ventricular wall segment
- Aortic atherosclerosis
- Arterial dissection
- Atrial fibrillation
- Atrial myxoma
- Brain injury (e.g., cerebrovascular impairment, neurological illness, trauma, tumor)
- Brain neoplasm
- Carotid stenosis
- Cerebral aneurysm
- Coagulopathy (e.g., sickle cell anemia)
- Dilated cardiomyopathy
- Disseminated intravascular coagulopathy
- Embolism
- Hypercholesterolemia
- Hypertension
- Infective endocarditis
- Mechanical prosthetic valve
- Mitral stenosis
- Pharmaceutical agent
- Recent myocardial infarction
- Sick sinus syndrome
- Substance abuse
- Treatment regimen

Original literature support available at www.nanda.org

00204

Ineffective peripheral **tissue perfusion**
(2008, 2010; LOE 2.1)

Definition
Decrease in blood circulation to the periphery that may compromise health.

Defining Characteristics

- Absence of peripheral pulses
- Alteration in motor functioning
- Alteration in skin characteristic (e.g., color, elasticity, hair, moisture, nails, sensation, temperature)
- Ankle-brachial index <0.90
- Capillary refill time >3 seconds
- Color does not return to lowered limb after 1 minute leg elevation
- Decrease in blood pressure in extremities
- Decrease in pain-free distances achieved in the 6-minute walk test
- Decrease in peripheral pulses
- Delay in peripheral wound healing
- Distance in the 6-minute walk test below normal range (400 m to 700 m in adults)
- Edema
- Extremity pain
- Femoral bruit
- Intermittent claudication
- Paresthesia
- Skin color pales with limb elevation

Related Factors

- Diabetes mellitus
- Hypertension
- Insufficient knowledge of aggravating factors (e.g., smoking, sedentary lifestyle, trauma, obesity, salt intake, immobility)
- Insufficient knowledge of disease process
- Sedentary lifestyle
- Smoking

Original literature support available at www.nanda.org

00228

Risk for ineffective peripheral **tissue perfusion**
(2010, 2013; LOE 2.1)

Definition
Vulnerable to a decrease in blood circulation to the periphery, which may compromise health.

Risk Factors

- Diabetes mellitus
- Endovascular procedure
- Excessive sodium intake
- Hypertension
- Insufficient knowledge of aggravating factors (e.g., smoking, sedentary lifestyle, trauma, obesity, salt intake, immobility)
- Insufficient knowledge of disease process
- Insufficient knowledge of risk factors
- Sedentary lifestyle
- Smoking
- Trauma

Original literature support available at www.nanda.org

00034

Dysfunctional **ventilatory weaning response**
(1992)

> ## Definition
> Inability to adjust to lowered levels of mechanical ventilator support that interrupts and prolongs the weaning process.

Defining Characteristics

Mild

- Breathing discomfort
- Fatigue
- Fear of machine malfunction
- Increase in focus on breathing
- Mild increase of respiratory rate over baseline
- Perceived need for increase in oxygen
- Restlessness
- Warmth

Moderate

- Abnormal skin color (e.g., pale, dusky, cyanosis)
- Apprehensiveness
- Decrease in air entry on auscultation
- Diaphoresis
- Facial expression of fear
- Hyperfocused on activities
- Impaired ability to cooperate
- Impaired ability to respond to coaching
- Increase in blood pressure from baseline (<20 mmHg)
- Increase in heart rate from baseline (<20 beats/min)
- Minimal use of respiratory accessory muscles
- Moderate increase in respiratory rate over baseline

Severe

- Abnormal skin color (e.g., pale, dusky, cyanosis)
- Adventitious breath sounds
- Agitation
- Asynchronized breathing with the ventilator
- Decrease in level of consciousness
- Deterioration in arterial blood gases from baseline
- Gasping breaths
- Increase in blood pressure from baseline (≥to 20 mmHg)

- Increase in heart rate from baseline (≥20 beats/min)
- Paradoxical abdominal breathing
- Profuse diaphoresis
- Shallow breathing
- Significant increase in respiratory rate above baseline
- Use of significant respiratory accessory muscles

Related Factors

Physiological
- Alteration in sleep pattern
- Ineffective airway clearance
- Inadequate nutrition
- Pain

Psychological
- Anxiety
- Decrease in motivation
- Fear
- Hopelessness
- Insufficient knowledge of weaning process
- Insufficient trust in healthcare professional
- Low self-esteem
- Powerlessness
- Uncertainty about ability to wean

Situational
- Environmental barrier (e.g., distractions, low nurse to patient ratio, unfamiliar healthcare staff)
- History of unsuccessful weaning attempt
- History of ventilator dependence > 4 days
- Inappropriate pace of weaning process
- Insufficient social support
- Uncontrolled episodic energy demands

00098

Impaired **home maintenance**
(1980)

Definition
Inability to independently maintain a safe growth-promoting immediate environment.

Defining Characteristics

- Difficulty maintaining a comfortable environment
- Excessive family responsibilities
- Financial crisis (e.g., debt, insufficient finances)
- Insufficient clothing
- Insufficient cooking equipment
- Insufficient equipment for maintaining home
- Insufficient linen
- Pattern of disease caused by unhygienic conditions
- Pattern of infection caused by unhygienic conditions
- Request for assistance with home maintenance
- Unsanitary environment

Related Factors

- Alteration in cognitive functioning
- Condition impacting ability to maintain home (e.g., disease, illness injury)
- Illness impacting ability to maintain home
- Injury impacting ability to maintain home
- Insufficient family organization
- Insufficient family planning
- Insufficient knowledge of home maintenance
- Insufficient knowledge of neighborhood resources
- Insufficient role model
- Insufficient support system

00108

Bathing self-care deficit
(1980, 1998, 2008; LOE 2.1)

> ## Definition
> Impaired ability to perform or complete bathing activities for self.

Defining Characteristics

- Impaired ability to dry body
- Impaired ability to access bathroom
- Impaired ability to access water
- Impaired ability to gather bathing supplies
- Impaired ability to regulate bath water
- Impaired ability to wash body

Related Factors

- Alteration in cognitive functioning
- Anxiety
- Decrease in motivation
- Environmental barrier
- Impaired ability to perceive body part
- Impaired ability to perceive spatial relationships
- Musculoskeletal impairment
- Neuromuscular impairment
- Pain
- Perceptual impairment
- Weakness

00109

Dressing self-care deficit
(1980, 1998, 2008; LOE 2.1)

Definition
Impaired ability to perform or complete dressing activities for self.

Defining Characteristics

- Decrease in motivation
- Discomfort
- Environmental barrier
- Fatigue
- Impaired ability to choose clothing
- Impaired ability to fasten clothing
- Impaired ability to gather clothing
- Impaired ability to maintain appearance
- Impaired ability to pick up clothing
- Impaired ability to put clothing on lower body
- Impaired ability to put clothing on upper body
- Impaired ability to put on various items of clothing (e.g., shirt, socks, shoes)
- Impaired ability to remove clothing item (e.g., shirt, socks, shoes)
- Impaired ability to use assistive device
- Impaired ability to use zipper
- Musculoskeletal impairment
- Neuromuscular impairment
- Pain

Related Factors

- Alteration in cognitive functioning
- Anxiety
- Perceptual impairment
- Weakness

00102

Feeding self-care deficit
(1980, 1998)

Definition
Impaired ability to perform or complete self-feeding activities.

Defining Characteristics

- Impaired ability to bring food to the mouth
- Impaired ability to chew food
- Impaired ability to get food onto utensil
- Impaired ability to handle utensils
- Impaired ability to manipulate food in mouth
- Impaired ability to open containers
- Impaired ability to pick up cup
- Impaired ability to prepare food
- Impaired ability to self-feed a complete meal
- Impaired ability to self-feed in an acceptable manner
- Impaired ability to swallow food
- Impaired ability to swallow sufficient amount of food
- Impaired ability to use assistive device

Related Factors

- Alteration in cognitive functioning
- Anxiety
- Decrease in motivation
- Discomfort
- Environmental barrier
- Fatigue
- Musculoskeletal impairment
- Neuromuscular impairment
- Pain
- Perceptual impairment
- Weakness

00110

Toileting self-care deficit
(1980, 1998, 2008; LOE 2.1)

Definition
Impaired ability to perform or complete self-toileting activities.

Defining Characteristics

- Impaired ability to complete toilet hygiene
- Impaired ability to flush toilet
- Impaired ability to manipulate clothing for toileting
- Impaired ability to reach toilet
- Impaired ability to rise from toilet
- Impaired ability to sit on toilet

Related Factors

- Alteration in cognitive functioning
- Anxiety
- Decrease in motivation
- Environmental barrier
- Fatigue
- Impaired ability to transfer
- Impaired mobility
- Musculoskeletal impairment
- Neuromuscular impairment
- Pain
- Perceptual impairment
- Weakness

00182

Readiness for enhanced **self-care**
(2006, 2013; LOE 2.1)

Definition
A pattern of performing activities for oneself to meet health-related goals, which can be strengthened.

Defining Characteristics

- Expresses desire to enhance independence with health
- Expresses desire to enhance independence with life
- Expresses desire to enhance independence with personal development

- Expresses desire to enhance independence with well-being
- Expresses desire to enhance knowledge of self-care strategies
- Expresses desire to enhance self-care

Original literature support available at www.nanda.org

00193

Self-neglect
(2008; LOE 2.1)

Definition
A constellation of culturally framed behaviors involving one or more self-care activities in which there is a failure to maintain a socially accepted standard of health and well-being (Gibbons, Lauder, & Ludwick, 2006).

Defining Characteristics

- Insufficient environmental hygiene
- Insufficient personal hygiene
- Nonadherence to health activity

Related Factors

- Alteration in cognitive functioning
- Capgras syndrome
- Deficient executive function
- Fear of institutionalization
- Frontal lobe dysfunction
- Functional impairment
- Inability to maintain control
- Learning disability
- Lifestyle choice
- Malingering
- Psychiatric disorder
- Psychotic disorder
- Stressors
- Substance abuse

Gibbons, S., Lauder, W., & Ludwick, R. (2006). Self-neglect: A proposed new NANDA diagnosis. *International Journal of Nursing Terminologies and Classification*, 17(1), 10–18.

Original literature support available at www.nanda.org

Domain 5
Perception/Cognition

DOMAIN 5. PERCEPTION/COGNITION
The human information processing system including attention, orientation, sensation, perception, cognition, and communication.

Class 1. Attention
Mental readiness to notice or observe

Code	Diagnosis	Page
00123	**Unilateral neglect**	251

Class 2. Orientation
Awareness of time, place, and person

None at this time		

Class 3. Sensation/perception
Receiving information through the senses of touch, taste, smell, vision, hearing, and kinesthesia, and the comprehension of sensory data resulting in naming, associating, and/or pattern recognition

None at this time		

Class 4. Cognition
Use of memory, learning, thinking, problem-solving, abstraction, judgment, insight, intellectual capacity, calculation, and language

Code	Diagnosis	Page
00128	Acute **confusion**	252

NANDA International, Inc. Nursing Diagnoses: Definitions & Classification 2015–2017, Tenth Edition. Edited by T. Heather Herdman and Shigemi Kamitsuru.
© 2014 NANDA International, Inc. Published 2014 by John Wiley & Sons, Ltd.
Companion website: www.wiley.com/go/nursingdiagnoses

Class 4. Cognition (continued)		
Code	**Diagnosis**	**Page**
00173	Risk for acute **confusion**	253
00129	Chronic **confusion**	254
00251	Labile **emotional control**	255
00222	Ineffective **impulse control**	256
00126	Deficient **knowledge**	257
00161	Readiness for enhanced **knowledge**	258
00131	Impaired **memory**	259

Class 5. Communication
Sending and receiving verbal and nonverbal information

Code	**Diagnosis**	**Page**
00157	Readiness for enhanced **communication**	260
00051	Impaired **verbal communication**	261

00123

Unilateral neglect
(1986, 2006; LOE 2.1)

Definition
Impairment in sensory and motor response, mental representation, and spatial attention of the body, and the corresponding environment, characterized by inattention to one side and overattention to the opposite side. Left-side neglect is more severe and persistent than right-side neglect.

Defining Characteristics

- Alteration in safety behavior on neglected side
- Disturbance of sound lateralization
- Failure to dress neglected side
- Failure to eat food from portion of plate on neglected side
- Failure to groom neglected side
- Failure to move eyes in the neglected hemisphere
- Failure to move head in the neglected hemisphere
- Failure to move limbs in the neglected hemisphere
- Failure to move trunk in the neglected hemisphere
- Failure to notice people approaching from the neglected side
- Hemianopsia
- Impaired performance on line cancellation, line bisection, and target cancellation tests
- Left hemiplegia from cerebrovascular accident
- Marked deviation of the eyes to stimuli on the non-neglected side
- Marked deviation of the trunk to stimuli on the non-neglected side
- Omission of drawing on the neglected side
- Perseveration
- Representational neglect (e.g., distortion of drawing on the neglected side)
- Substitution of letters to form alternative words when reading
- Transfer of pain sensation to the non-neglected side
- Unaware of positioning of neglected limb
- Unilateral visuospatial neglect
- Use of vertical half of page only when writing

Related Factors

- Brain injury (e.g., cerebrovascular impairment, neurological illness, trauma, tumor)

Original literature support available at www.nanda.org

00128

Acute **confusion**
(1994, 2006; LOE 2.1)

Definition
Abrupt onset of reversible disturbances of consciousness, attention, cognition, and perception that develop over a short period of time.

Defining Characteristics

- Agitation
- Alteration in cognitive functioning
- Alteration in level of consciousness
- Alteration in psychomotor functioning
- Hallucinations
- Inability to initiate goal-directed behavior
- Inability to initiate purposeful behavior
- Insufficient follow-through with goal-directed behavior
- Insufficient follow-through with purposeful behavior
- Misperception
- Restlessness

Related Factors

- Age ≥ 60 years
- Alteration in sleep-wake cycle
- Delirium
- Dementia
- Substance abuse

Original literature support available at www.nanda.org

00173

Risk for acute **confusion**
(2006, 2013; LOE 2.2)

Definition
Vulnerable to reversible disturbances of consciousness, attention, cognition, and perception that develop over a short period of time, which may compromise health.

Risk Factors

- Age ≥ 60 years
- Alteration in cognitive functioning
- Alteration in sleep-wake cycle
- Dehydration
- Dementia
- History of cerebral vascular accident
- Impaired metabolic functioning (e.g., azotemia, decreased hemoglobin, electrolyte imbalance, increase in blood urea nitrogen/creatinine)
- Impaired mobility
- Inappropriate use of restraints
- Infection
- Male gender
- Malnutrition
- Pain
- Pharmaceutical agent
- Sensory deprivation
- Substance abuse
- Urinary retention

Original literature support available at www.nanda.org

00129

Chronic **confusion**
(1994)

Definition
Irreversible, longstanding, and/or progressive deterioration of intellect and personality characterized by decreased ability to interpret environmental stimuli and decreased capacity for intellectual thought processes, and manifested by disturbances of memory, orientation, and behavior.

Defining Characteristics

- Alteration in interpretation
- Alteration in long-term memory
- Alteration in personality
- Alteration in response to stimuli
- Alteration in short-term memory
- Chronic cognitive impairment
- Impaired social functioning
- Normal level of consciousness
- Organic brain disorder
- Progressive alteration in cognitive functioning

Related Factors

- Alzheimer's disease
- Brain injury (e.g., cerebrovascular impairment, neurological illness, trauma, tumor)
- Cerebral vascular accident
- Korsakoff's psychosis
- Multi-infarct dementia

00251

Labile emotional control
(2013; LOE 2.1)

Definition
Uncontrollable outbursts of exaggerated and involuntary emotional expression.

Defining Characteristics

- Absence of eye contact
- Difficulty in use of facial expressions
- Embarrassment regarding emotional expression
- Excessive crying without feeling sadness
- Excessive laughing without feeling happiness
- Expression of emotion incongruent with triggering factor
- Involuntary crying
- Involuntary laughing
- Tearfulness
- Uncontrollable crying
- Uncontrollable laughing
- Withdrawal from occupational situation
- Withdrawal from social situation

Related Factors

- Alternation in self-esteem
- Brain injury
- Emotional disturbance
- Fatigue
- Functional impairment
- Insufficient knowledge about symptom control
- Insufficient knowledge of disease
- Insufficient muscle strength
- Mood disorder
- Musculoskeletal impairment
- Pharmaceutical agent
- Physical disability
- Psychiatric disorder
- Social distress
- Stressors
- Substance abuse

Original literature support available at www.nanda.org

00222

Ineffective **impulse control**
(2010; LOE 2.1)

Definition
A pattern of performing rapid, unplanned reactions to internal or external stimuli without regard for the negative consequences of these reactions to the impulsive individual or to others.

Defining Characteristics

- Acting without thinking
- Asking personal questions despite discomfort of others
- Gambling addiction
- Inability to save money or regulate finances
- Inappropriate sharing of personal details
- Irritability
- Overly familiar with strangers
- Sensation seeking
- Sexual promiscuity
- Temper outbursts
- Violent behavior

Related Factors

- Alteration in cognitive functioning
- Alteration in development
- Hopelessness
- Mood disorder
- Organic brain disorder
- Personality disorder
- Smoking
- Substance abuse

Original literature support available at www.nanda.org

00126

Deficient knowledge
(1980)

Definition
Absence or deficiency of cognitive information related to a specific topic.

Defining Characteristics

- Inaccurate follow-through of instruction
- Inaccurate performance on a test
- Inappropriate behavior (e.g., hysterical, hostile, agitated, apathetic)
- Insufficient knowledge

Related Factors

- Alteration in cognitive functioning
- Alteration in memory
- Insufficient information
- Insufficient interest in learning
- Insufficient knowledge of resources
- Misinformation presented by others

00161

Readiness for enhanced **knowledge**
(2002, 2013; LOE 2.1)

Definition
A pattern of cognitive information related to a specific topic, or its acquisition, which can be strengthened.

Defining Characteristics

- Expresses desire to enhance learning

00131

Impaired **memory**
(1994)

Definition
Inability to remember or recall bits of information or behavioral skills.

Defining Characteristics

- Forgetfulness
- Forgets to perform a behavior at scheduled time
- Inability to learn new information
- Inability to learn new skill
- Inability to perform a previously learned skill
- Inability to recall events
- Inability to recall factual information
- Inability to recall if a behavior was performed
- Inability to retain new information

Related Factors

- Alteration in fluid volume
- Anemia
- Decrease in cardiac output
- Distractions in the environment
- Electrolyte imbalance
- Hypoxia
- Neurological impairment (e.g., positive EEG, head trauma, seizure disorders)

5. Perception/Cognition

00157

Readiness for enhanced **communication**
(2002, 2013; LOE 2.1)

Definition
A pattern of exchanging information and ideas with others, which can be strengthened.

Defining Characteristics

- Expresses desire to enhance communication

00051

Impaired **verbal communication**
(1983, 1996, 1998)

Definition
Decreased, delayed, or absent ability to receive, process, transmit, and/ or use a system of symbols.

Defining Characteristics

- Absence of eye contact
- Difficulty comprehending communication
- Difficulty expressing thoughts verbally (e.g., aphasia, dysphasia, apraxia, dyslexia)
- Difficulty forming sentences
- Difficulty forming words (e.g., aphonia, dyslalia, dysarthria)
- Difficulty in selective attending
- Difficulty in use of body expressions
- Difficulty in use of facial expressions
- Difficulty maintaining communication
- Difficulty speaking
- Difficulty verbalizing
- Disoriented to person
- Disoriented to place
- Disoriented to time
- Does not speak
- Dyspnea
- Inability to speak
- Inability to speak language of caregiver
- Inability to use body expressions
- Inability to use facial expressions
- Inappropriate verbalization
- Partial visual deficit
- Refusal to speak
- Slurred speech
- Stuttering
- Total visual deficit

Related Factors

- Absence of significant other
- Alteration in development
- Alteration in perception
- Alteration in self-concept
- Central nervous system impairment
- Cultural incongruence
- Emotional disturbance
- Environmental barrier
- Insufficient information
- Insufficient stimuli
- Low self-esteem
- Oropharyngeal defect

- Physical barrier (e.g., tracheostomy, intubation)
- Physiological condition (e.g., brain tumor, decreased circulation to brain, weakened musculoskeletal system)

- Psychotic disorder
- Treatment regimen
- Vulnerability

Domain 6
Self-Perception

DOMAIN 6. SELF-PERCEPTION		
Awareness about the self		

Class 1. Self-concept
The perception(s) about the total self

Code	Diagnosis	Page
00185	Readiness for enhanced **hope**	265
00124	**Hope**lessness	266
00174	Risk for compromised **human dignity**	267
00121	Disturbed **personal identity**	268
00225	Risk for disturbed **personal identity**	269
00167	Readiness for enhanced **self-concept**	270

Class 2. Self-esteem
Assessment of one's own worth, capability, significance, and success

Code	Diagnosis	Page
00119	Chronic low **self-esteem**	271
00224	Risk for chronic low **self-esteem**	272
00120	Situational low **self-esteem**	273
00153	Risk for situational low **self-esteem**	274

Class 3. Body image
A mental image of one's own body

Code	Diagnosis	Page
00118	Disturbed **body image**	275

NANDA International, Inc. Nursing Diagnoses: Definitions & Classification 2015–2017,
Tenth Edition. Edited by T. Heather Herdman and Shigemi Kamitsuru.
© 2014 NANDA International, Inc. Published 2014 by John Wiley & Sons, Ltd.
Companion website: www.wiley.com/go/nursingdiagnoses

00185

Readiness for enhanced **hope**
(2006, 2013; LOE 2.1)

Definition

A pattern of expectations and desires for mobilizing energy on one's own behalf, which can be strengthened.

Defining Characteristics

- Expresses desire to enhance ability to set achievable goals
- Expresses desire to enhance belief in possibilities
- Expresses desire to enhance congruency of expectation with goal
- Expresses desire to enhance connectedness with others
- Expresses desire to enhance hope
- Expresses desire to enhance problem-solving to meet goal
- Expresses desire to enhance sense of meaning in life
- Expresses desire to enhance spirituality

00124

Hopelessness
(1986)

Definition
Subjective state in which an individual sees limited or no alternatives or personal choices available and is unable to mobilize energy on own behalf.

Defining Characteristics

- Alteration in sleep pattern
- Decrease in affect
- Decrease in appetite
- Decrease in initiative
- Decrease in response to stimuli
- Decrease in verbalization
- Despondent verbal cues (e.g., "I can't," sighing)
- Inadequate involvement in care
- Passivity
- Poor eye contact
- Shrugging in response to speaker
- Turning away from speaker

Related Factors

- Chronic stress
- Deterioration in physiological condition
- History of abandonment
- Loss of belief in spiritual power
- Loss of belief in transcendent values
- Prolonged activity restriction
- Social isolation

00174

Risk for compromised **human dignity**
(2006, 2013; LOE 2.1)

Definition
Vulnerable for perceived loss of respect and honor, which may compromise health.

Risk Factors

- Cultural incongruence
- Dehumanizing treatment
- Disclosure of confidential information
- Exposure of the body
- Humiliation
- Insufficient comprehension of health information
- Intrusion by clinician
- Invasion of privacy
- Limited decision-making experience
- Loss of control over body function
- Stigmatization

Original literature support available at www.nanda.org

6. Self-Perception

00121

Disturbed **personal identity**
(1978, 2008; LOE 2.1)

Definition
Inability to maintain an integrated and complete perception of self.

Defining Characteristics

- Alteration in body image
- Confusion about cultural values
- Confusion about goals
- Confusion about ideological values
- Delusional description of self
- Feeling of emptiness
- Feeling of strangeness
- Fluctuating feelings about self
- Gender confusion
- Inability to distinguish between internal and external stimuli
- Inconsistent behavior
- Ineffective coping strategies
- Ineffective relationships
- Ineffective role performance

Related Factors

- Alteration in social role
- Cult indoctrination
- Cultural incongruence
- Developmental transition
- Discrimination
- Dissociative identity disorder
- Dysfunctional family processes
- Exposure to toxic chemical
- Low self-esteem
- Manic states
- Organic brain disorder
- Perceived prejudice
- Pharmaceutical agent
- Psychiatric disorder
- Situational crisis
- Stages of growth

Original literature support available at www.nanda.org

6. Self-Perception

00225

Risk for disturbed **personal identity**
(2010, 2013; LOE 2.1)

Definition
Vulnerable to the inability to maintain an integrated and complete perception of self, which may compromise health.

Risk Factors

- Alteration in social role
- Cult indoctrination
- Cultural incongruence
- Developmental transition
- Discrimination
- Dissociative identity disorder
- Dysfunctional family processes
- Exposure to toxic chemical
- Low self-esteem
- Manic states
- Organic brain disorder
- Perceived prejudice
- Pharmaceutical agent
- Psychiatric disorder
- Situational crisis
- Stages of growth

Original literature support available at www.nanda.org

6. Self-Perception

00167

Readiness for enhanced **self-concept**
(2002, 2013; LOE 2.1)

Definition
A pattern of perceptions or ideas about the self, which can be strengthened.

Defining Characteristics

- Acceptance of limitations
- Acceptance of strengths
- Actions congruent with verbal expressions
- Confidence in abilities
- Expresses desire to enhance role performance
- Expresses desire to enhance self-concept
- Satisfaction with body image
- Satisfaction with personal identity
- Satisfaction with sense of worth
- Satisfaction with thoughts about self

6. Self-Perception

00119

Chronic low **self-esteem**
(1988, 1996, 2008; LOE 2.1)

Definition
Longstanding negative self-evaluating/feelings about self or self-capabilities.

Defining Characteristics

- Dependent on others' opinions
- Exaggerates negative feedback about self
- Excessive seeking of reassurance
- Guilt
- Hesitant to try new experiences
- Indecisive behavior
- Nonassertive behavior
- Overly conforming
- Passivity
- Poor eye contact
- Rejection of positive feedback
- Repeatedly unsuccessful in life events
- Shame
- Underestimates ability to deal with situation

Related Factors

- Cultural incongruence
- Exposure to traumatic situation
- Inadequate belonging
- Inadequate respect from others
- Ineffective coping with loss
- Insufficient group membership
- Psychiatric disorder
- Receiving insufficient affection
- Receiving insufficient approval from others
- Repeated failures
- Repeated negative reinforcement
- Spiritual incongruence

Original literature support available at www.nanda.org

00224

Risk for chronic low **self-esteem**
(2010, 2013; LOE 2.1)

Definition
Vulnerable to longstanding negative self-evaluating/feelings about self or self-capabilities, which may compromise health.

Risk Factors

- Cultural incongruence
- Exposure to traumatic situation
- Inadequate affection received
- Inadequate group membership
- Inadequate respect from others
- Ineffective coping with loss
- Insufficient feeling of belonging
- Psychiatric disorder
- Repeated failures
- Repeated negative reinforcement
- Spiritual incongruence

Original literature support available at www.nanda.org

00120
Situational low **self-esteem**
(1988, 1996, 2000)

Definition
Development of a negative perception of self-worth in response to a current situation.

Defining Characteristics

- Helplessness
- Indecisive behavior
- Nonassertive behavior
- Purposelessness
- Self-negating verbalizations
- Situational challenge to self-worth
- Underestimates ability to deal with situation

Related Factors

- Alteration in body image
- Alteration in social role
- Behavior inconsistent with values
- Developmental transition
- Functional impairment
- History of loss
- History of rejection
- Inadequate recognition
- Pattern of failure

6. Self-Perception

00153

Risk for situational low **self-esteem**
(2000, 2013)

Definition
Vulnerable to developing a negative perception of self-worth in response to a current situation, which may compromise health.

Risk Factors

- Alteration in body image
- Alteration in social role
- Behavior inconsistent with values
- Decrease in control over environment
- Developmental transition
- Functional impairment
- History of abandonment
- History of abuse (e.g., physical, psychological, sexual)
- History of loss
- History of neglect
- History of rejection
- Inadequate recognition
- Pattern of failure
- Pattern of helplessness
- Physical illness
- Unrealistic self-expectations

00118

Disturbed **body image**
(1973, 1998)

Definition
Confusion in mental picture of one's physical self.

Defining Characteristics

- Absence of body part
- Alteration in body function
- Alteration in body structure
- Alteration in view of one's body (e.g., appearance, structure, function)
- Avoids looking at one's body
- Avoids touching one's body
- Behavior of acknowledging one's body
- Behavior of monitoring one's body
- Change in ability to estimate spatial relationship of body to environment
- Change in lifestyle
- Change in social involvement
- Depersonalization of body part by use of impersonal pronouns
- Depersonalization of loss by use of impersonal pronouns
- Emphasis on remaining strengths
- Extension of body boundary (e.g., includes external object)
- Fear of reaction by others
- Focus on past appearance
- Focus on past function
- Focus on previous strength
- Heightened achievement
- Hiding of body part
- Negative feeling about body
- Nonverbal response to change in body (e.g., appearance, structure, function)
- Nonverbal response to perceived change in body (e.g., appearance, structure, function)
- Overexposure of body part
- Perceptions that reflect an altered view of one's body appearance
- Personalization of body part by name
- Personalization of loss by name
- Preoccupation with change
- Preoccupation with loss
- Refusal to acknowledge change
- Trauma to nonfunctioning body part

6. Self-Perception

Related Factors

- Alteration in body function (due to anomaly, disease, medication, pregnancy, radiation, surgery, trauma, etc.)
- Alteration in cognitive functioning
- Alteration in self-perception
- Cultural incongruence
- Developmental transition
- Illness
- Impaired psychosocial functioning
- Injury
- Spiritual incongruence
- Surgical procedure
- Trauma
- Treatment regimen

DOMAIN 7. ROLE RELATIONSHIPS

The positive and negative connections or associations between people or groups of people and the means by which those connections are demonstrated

Class 1. Caregiving Roles
Socially expected behavior patterns by people providing care who are not healthcare professionals

Code	Diagnosis	Page
00061	Caregiver **role strain**	279
00062	Risk for caregiver **role strain**	282
00056	Impaired **parenting**	283
00164	Readiness for enhanced **parenting**	286
00057	Risk for impaired **parenting**	287

Class 2. Family Relationships
Associations of people who are biologically related or related by choice

Code	Diagnosis	Page
00058	Risk for impaired **attachment**	289
00063	Dysfunctional **family processes**	290
00060	Interrupted **family processes**	293
00159	Readiness for enhanced **family processes**	294

NANDA International, Inc. Nursing Diagnoses: Definitions & Classification 2015–2017,
Tenth Edition. Edited by T. Heather Herdman and Shigemi Kamitsuru.
© 2014 NANDA International, Inc. Published 2014 by John Wiley & Sons, Ltd.
Companion website: www.wiley.com/go/nursingdiagnoses

Class 3. Role Performance *Quality of functioning in socially expected behavior patterns*		
Code	**Diagnosis**	**Page**
00223	Ineffective **relationship**	295
00207	Readiness for enhanced **relationship**	296
00229	Risk for ineffective **relationship**	297
00064	Parental **role conflict**	298
00055	Ineffective **role performance**	299
00052	Impaired **social interaction**	301

00061

Caregiver **role strain**
(1992, 1998, 2000)

Definition
Difficulty in performing family/significant other caregiver role.

Defining Characteristics

Caregiving Activities
- Apprehensiveness about future ability to provide care
- Apprehensiveness about future health of care receiver
- Apprehensiveness about potential institutionalization of care receiver
- Apprehensiveness about well-being of care receiver if unable to provide care
- Difficulty completing required tasks
- Difficulty performing required tasks
- Dysfunctional change in caregiving activities
- Preoccupation with care routine

Caregiver Health Status: Physiological
- Cardiovascular disease
- Diabetes mellitus
- Fatigue
- Gastrointestinal distress
- Headache
- Hypertension
- Rash
- Weight change

Caregiver Health Status: Emotional
- Alteration in sleep pattern
- Anger
- Depression
- Emotional vacillation
- Frustration
- Impatience
- Ineffective coping strategies
- Insufficient time to meet personal needs
- Nervousness
- Somatization
- Stressors

Caregiver Health Status: Socioeconomic
- Change in leisure activities
- Low work productivity
- Refusal of career advancement
- Social isolation

Caregiver–Care Receiver Relationship
- Difficulty watching care receiver with illness
- Grieving of changes in relationship with care receiver
- Uncertainty about changes in relationship with care receiver

Family Processes
- Concern about family member(s)
- Family conflict

Related Factors

Care Receiver Health Status
- Alteration in cognitive functioning
- Chronic illness
- Codependency
- Dependency
- Illness severity
- Increase in care needs
- Problematic behavior
- Psychiatric disorder
- Substance abuse
- Unpredictability of illness trajectory
- Unstable health condition

Caregiver Health Status
- Alteration in cognitive functioning
- Codependency
- Ineffective coping strategies
- Insufficient fulfillment of others' expectations
- Insufficient fulfillment of self-expectations
- Physical conditions
- Substance abuse
- Unrealistic self-expectations

Caregiver–Care Receiver Relationship
- Abusive relationship
- Care receiver's condition inhibits conversation
- Pattern of ineffective relationships
- Unrealistic care receiver expectations
- Violent relationship

Caregiving Activities
- Around-the-clock care responsibilities
- Change in nature of care activities
- Complexity of care activities
- Duration of caregiving
- Excessive caregiving activities
- Recent discharge home with significant care needs
- Unpredictability of care situation

Family Processes
- Pattern of family dysfunction
- Pattern of ineffective family coping

Resources
- Caregiver not developmentally ready for caregiver role
- Difficulty accessing assistance
- Difficulty accessing community resources
- Difficulty accessing support
- Financial crisis (e.g., debt, insufficient finances)
- Inexperience with caregiving
- Insufficient assistance
- Insufficient caregiver privacy
- Insufficient community resources (e.g., respite, recreation, social support)
- Insufficient emotional resilience
- Insufficient energy
- Insufficient equipment for providing care
- Insufficient knowledge about community resources
- Insufficient physical environment for providing care
- Insufficient social support
- Insufficient time
- Insufficient transportation

Socioeconomic
- Alienation
- Competing role commitments
- Insufficient recreation
- Social isolation

00062

Risk for caregiver **role strain**
(1992, 2010, 2013; LOE 2.1)

Definition
Vulnerable to difficulty in performing the family/significant other caregiver role, which may compromise health.

Risk Factors

- Alteration in cognitive functioning in care receiver
- Care receiver discharged home with significant needs
- Care receiver exhibits bizarre behavior
- Care receiver exhibits deviant behavior
- Caregiver health impairment
- Caregiver isolation
- Caregiver not developmentally ready for caregiver role
- Caregiver's competing role commitments
- Caregiving task complexity
- Codependency
- Congenital disorder
- Developmental delay
- Developmental delay of caregiver
- Excessive caregiving activities
- Exposure to violence
- Extended duration of caregiving required
- Family isolation
- Female caregiver
- Illness severity of care receiver
- Inadequate physical environment for providing care
- Ineffective caregiver coping pattern
- Ineffective family adaptation
- Inexperience with caregiving
- Instability in care receiver's health
- Insufficient caregiver recreation
- Insufficient respite for caregiver
- Partner as caregiver
- Pattern of family dysfunction prior to the caregiving situation
- Pattern of ineffective relationship between caregiver and care receiver
- Prematurity
- Presence of abuse (e.g., physical, psychological, sexual)
- Psychological disorder in caregiver
- Psychological disorder in care receiver
- Stressors
- Substance abuse
- Unpredictability of illness trajectory

00056

Impaired **parenting**
(1978, 1998)

Definition

Inability of the primary caretaker to create, maintain, or regain an environment that promotes the optimum growth and development of the child.

Defining Characteristics

Infant or Child

- Behavior disorder (e.g., attention deficit, oppositional defiant)
- Delay in cognitive development
- Diminished separation anxiety
- Failure to thrive
- Frequent accidents
- Frequent illness
- History of abuse (e.g., physical, psychological, sexual)
- History of trauma (e.g., physical, psychological, sexual)
- Impaired social functioning
- Insufficient attachment behavior
- Low academic performance
- Runaway

Parental

- Abandonment
- Decrease in ability to manage child
- Decrease in cuddling
- Deficient parent-child interaction
- Frustration with child
- History of childhood abuse (e.g., physical, psychological, sexual)
- Hostility
- Inadequate child health maintenance
- Inappropriate care-taking skills
- Inappropriate child-care arrangements
- Inappropriate stimulation (e.g., visual, tactile, auditory)
- Inconsistent behavior management
- Inconsistent care
- Inflexibility in meeting needs of child
- Neglects needs of child
- Perceived inability to meet child's needs
- Perceived role inadequacy
- Punitive
- Rejection of child
- Speaks negatively about child
- Unsafe home environment

7. Role Relationships

Related Factors

Infant or Child
- Alteration in perceptual abilities
- Behavior disorder (e.g., attention deficit, oppositional defiant)
- Chronic illness
- Developmental delay
- Difficult temperament
- Disabling condition
- Gender other than desired
- Multiple births
- Parent-child separation
- Prematurity
- Temperament conflicts with parental expectations

Knowledge
- Alteration in cognitive functioning
- Ineffective communication skills
- Insufficient cognitive readiness for parenting
- Insufficient knowledge about child development
- Insufficient knowledge about child health maintenance
- Insufficient knowledge about parenting skills
- Insufficient response to infant cues
- Low educational level
- Preference for physical punishment
- Unrealistic expectations

Physiological
- Physical illness

Psychological
- Alteration in sleep pattern
- Closely spaced pregnancies
- Depression
- Difficult birthing process
- Disabling condition
- High number of pregnancies
- History of mental illness
- History of substance abuse
- Insufficient prenatal care
- Sleep deprivation
- Young parental age

Social
- Change in family unit
- Compromised home environment
- Conflict between partners
- Economically disadvantaged
- Father of child not involved
- History of abuse (e.g., physical, psychological, sexual)
- History of being abusive
- Inability to put child's needs before own
- Inadequate child-care arrangements
- Ineffective coping strategies
- Insufficient family cohesiveness

- Insufficient parental role model
- Insufficient problem-solving skills
- Insufficient resources (e.g., financial, social, knowledge)
- Insufficient social support
- Insufficient transportation
- Insufficient valuing of parenthood
- Legal difficulty
- Low self-esteem
- Mother of child not involved
- Relocation
- Single parent
- Social isolation
- Stressors
- Unemployment
- Unplanned pregnancy
- Unwanted pregnancy
- Work difficulty

7. Role Relationships

00164

Readiness for enhanced **parenting**
(2002, 2013; LOE 2.1)

Definition
A pattern of providing an environment for children or other dependent person(s) to nurture growth and development, which can be strengthened.

Defining Characteristics

- Children express desire to enhance home environment
- Expresses desire to enhance parenting
- Parent expresses desire to enhance emotional support of children
- Parent expresses desire to enhance emotional support of other dependent person

00057

Risk for impaired **parenting**
(1978, 1998, 2013)

Definition
Vulnerable to inability of the primary caretaker to create, maintain, or regain an environment that promotes the optimum growth and development of the child, which may compromise the well-being of the child.

Risk Factors

Infant or Child
- Alteration in perceptual abilities
- Behavior disorder (e.g., attention deficit, oppositional defiant)
- Developmental delay
- Difficult temperament
- Disabling condition
- Gender other than desired
- Illness
- Multiple births
- Prematurity
- Prolonged separation from parent
- Temperament conflicts with parental expectations

Knowledge
- Alteration in cognitive functioning
- Ineffective communication skills
- Insufficient cognitive readiness for parenting
- Insufficient knowledge about child development
- Insufficient knowledge about child health maintenance
- Insufficient knowledge about parenting skills
- Insufficient response to infant cues
- Low educational level
- Preference for physical punishment
- Unrealistic expectations

Physiological
- Physical illness

Psychological
- Closely spaced pregnancies
- Depression
- Difficult birthing process
- Disabling condition

- High number of pregnancies
- History of mental illness
- History of substance abuse
- Nonrestorative sleep pattern (i.e., due to caregiver

responsibilities, parenting practices, sleep partner)
- Sleep deprivation
- Young parental age

Social
- Change in family unit
- Compromised home environment
- Conflict between partners
- Economically disadvantaged
- Father of child not involved
- History of abuse (e.g., physical, psychological, sexual)
- History of being abusive
- Inadequate child-care arrangements
- Ineffective coping strategies
- Insufficient access to resources
- Insufficient family cohesiveness
- Insufficient parental role model
- Insufficient prenatal care
- Insufficient problem-solving skills
- Insufficient resources (e.g., financial, social, knowledge)
- Insufficient social support
- Insufficient transportation
- Insufficient valuing of parenthood
- Late-term prenatal care
- Legal difficulty
- Low self-esteem
- Mother of child not involved
- Parent-child separation
- Relocation
- Role strain
- Single parent
- Social isolation
- Stressors
- Unemployment
- Unplanned pregnancy
- Unwanted pregnancy
- Work difficulty

00058

Risk for impaired **attachment**
(1994, 2008, 2013; LOE 2.1)

Definition
Vulnerable to disruption of the interactive process between parent/ significant other and child that fosters the development of a protective and nurturing reciprocal relationship.

Risk Factors

- Anxiety
- Child's illness prevents effective initiation of parental contact
- Disorganized infant behavior
- Inability of parent to meet personal needs
- Insufficient privacy
- Parental conflict resulting from disorganized infant behavior
- Parent-child separation
- Physical barrier (e.g., infant in isolette)
- Prematurity
- Substance abuse

00063

Dysfunctional **family processes**
(1994, 2008; LOE 2.1)

Definition
Psychosocial, spiritual, and physiological functions of the family unit are chronically disorganized, which leads to conflict, denial of problems, resistance to change, ineffective problem-solving, and a series of self-perpetuating crises.

Defining Characteristics

Behavioral

- Agitation
- Alteration in concentration
- Blaming
- Broken promises
- Chaos
- Complicated grieving
- Conflict avoidance
- Contradictory communication pattern
- Controlling communication pattern
- Criticizing
- Decrease in physical contact
- Denial of problems
- Dependency
- Difficulty having fun
- Difficulty with intimate relationship
- Difficulty with life-cycle transition
- Disturbance in academic performance in children
- Enabling substance use pattern
- Escalating conflict
- Failure to accomplish developmental tasks
- Harsh self-judgment
- Immaturity
- Inability to accept a wide range of feelings
- Inability to accept help
- Inability to adapt to change
- Inability to deal constructively with traumatic experiences
- Inability to express a wide range of feelings
- Inability to meet the emotional needs of its members
- Inability to meet the security needs of its members
- Inability to meet the spiritual needs of its members
- Inability to receive help appropriately
- Inappropriate anger expression
- Ineffective communication skills
- Insufficient knowledge about substance abuse
- Insufficient problem-solving skills

- Lying
- Manipulation
- Nicotine addiction
- Orientation favors tension relief rather than goal attainment
- Paradoxical communication pattern
- Power struggles
- Rationalization
- Refusal to get help
- Seeking of affirmation

- Seeking of approval
- Self-blame
- Social isolation
- Special occasions centered on substance use
- Stress-related physical illness
- Substance abuse
- Unreliable behavior
- Verbal abuse of children
- Verbal abuse of parent
- Verbal abuse of partner

Feelings
- Abandonment
- Anger
- Anxiety
- Confuses love and pity
- Confusion
- Depression
- Dissatisfaction
- Distress
- Embarrassment
- Emotional isolation
- Emotionally controlled by others
- Failure
- Fear
- Feeling different from others
- Feeling misunderstood
- Feeling unloved
- Frustration
- Guilt
- Hopelessness
- Hostility

- Hurt
- Insecurity
- Lingering resentment
- Loneliness
- Loss
- Loss of identity
- Low self-esteem
- Mistrust
- Moodiness
- Powerlessness
- Rejection
- Repressed emotions
- Shame
- Surgical procedure
- Taking responsibility for substance abuser's behavior
- Tension
- Unhappiness
- Vulnerability
- Worthlessness

Roles and Relationships
- Change in role function
- Chronic family problems
- Closed communication system
- Conflict between partners
- Deterioration in family relationships

- Diminished ability of family members to relate to each other for mutual growth and maturation
- Disrupted family rituals
- Disrupted family roles

- Disturbance in family dynamics
- Economically disadvantaged
- Family denial
- Inconsistent parenting
- Ineffective communication with partner
- Insufficient cohesiveness
- Insufficient family respect for autonomy of its members
- Insufficient family respect for individuality of its members
- Insufficient relationship skills
- Intimacy dysfunction
- Neglect of obligation to family member
- Pattern of rejection
- Perceived insufficient parental support
- Triangulating family relationships

Related Factors

- Addictive personality
- Biological factors
- Family history of resistance to treatment
- Family history of substance abuse
- Genetic predisposition to substance abuse
- Ineffective coping strategies
- Insufficient problem-solving skills
- Substance abuse

00060

Interrupted **family processes**
(1982, 1998)

Definition
Change in family relationships and/or functioning.

Defining Characteristics

- Alteration in availability for affective responsiveness
- Alteration in family conflict resolution
- Alteration in family satisfaction
- Alteration in intimacy
- Alteration in participation for problem-solving
- Assigned tasks change
- Change in communication pattern
- Change in somatization
- Change in stress-reduction behavior
- Changes in expressions of conflict with community resources
- Changes in expressions of isolation from community resources
- Changes in participation for decision-making
- Changes in relationship pattern
- Decrease in available emotional support
- Decrease in mutual support
- Ineffective task completion
- Power alliance change
- Ritual change

Related Factors

- Alteration in family finances
- Change in family social status
- Changes in interaction with community
- Developmental crisis
- Developmental transition
- Power shift among family members
- Shift in family roles
- Shift in health status of a family member
- Situational crisis
- Situational transition

7. Role Relationships

00159

Readiness for enhanced **family processes**
(2002, 2013; LOE 2.1)

Definition

A pattern of family functioning to support the well-being of family members, which can be strengthened.

Defining Characteristics

- Expresses desire to enhance balance between autonomy and cohesiveness
- Expresses desire to enhance communication pattern
- Expresses desire to enhance energy level of family to support activities of daily living
- Expresses desire to enhance family adaptation to change
- Expresses desire to enhance family dynamics
- Expresses desire to enhance family resilience

- Expresses desire to enhance growth of family members
- Expresses desire to enhance interdependence with community
- Expresses desire to enhance maintenance of boundaries between family members
- Expresses desire to enhance respect for family members
- Expresses desire to enhance safety of family members

00223

Ineffective **relationship**
(2010; LOE 2.1)

Definition
A pattern of mutual partnership that is insufficient to provide for each other's needs.

Defining Characteristics

- Delay in meeting of developmental goals appropriate for family life-cycle stage
- Dissatisfaction with complementary relationship between partners
- Dissatisfaction with emotional need fulfillment between partners
- Dissatisfaction with idea sharing between partners
- Dissatisfaction with information sharing between partners
- Dissatisfaction with physical need fulfillment between partners
- Inadequate understanding of partner's compromised functioning (e.g., physical, psychological, social)
- Insufficient balance in autonomy between partners
- Insufficient balance in collaboration between partners
- Insufficient mutual respect between partners
- Insufficient mutual support in daily activities between partners
- Partner not identified as support person
- Unsatisfying communication with partner

Related Factors

- Alteration in cognitive functioning in one partner
- Developmental crisis
- History of domestic violence
- Incarceration of one partner
- Ineffective communication skills
- Stressors
- Substance abuse
- Unrealistic expectations

Original literature support available at www.nanda.org

7. Role Relationships

00207

Readiness for enhanced **relationship**
(2006, 2013; LOE 2.1)

Definition

A pattern of mutual partnership to provide for each other's needs, which can be strengthened.

Defining Characteristics

- Expresses desire to enhance autonomy between partners
- Expresses desire to enhance collaboration between partners
- Expresses desire to enhance communication between partners
- Expresses desire to enhance emotional need fulfillment for each partner
- Expresses desire to enhance mutual respect between partners
- Expresses desire to enhance satisfaction with complementary relationship between partners
- Expresses desire to enhance satisfaction with emotional need fulfillment for each partner
- Expresses desire to enhance satisfaction with idea sharing between partners
- Expresses desire to enhance satisfaction with information sharing between partners
- Expresses desire to enhance satisfaction with physical need fulfillment for each partner
- Expresses desire to enhance understanding of partner's functional deficit (e.g., physical, psychological, social)

Original literature support available at www.nanda.org

00229

Risk for ineffective **relationship**
(2010, 2013; LOE 2.1)

Definition
Vulnerable to developing a pattern that is insufficient for providing a mutual partnership to provide for each other's needs.

Risk Factors

- Alteration in cognitive functioning in one partner
- Developmental crisis
- History of domestic violence
- Incarceration of one partner
- Ineffective communication skills
- Stressors
- Substance abuse
- Unrealistic expectations

Original literature support available at www.nanda.org

7. Role Relationships

00064

Parental role conflict
(1988)

Definition
Parental experience of role confusion and conflict in response to crisis.

Defining Characteristics

- Anxiety
- Concern about change in parental role
- Concern about family (e.g., functioning, communication, health)
- Disruption in caregiver routines
- Fear
- Frustration
- Guilt
- Perceived inadequacy to provide for child's needs (e.g., physical, emotional)
- Perceived loss of control over decisions relating to child
- Reluctance to participate in usual caregiver activities

Related Factors

- Change in marital status
- Home care of a child with special needs
- Interruptions in family life due to home care regimen (e.g., treatments, caregivers, lack of respite)
- Intimidated by invasive modalities (e.g., intubation)
- Intimidated by restrictive modalities (e.g., isolation)
- Living in nontraditional setting (e.g., foster, group or institutional care)
- Parent–child separation

00055

Ineffective **role performance**
(1978, 1996, 1998)

Definition
A pattern of behavior and self-expression that does not match the environmental context, norms, and expectations.

Defining Characteristics

- Alteration in role perception
- Anxiety
- Change in capacity to resume role
- Change in others' perception of role
- Change in self-perception of role
- Change in usual pattern of responsibility
- Depression
- Discrimination
- Domestic violence
- Harassment
- Inappropriate developmental expectations
- Ineffective adaptation to change
- Ineffective coping strategies
- Ineffective role performance
- Insufficient confidence
- Insufficient external support for role enactment
- Insufficient knowledge of role requirements
- Insufficient motivation
- Insufficient opportunity for role enactment
- Insufficient self-management
- Insufficient skills
- Pessimism
- Powerlessness
- Role ambivalence
- Role conflict
- Role confusion
- Role denial
- Role dissatisfaction
- Role strain
- System conflict
- Uncertainty

Related Factors

Knowledge
- Insufficient role model
- Insufficient role preparation (e.g., role transition, skill rehearsal, validation)
- Low educational level
- Unrealistic role expectations

7. Role Relationships

Physiological
- Alteration in body image
- Depression
- Fatigue
- Low self-esteem
- Mental health issue (e.g., depression, psychosis, personality disorder, substance abuse)
- Neurological defect
- Pain
- Physical illness
- Substance abuse

Social
- Conflict
- Developmental level inappropriate for role expectation
- Domestic violence
- Economically disadvantaged
- High demands of job schedule
- Inappropriate linkage with the healthcare system
- Insufficient resources (e.g., financial, social, knowledge)
- Insufficient rewards
- Insufficient role socialization
- Insufficient support system
- Stressors
- Young age

00052

Impaired **social interaction**
(1986)

Insufficient or excessive quantity or ineffective quality of social exchange.

Defining Characteristics

- Discomfort in social situations
- Dissatisfaction with social engagement (e.g., belonging, caring, interest, shared history)
- Dysfunctional interaction with others
- Family reports change in interaction (e.g., style, pattern)
- Impaired social functioning

Related Factors

- Absence of significant other
- Communication barrier
- Disturbance in self-concept
- Disturbance in thought processes
- Environmental barrier
- Impaired mobility
- Insufficient knowledge about how to enhance mutuality
- Insufficient skills to enhance mutuality
- Sociocultural dissonance
- Therapeutic isolation

7. Role Relationships

DOMAIN 8. SEXUALITY

Sexual identity, sexual function, and reproduction

Class 1. Sexual identity
The state of being a specific person in regard to sexuality and/or gender

Code	Diagnosis	Page
None at present time		

Class 2. Sexual function
The capacity or ability to participate in sexual activities

Code	Diagnosis	Page
00059	**Sexual dysfunction**	305
00065	Ineffective **sexuality pattern**	306

Class 3. Reproduction
Any process by which human beings are produced

Code	Diagnosis	Page
00221	Ineffective **childbearing process**	307
00208	Readiness for enhanced **childbearing process**	309
00227	Risk for ineffective **childbearing process**	310
00209	Risk for disturbed **maternal–fetal dyad**	311

NANDA International, Inc. Nursing Diagnoses: Definitions & Classification 2015–2017,
Tenth Edition. Edited by T. Heather Herdman and Shigemi Kamitsuru.
© 2014 NANDA International, Inc. Published 2014 by John Wiley & Sons, Ltd.
Companion website: www.wiley.com/go/nursingdiagnoses

00059

Sexual dysfunction
(1980, 2006; LOE 2.1)

Definition
A state in which an individual experiences a change in sexual function during the sexual response phases of desire, excitation, and/or orgasm, which is viewed as unsatisfying, unrewarding, or inadequate.

Defining Characteristics

- Alteration in sexual activity
- Alteration in sexual excitation
- Alteration in sexual satisfaction
- Change in interest toward others
- Change in self-interest
- Change in sexual role

- Decrease in sexual desire
- Perceived sexual limitation
- Seeks confirmation of desirability
- Undesired change in sexual function

Related Factors

- Absence of privacy
- Absence of significant other
- Alteration in body function (due to anomaly, disease, medication, pregnancy, radiation, surgery, trauma, etc.)
- Alteration in body structure (due to anomaly, disease, pregnancy, radiation, surgery, trauma, etc.)
- Inadequate role model

- Insufficient knowledge about sexual function
- Misinformation about sexual function
- Presence of abuse (e.g., physical, psychological, sexual)
- Psychosocial abuse (e.g., controlling, manipulation, verbal abuse)
- Value conflict
- Vulnerability

Original literature support available at www.nanda.org

8. Sexuality

00065

Ineffective **sexuality pattern**
(1986, 2006; LOE 2.1)

Definition
Expressions of concern regarding own sexuality.

Defining Characteristics

- Alteration in relationship with significant other
- Alteration in sexual activity
- Alteration in sexual behavior
- Change in sexual role
- Difficulty with sexual activity
- Difficulty with sexual behavior
- Value conflict

Related Factors

- Absence of privacy
- Absence of significant other
- Conflict about sexual orientation
- Conflict about variant preference
- Fear of pregnancy
- Fear of sexually transmitted infection
- Impaired relationship with a significant other
- Inadequate role model
- Insufficient knowledge about alternatives related to sexuality
- Skill deficit about alternatives related to sexuality

Original literature support available at www.nanda.org

00221

Ineffective **childbearing process**
(2010; LOE 2.1)

Definition
Pregnancy and childbirth process and care of the newborn that does not match the environmental context, norms, and expectations.

Defining Characteristics

During Pregnancy
- Inadequate prenatal care
- Inadequate prenatal lifestyle (e.g., elimination, exercise, nutrition, personal hygiene, sleep)
- Inadequate preparation of newborn care items
- Inadequate preparation of the home environment

- Ineffective management of unpleasant symptoms in pregnancy
- Insufficient access of support system
- Insufficient respect for unborn baby
- Unrealistic birth plan

During Labor and Delivery
- Decrease in proactivity during labor and delivery
- Inadequate lifestyle for stage of labor (e.g., elimination, exercise, nutrition, personal hygiene, sleep)

- Inappropriate response to onset of labor
- Insufficient access of support system
- Insufficient attachment behavior

After Birth
- Inadequate baby care techniques
- Inadequate postpartum lifestyle (e.g., elimination, exercise, nutrition, personal hygiene, sleep)
- Inappropriate baby feeding techniques

- Inappropriate breast care
- Insufficient access of support system
- Insufficient attachment behavior
- Unsafe environment for an infant

8. Sexuality

- Domestic violence
- Inconsistent prenatal health visits
- Insufficient knowledge of childbearing process
- Inadequate maternal nutrition
- Insufficient parental role model
- Insufficient prenatal care

- Insufficient support system
- Low maternal confidence
- Maternal powerlessness
- Maternal psychological distress
- Substance abuse
- Unplanned pregnancy
- Unrealistic birth plan
- Unsafe environment
- Unwanted pregnancy

Original literature support available at www.nanda.org

00208

Readiness for enhanced **childbearing process**
(2008, 2013; LOE 2.1)

Definition
A pattern of preparing for and maintaining a healthy pregnancy, child-birth process, and care of the newborn for ensuring well-being, which can be strengthened.

Defining Characteristics

During Pregnancy
- Expresses desire to enhance knowledge of childbearing process
- Expresses desire to enhance management of unpleasant pregnancy symptoms
- Expresses desire to enhance prenatal lifestyle (e.g., elimination, exercise, nutrition, personal hygiene, sleep)
- Expresses desire to enhance preparation for newborn

During Labor and Delivery
- Expresses desire to enhance lifestyle appropriate for stage of labor (e.g., elimination, exercise, nutrition, personal hygiene, sleep)
- Expresses desire to enhance proactivity during labor and delivery

After Birth
- Expresses desire to enhance attachment behavior
- Expresses desire to enhance baby care techniques
- Expresses desire to enhance baby feeding techniques
- Expresses desire to enhance breast care
- Expresses desire to enhance environmental safety for the baby
- Expresses desire to enhance postpartum lifestyle (e.g., elimination, exercise, nutrition, personal hygiene, sleep)
- Expresses desire to enhance use of support system

Original literature support available at www.nanda.org

8. Sexuality

00227

Risk for ineffective **childbearing process**
(2010, 2013; LOE 2.1)

Definition
Vulnerable to not matching environmental context, norms and expectations of pregnancy, childbirth process, and the care of the newborn.

Risk Factors

- Domestic violence
- Inconsistent prenatal health visits
- Insufficient cognitive readiness for parenting
- Insufficient knowledge of childbearing process
- Inadequate maternal nutrition
- Insufficient parental role model
- Insufficient prenatal care
- Insufficient support system
- Low maternal confidence
- Maternal powerlessness
- Maternal psychological distress
- Substance abuse
- Unplanned pregnancy
- Unrealistic birth plan
- Unwanted pregnancy

Original literature support available at www.nanda.org

00209

Risk for disturbed **maternal–fetal dyad**
(2008, 2013; LOE 2.1)

Definition
Vulnerable to disruption of the symbiotic maternal-fetal dyad as a result of comorbid or pregnancy-related conditions, which may compromise health.

Risk Factors

- Alteration in glucose metabolism (e.g., diabetes mellitus, steroid use)
- Compromised fetal oxygen transport (due to anemia, asthma, cardiac disease, hypertension, seizures, premature labor, hemorrhage, etc.)
- Inadequate prenatal care
- Pregnancy complication (e.g., premature rupture of membranes, placenta previa/ abruption, multiple gestation)
- Presence of abuse (e.g., physical, psychological, sexual)
- Substance abuse
- Treatment regimen

Original literature support available at www.nanda.org

8. Sexuality

DOMAIN 9. COPING/STRESS TOLERANCE		
Contending with life events/life processes		

Class 1. Post-trauma responses
Reactions occurring after physical or psychological trauma

Code	Diagnosis	Page
00141	**Post-trauma syndrome**	315
00145	Risk for **post-trauma syndrome**	317
00142	**Rape-trauma syndrome**	318
00114	**Relocation stress syndrome**	319
00149	Risk for **relocation stress syndrome**	320

Class 2. Coping responses
The process of managing environmental stress

Code	Diagnosis	Page
00199	Ineffective **activity planning**	321
00226	Risk for ineffective **activity planning**	322
00146	**Anxiety**	323
00071	Defensive **coping**	325
00069	Ineffective **coping**	326
00158	Readiness for enhanced **coping**	327
00077	Ineffective community **coping**	328
00076	Readiness for enhanced community **coping**	329

NANDA International, Inc. Nursing Diagnoses: Definitions & Classification 2015–2017,
Tenth Edition. Edited by T. Heather Herdman and Shigemi Kamitsuru.
© 2014 NANDA International, Inc. Published 2014 by John Wiley & Sons, Ltd.
Companion website: www.wiley.com/go/nursingdiagnoses

Class 2. Coping responses (continued)

Code	Diagnosis	Page
00074	Compromised family **coping**	330
00073	Disabled family **coping**	332
00075	Readiness for enhanced family **coping**	333
00147	**Death anxiety**	334
00072	Ineffective **denial**	335
00148	**Fear**	336
00136	**Grieving**	338
00135	Complicated **grieving**	339
00172	Risk for complicated **grieving**	340
00241	Impaired **mood regulation**	341
00187	Readiness for enhanced **power**	342
00125	**Power**lessness	343
00152	Risk for **power**lessness	344
00210	Impaired **resilience**	345
00212	Readiness for enhanced **resilience**	346
00211	Risk for impaired **resilience**	347
00137	Chronic **sorrow**	348
00177	**Stress** overload	349

Class 3. Neurobehavioral stress
Behavioral responses reflecting nerve and brain function

Code	Diagnosis	Page
00049	Decreased intracranial **adaptive capacity**	350
00009	**Autonomic dysreflexia**	351
00010	Risk for **autonomic dysreflexia**	352
00116	**Disorganized** infant **behavior**	354
00117	Readiness for enhanced **organized** infant **behavior**	356
00115	Risk for **disorganized** infant **behavior**	357

00141

Post-trauma syndrome
(1986, 1998, 2010; LOE 2.1)

Definition
Sustained maladaptive response to a traumatic, overwhelming event.

Defining Characteristics

- Aggression
- Alienation
- Alteration in concentration
- Alteration in mood
- Anger
- Anxiety
- Avoidance behaviors
- Compulsive behavior
- Denial
- Depression
- Dissociative amnesia
- Enuresis
- Exaggerated startle response
- Fear
- Flashbacks
- Gastrointestinal irritation
- Grieving
- Guilt
- Headache
- Heart palpitations
- History of detachment
- Hopelessness
- Horror
- Hypervigilence
- Intrusive dreams
- Intrusive thoughts
- Irritability
- Neurosensory irritability
- Nightmares
- Panic attacks
- Rage
- Reports feeling numb
- Repression
- Shame
- Substance abuse

Related Factors

- Destruction of one's home
- Event outside the range of usual human experience
- Exposure to disaster (natural or man-made)
- Exposure to epidemic
- Exposure to event involving multiple deaths
- Exposure to war
- History of abuse (e.g., physical, psychological, sexual)
- History of being a prisoner of war

- History of criminal victimization
- History of torture
- Self-injurious behavior
- Serious accident (e.g., industrial, motor vehicle)
- Serious injury to loved one
- Serious threat to loved one
- Serious threat to self
- Witnessing mutilation
- Witnessing violent death

9. Coping/Stress Tolerance

00145

Risk for **post-trauma syndrome**
(1998, 2013)

Definition
Vulnerable to sustained maladaptive response to a traumatic, over-whelming event, which may compromise health.

Risk Factors

- Diminished ego strength
- Displacement from home
- Duration of traumatic event
- Environment not conducive to needs
- Exaggerated sense of responsibility
- Human service occupations (e.g., police, fire, rescue, corrections, emergency room, mental health)
- Insufficient social support
- Perceives event as traumatic
- Survivor role

00142

Rape-trauma syndrome
(1980, 1998)

Definition
Sustained maladaptive response to a forced, violent, sexual penetration against the victim's will and consent.

Defining Characteristics

- Aggression
- Agitation
- Alteration in sleep pattern
- Anger
- Anxiety
- Change in relationship(s)
- Confusion
- Denial
- Dependency
- Depression
- Disorganization
- Dissociative identity disorder
- Embarrassment
- Fear
- Guilt
- Helplessness
- History of suicide attempt
- Humiliation
- Hyperalertness
- Impaired decision-making
- Low self-esteem
- Mood swings
- Muscle spasm
- Muscle tension
- Nightmares
- Paranoia
- Perceived vulnerability
- Phobias
- Physical trauma
- Powerlessness
- Self-blame
- Sexual dysfunction
- Shame
- Shock
- Substance abuse
- Thoughts of revenge

Related Factors

- Rape

00114

Relocation stress syndrome
(1992, 2000)

Definition
Physiological and/or psychosocial disturbance following transfer from one environment to another.

Defining Characteristics

- Alienation
- Aloneness
- Alteration in sleep pattern
- Anger
- Anxiety
- Concern about relocation
- Dependency
- Depression
- Fear
- Frustration
- Increase in illness
- Increase in physical symptoms
- Increase in verbalization of needs
- Insecurity
- Loneliness
- Loss of identity
- Loss of self-worth
- Low self-esteem
- Pessimism
- Unwillingness to move
- Withdrawal
- Worried

Related Factors

- Compromised health status
- History of loss
- Impaired psychosocial functioning
- Ineffective coping strategies
- Insufficient predeparture counseling
- Insufficient support system
- Language barrier
- Move from one environment to another
- Powerlessness
- Social isolation
- Unpredictability of experience

9. Coping/Stress Tolerance

00149

Risk for **relocation stress syndrome**
(2000, 2013)

Definition
Vulnerable to physiological and/or psychosocial disturbance following transfer from one environment to another that may compromise health.

Risk Factors

- Compromised health status
- Deficient mental competence
- History of loss
- Ineffective coping strategies
- Insufficient predeparture counseling
- Insufficient support system
- Move from one environment to another
- Powerlessness
- Significant environmental change
- Unpredictability of experience

00199

Ineffective **activity planning**
(2008; LOE 2.2)

Definition
Inability to prepare for a set of actions fixed in time and under certain conditions.

Defining Characteristics

- Absence of plan
- Excessive anxiety about a task to be undertaken
- Fear about a task to be undertaken
- Insufficient organizational skills
- Insufficient resources (e.g., financial, social, knowledge)
- Pattern of failure
- Pattern of procrastination
- Unmet goals for chosen activity
- Worried about a task to be undertaken

Related Factors

- Flight behavior when faced with proposed solution
- Hedonism
- Insufficient information-processing ability
- Insufficient social support
- Unrealistic perception of event
- Unrealistic perception of personal abilities

Original literature support available at www.nanda.org

9. Coping/Stress Tolerance

00226

Risk for ineffective **activity planning**
(2010, 2013; LOE 2.1)

Definition
Vulnerable to an inability to prepare for a set of actions fixed in time and under certain conditions, which may compromise health.

Risk Factors

- Flight behavior when faced with proposed solution
- Hedonism
- Insufficient information processing ability
- Insufficient social support
- Pattern of procrastination
- Unrealistic perception of event
- Unrealistic perception of personal abilities

Original literature support available at www.nanda.org

00146

Anxiety
(1973, 1982, 1998)

Definition
Vague, uneasy feeling of discomfort or dread accompanied by an autonomic response (the source is often nonspecific or unknown to the individual); a feeling of apprehension caused by anticipation of danger. It is an alerting sign that warns of impending danger and enables the individual to take measures to deal with that threat.

Defining Characteristics

Behavioral

- Decrease in productivity
- Extraneous movement
- Fidgeting
- Glancing about
- Hypervigilence
- Insomnia
- Poor eye contact
- Restlessness
- Scanning behavior
- Worried about change in life event

Affective

- Anguish
- Apprehensiveness
- Distress
- Fear
- Feeling of inadequacy
- Helplessness
- Increase in wariness
- Irritability
- Jitteriness
- Overexcitement
- Rattled
- Regretful
- Self-focused
- Uncertainty
- Worried

Physiological

- Facial tension
- Hand tremors
- Increase in perspiration
- Increase in tension
- Shakiness
- Trembling
- Voice quivering

9. Coping/Stress Tolerance

Sympathetic
- Alteration in respiratory pattern
- Anorexia
- Brisk reflexes
- Cardiovascular excitation
- Diarrhea
- Dry mouth
- Facial flushing
- Heart palpitations
- Increase in blood pressure
- Increase in heart rate
- Increase in respiratory rate
- Pupil dilation
- Superficial vasoconstriction
- Twitching
- Weakness

Parasympathetic
- Abdominal pain
- Alteration in sleep pattern
- Decrease in heart rate
- Decreased blood pressure
- Diarrhea
- Faintness
- Fatigue
- Nausea
- Tingling in extremities
- Urinary frequency
- Urinary hesitancy
- Urinary urgency

Cognitive
- Alteration in attention
- Alteration in concentration
- Awareness of physiological symptoms
- Blocking of thoughts
- Confusion
- Decrease in perceptual field
- Diminished ability to learn
- Diminished ability to problem-solve
- Fear
- Forgetfulness
- Preoccupation
- Rumination
- Tendency to blame others

Related Factors

- Conflict about life goals
- Exposure to toxin
- Family history of anxiety
- Heredity
- Interpersonal contagion
- Interpersonal transmission
- Major change (e.g., economic status, environment, health status, role function, role status)
- Maturational crisis
- Situational crisis
- Stressors
- Substance abuse
- Threat of death
- Threat to current status
- Unmet needs
- Value conflict

00071

Defensive **coping**
(1988, 2008; LOE 2.1)

Definition
Repeated projection of falsely positive self-evaluation based on a self-protective pattern that defends against underlying perceived threats to positive self-regard.

Defining Characteristics

- Alteration in reality testing
- Denial of problems
- Denial of weaknesses
- Difficulty establishing relationships
- Difficulty maintaining relationship(s)
- Grandiosity
- Hostile laughter
- Hypersensitivity to a discourtesy
- Hypersensitivity to criticism
- Insufficient follow through with treatment
- Insufficient participation in treatment
- Projection of blame
- Projection of responsibility
- Rationalization of failures
- Reality distortion
- Ridicule of others
- Superior attitude toward others

Related Factors

- Conflict between self-perception and value system
- Fear of failure
- Fear of humiliation
- Fear of repercussions
- Insufficient confidence in others
- Insufficient resilience
- Insufficient self-confidence
- Insufficient support system
- Uncertainty
- Unrealistic self-expectations

Original literature support available at www.nanda.org

9. Coping/Stress Tolerance

00069

Ineffective **coping**
(1978, 1998)

Definition
Inability to form a valid appraisal of the stressors, inadequate choices of practiced responses, and/or inability to use available resources.

Defining Characteristics

- Alteration in concentration
- Alteration in sleep pattern
- Change in communication pattern
- Destructive behavior toward others
- Destructive behavior toward self
- Difficulty organizing information
- Fatigue
- Frequent illness
- Inability to ask for help
- Inability to attend to information
- Inability to deal with a situation
- Inability to meet basic needs
- Inability to meet role expectation
- Ineffective coping strategies
- Insufficient access of social support
- Insufficient goal-directed behavior
- Insufficient problem resolution
- Insufficient problem-solving skills
- Risk-taking behavior
- Substance abuse

Related Factors

- Gender differences in coping strategies
- High degree of threat
- Inability to conserve adaptive energies
- Inaccurate threat appraisal
- Inadequate confidence in ability to deal with a situation
- Inadequate opportunity to prepare for stressor
- Inadequate resources
- Ineffective tension release strategies
- Insufficient sense of control
- Insufficient social support
- Maturational crisis
- Situational crisis
- Uncertainty

00158

Readiness for enhanced **coping**
(2002, 2013; LOE 2.1)

Definition
A pattern of cognitive and behavioral efforts to manage demands related to well-being, which can be strengthened.

Defining Characteristics

- Awareness of possible environmental change
- Expresses desire to enhance knowledge of stress management strategies
- Expresses desire to enhance management of stressors
- Expresses desire to enhance social support
- Expresses desire to enhance use of emotion-oriented strategies
- Expresses desire to enhance use of problem-oriented strategies
- Expresses desire to enhance use of spiritual resource

9. Coping/Stress Tolerance

00077

Ineffective community **coping**
(1994, 1998)

Definition
A pattern of community activities for adaptation and problem-solving that is unsatisfactory for meeting the demands or needs of the community.

Defining Characteristics

- Community does not meet expectations of its members
- Deficient community participation
- Elevated community illness rate
- Excessive community conflict
- Excessive stress
- High incidence of community problems (e.g., homicides, vandalism, terrorism, robbery, abuse, unemployment, poverty, militancy, mental illness)
- Perceived community powerlessness
- Perceived community vulnerability

Related Factors

- Exposure to disaster (natural or man-made)
- History of disaster (e.g., natural, man-made)
- Inadequate resources for problem-solving
- Insufficient community resources (e.g., respite, recreation, social support)
- Nonexistent community systems

00076

Readiness for enhanced community **coping**
(1994, 2013)

Definition
A pattern of community activities for adaptation and problem-solving for meeting the demands or needs of the community, which can be strengthened.

Defining Characteristics

- Expresses desire to enhance availability of community recreation programs
- Expresses desire to enhance availability of community relaxation programs
- Expresses desire to enhance communication among community members
- Expresses desire to enhance communication between aggregates and larger community
- Expresses desire to enhance community planning for predictable stressors
- Expresses desire to enhance community resources for managing stressors
- Expresses desire to enhance community responsibility for stress management
- Expresses desire to enhance problem-solving for identified issue

9. Coping/Stress Tolerance

00074

Compromised family coping
(1980, 1996)

Definition

A usually supportive primary person (family member, significant other, or close friend) provides insufficient, ineffective, or compromised support, comfort, assistance, or encouragement that may be needed by the client to manage or master adaptive tasks related to his or her health challenge.

Defining Characteristics

- Assistive behaviors by support person produce unsatisfactory results
- Client complaint about support person's response to health problem
- Client concern about support person's response to health problem
- Limitation in communication between support person and client
- Protective behavior by support person incongruent with client's abilities
- Protective behavior by support person incongruent with client's need for autonomy
- Support person reports inadequate understanding that interferes with effective behaviors
- Support person reports insufficient knowledge that interferes with effective behaviors
- Support person reports preoccupation with own reaction to client's need
- Support person withdraws from client

Related Factors

- Coexisting situations affecting the support person
- Developmental crisis experienced by support person
- Exhaustion of support person's capacity
- Family disorganization
- Family role change
- Insufficient information available to support person
- Insufficient reciprocal support
- Insufficient support given by client to support person
- Insufficient understanding of information by support person
- Misinformation obtained by support person
- Misunderstanding of information by support person
- Preoccupation by support person with concern outside of family
- Prolonged disease that exhausts capacity of support person
- Situational crisis faced by support person

9. Coping/Stress Tolerance

00073

Disabled family coping
(1980, 1996, 2008; LOE 2.1)

Definition
Behavior of primary person (family member, significant other, or close friend) that disables his or her capacities and the client's capacities to effectively address tasks essential to either person's adaptation to the health challenge.

Defining Characteristics

- Abandonment
- Adopts illness symptoms of client
- Aggression
- Agitation
- Client dependence
- Depression
- Desertion
- Disregard for client's needs
- Distortion of reality about client's health problem
- Family behaviors detrimental to well-being
- Hostility
- Impaired ability to structure a meaningful life
- Impaired individualism
- Intolerance
- Neglect of basic needs of client
- Neglect of relationship with family member
- Neglect of treatment regimen
- Performing routines without regard for client's needs
- Prolonged hyperfocus on client
- Psychosomatic symptoms
- Rejection

Related Factors

- Ambivalent family relationships
- Chronically unexpressed feelings by support person
- Differing coping styles between support person and client
- Differing coping styles between support persons
- Inconsistent management of family's resistance to treatment

00075

Readiness for enhanced family **coping**
(1980, 2013)

Definition

A pattern of management of adaptive tasks by primary person (family member, significant other, or close friend) involved with the client's health change, which can be strengthened.

Defining Characteristics

- Expresses desire to acknowledge growth impact of crisis
- Expresses desire to choose experiences that optimize wellness
- Expresses desire to enhance connection with others who have experienced a similar situation
- Expresses desire to enhance enrichment of lifestyle
- Expresses desire to enhance health promotion

9. Coping/Stress Tolerance

00147

Death anxiety
(1998, 2006; LOE 2.1)

Definition
Vague, uneasy feeling of discomfort or dread generated by perceptions of a real or imagined threat to one's existence.

Defining Characteristics

- Concern about strain on the caregiver
- Deep sadness
- Fear of developing terminal illness
- Fear of loss of mental abilities when dying
- Fear of pain related to dying
- Fear of premature death
- Fear of prolonged dying process
- Fear of suffering related to dying
- Fear of the dying process
- Negative thoughts related to death and dying
- Powerlessness
- Worried about the impact of one's death on significant other

Related Factors

- Anticipation of adverse consequences of anesthesia
- Anticipation of impact of death on others
- Anticipation of pain
- Anticipation of suffering
- Confronting the reality of terminal disease
- Discussions on the topic of death
- Experiencing dying process
- Near-death experience
- Nonacceptance of own mortality
- Observations related to death
- Perceived imminence of death
- Uncertainty about encountering a higher power
- Uncertainty about life after death
- Uncertainty about the existence of a higher power
- Uncertainty of prognosis

Original literature support available at www.nanda.org

9. Coping/Stress Tolerance

00072

Ineffective **denial**
(1988, 2006; LOE 2.1)

Definition
Conscious or unconscious attempt to disavow the knowledge or meaning of an event to reduce anxiety and/or fear, leading to the detriment of health.

Defining Characteristics

- Delay in seeking healthcare
- Denies fear of death
- Denies fear of invalidism
- Displaces fear of impact of the condition
- Displaces source of symptoms
- Does not admit impact of disease on life
- Does not perceive relevance of danger
- Does not perceive relevance of symptoms
- Inappropriate affect
- Minimizes symptoms
- Refusal of healthcare
- Use of dismissive gestures when speaking of distressing event
- Use of dismissive comments when speaking of distressing event
- Use of treatment not advised by healthcare professional

Related Factors

- Anxiety
- Excessive stress
- Fear of death
- Fear of losing autonomy
- Fear of separation
- Ineffective coping strategies
- Insufficient emotional support
- Insufficient sense of control
- Perceived inadequacy in dealing with strong emotions
- Threat of unpleasant reality

Original literature support available at www.nanda.org

9. Coping/Stress Tolerance

00148

Fear
(1980, 1996, 2000)

Definition
Response to perceived threat that is consciously recognized as a danger.

Defining Characteristics

- Apprehensiveness
- Decrease in self-assurance
- Excitedness
- Feeling dread
- Feeling of fear
- Feeling of panic
- Feeling of terror
- Feeling of alarm

- Increase in blood pressure
- Increase in tension
- Jitteriness
- Muscle tension
- Nausea
- Pallor
- Pupil dilation
- Vomiting

Cognitive
- Decrease in learning ability
- Decrease in problem-solving ability
- Decrease in productivity

- Identifies object of fear
- Stimulus believed to be a threat

Behaviors
- Attack behaviors
- Avoidance behaviors
- Focus narrowed to the source of fear

- Impulsiveness
- Increase in alertness

Physiological
- Anorexia
- Change in physiological response (e.g., blood pressure, heart rate, respiratory rate, oxygen saturation, and end-tital CO_2)

- Diarrhea
- Dry mouth
- Dyspnea
- Fatigue
- Increase in perspiration
- Increase in respiratory rate

9. Coping/Stress Tolerance

Related Factors

- Innate releasing mechanism to external stimuli (e.g., neurotransmitters)
- Innate response to stimuli (e.g., sudden noise, height)
- Language barrier
- Learned response
- Phobic stimulus
- Sensory deficit (e.g., visual, hearing)
- Separation from support system
- Unfamiliar setting

00136

Grieving
(1980, 1996, 2006; LOE 2.1)

Definition
A normal complex process that includes emotional, physical, spiritual, social, and intellectual responses and behaviors by which individuals, families, and communities incorporate an actual, anticipated, or perceived loss into their daily lives.

Defining Characteristics

- Alteration in activity level
- Alteration in dream pattern
- Alteration in immune functioning
- Alteration in neuroendocrine functioning
- Alteration in sleep pattern
- Anger
- Blaming
- Despair
- Detachment
- Disorganization
- Finding meaning in a loss
- Guilt about feeling relieved
- Maintaining a connection to the deceased
- Pain
- Panic behavior
- Personal growth
- Psychological distress
- Suffering

Related Factors

- Anticipatory loss of significant object (e.g., possession, job, status)
- Anticipatory loss of significant other
- Death of significant other
- Loss of significant object (e.g., possession, job, status, home, body part)

Original literature support available at www.nanda.org

00135

Complicated **grieving**
(1980, 1986, 2004, 2006; LOE 2.1)

Definition
A disorder that occurs after the death of a significant other, in which the experience of distress accompanying bereavement fails to follow normative expectations and manifests in functional impairment.

Defining Characteristics

- Anger
- Anxiety
- Avoidance of grieving
- Decrease in functioning in life roles
- Depression
- Disbelief
- Distress about the deceased person
- Excessive stress
- Experiencing symptoms the deceased experienced
- Fatigue
- Feeling dazed
- Feeling of detachment from others
- Feeling of shock
- Feeling stunned
- Feelings of emptiness
- Insufficient sense of well-being
- Longing for the deceased person
- Low levels of intimacy
- Mistrust
- Nonacceptance of a death
- Persistent painful memories
- Preoccupation with thoughts about a deceased person
- Rumination
- Searching for a deceased person
- Self-blame
- Separation distress
- Traumatic distress
- Yearning for deceased person

Related Factors

- Death of significant other
- Emotional disturbance
- Insufficient social support

Original literature support available at www.nanda.org

9. Coping/Stress Tolerance

00172

Risk for complicated **grieving**
(2004, 2006, 2013; LOE 2.1)

Definition
Vulnerable to a disorder that occurs after death of a significant other in which the experience of distress accompanying bereavement fails to follow normative expectations and manifests in functional impairment, which may compromise health.

Risk Factors

- Death of significant other
- Emotional disturbance
- Insufficient social support

Original literature support available at www.nanda.org

00241

Impaired **mood regulation**
(2013; LOE 2.1)

Definition

A mental state characterized by shifts in mood or affect and which is comprised of a constellation of affective, cognitive, somatic, and/or physiological manifestations varying from mild to severe.

Defining Characteristics

- Changes in verbal behavior
- Disinhibition
- Dysphoria
- Excessive guilt
- Excessive self-awareness
- Excessive self-blame
- Flight of thoughts
- Hopelessness
- Impaired concentration
- Influenced self-esteem
- Irritability
- Psychomotor agitation
- Psychomotor retardation
- Sad affect
- Withdrawal

Related Factors

- Alteration in sleep pattern
- Anxiety
- Appetite change
- Chronic illness
- Functional impairment
- Hypervigilance
- Impaired social functioning
- Loneliness
- Pain
- Psychosis
- Recurrent thoughts of death
- Recurrent thoughts of suicide
- Social isolation
- Substance misuse
- Weight change

Original literature support available at www.nanda.org

00187

Readiness for enhanced **power**
(2006, 2013; LOE 2.1)

Definition

A pattern of participating knowingly in change for well-being, which can be strengthened.

Defining Characteristics

- Expresses desire to enhance awareness of possible changes
- Expresses desire to enhance identification of choices that can be made for change
- Expresses desire to enhance independence with actions for change
- Expresses desire to enhance involvement in change
- Expresses desire to enhance knowledge for participation in change
- Expresses desire to enhance participation in choices for daily living
- Expresses desire to enhance participation in choices for health
- Expresses desire to enhance power

Original literature support available at www.nanda.org

00125

Powerlessness
(1982, 2010; LOE 2.1)

Definition
The lived experience of lack of control over a situation, including a perception that one's actions do not significantly affect an outcome.

Defining Characteristics

- Alienation
- Dependency
- Depression
- Doubt about role performance
- Frustration about inability to perform previous activities
- Inadequate participation in care
- Insufficient sense of control
- Shame

Related Factors

- Complex treatment regimen
- Dysfunctional institutional environment
- Insufficient interpersonal interactions

Original literature support available at www.nanda.org

00152

Risk for **power**lessness
(2000, 2010, 2013; LOE 2.1)

Definition
Vulnerable to the lived experience of lack of control over a situation, including apperception that one's actions do not significantly affect the outcome, which may compromise health.

Risk Factors

- Anxiety
- Caregiver role
- Economically disadvantaged
- Illness
- Ineffective coping strategies
- Insufficient knowledge to manage a situation
- Insufficient social support

- Low self-esteem
- Pain
- Progressive illness
- Social marginalization
- Stigmatization
- Unpredictability of illness trajectory

Original literature support available at www.nanda.org

00210

Impaired **resilience**
(2008, 2013; LOE 2.1)

Definition
Decreased ability to sustain a pattern of positive responses to an adverse situation or crisis.

Defining Characteristics

- Decrease interest in academic activities
- Decrease interest in vocational activities
- Depression
- Guilt
- Impaired health status
- Ineffective coping strategies
- Low self-esteem
- Renewed elevation of distress
- Shame
- Social isolation

Related Factors

- Community violence
- Demographics that increase chance of maladjustment
- Economically disadvantaged
- Ethnic minority status
- Exposure to violence
- Female gender
- Inconsistent parenting
- Insufficient impulse control
- Large family size
- Low intellectual ability
- Low maternal educational level
- Parental mental illness
- Perceived vulnerability
- Psychological disorder
- Substance abuse

Original literature support available at www.nanda.org

00212

Readiness for enhanced **resilience**
(2008, 2013; LOE 2.1)

Definition

A pattern of positive responses to an adverse situation or crisis, which can be strengthened.

Defining Characteristics

- Demonstrates positive outlook
- Exposure to a crisis
- Expresses desire to enhance available resources
- Expresses desire to enhance communication skills
- Expresses desire to enhance environmental safety
- Expresses desire to enhance goal-setting
- Expresses desire to enhance involvement in activities
- Expresses desire to enhance own responsibility for action
- Expresses desire to enhance progress toward goal
- Expresses desire to enhance relationships with others
- Expresses desire to enhance resilience
- Expresses desire to enhance self-esteem
- Expresses desire to enhance sense of control
- Expresses desire to enhance support system
- Expresses desire to enhance use of conflict management strategies
- Expresses desire to enhance use of coping skills
- Expresses desire to enhance use of resource

Original literature support available at www.nanda.org

00211

Risk for impaired **resilience**
(2008, 2013; LOE 2.1)

___

Definition
Vulnerable to decreased ability to sustain a pattern of positive response to an adverse situation or crisis, which may compromise health.

Risk Factors

- Chronicity of existing crisis
- Multiple coexisting adverse situations
- New crisis (e.g., unplanned pregnancy, loss of housing, death of family member)

Original literature support available at www.nanda.org

00137

Chronic **sorrow**
(1998)

Definition
Cyclical, recurring, and potentially progressive pattern of pervasive sadness experienced (by a parent, caregiver, individual with chronic illness or disability) in response to continual loss, throughout the trajectory of an illness or disability.

Defining Characteristics

- Feelings that interfere with well-being (e.g., personal, social)
- Overwhelming negative feelings
- Sadness (e.g., periodic, recurrent)

Related Factors

- Chronic disability (e.g., physical, mental)
- Chronic illness
- Crisis in disability management
- Crisis in illness management
- Crisis related to developmental stage
- Death of significant other
- Length of time as a caregiver
- Missed milestones
- Missed opportunities

00177

Stress overload
(2006; LOE 3.2)

Definition
Excessive amounts and types of demands that require action.

Defining Characteristics

- Excessive stress
- Feeling of pressure
- Impaired decision-making
- Impaired functioning
- Increase in anger
- Increase in anger behavior
- Increase in impatience
- Negative impact from stress (e.g., physical symptoms, psychological distress, feeling sick)
- Tension

Related Factors

- Excessive stress
- Insufficient resources (e.g., financial, social, knowledge)
- Repeated stressors
- Stressors

Original literature support available at www.nanda.org

00049

Decreased intracranial **adaptive capacity**
(1994)

Definition
Intracranial fluid dynamic mechanisms that normally compensate for increases in intracranial volumes are compromised, resulting in repeated disproportionate increases in intracranial pressure (ICP) in response to a variety of noxious and non-noxious stimuli.

Defining Characteristics

- Baseline intracranial pressure (ICP) ≥ 10 mmHg
- Disproportionate increase in intracranial pressure (ICP) following stimuli
- Elevated P2 ICP waveform
- Repeated increase in intracranial pressure (ICP) ≥ 10 mmHg for ≥ 5 minutes following external stimuli
- Volume-pressure response test variation (volume: pressure ratio 2, pressure-volume index < 10)
- Wide-amplitude ICP waveform

Related Factors

- Brain injury (e.g., cerebrovascular impairment, neurological illness, trauma, tumor)
- Decreased cerebral perfusion ≥ 50–60 mmHg
- Sustained increase in intracranial pressure (ICP) of 10–15 mmHg
- Systemic hypotension with intracranial hypertension

00009

Autonomic dysreflexia
(1988)

Definition
Life-threatening, uninhibited sympathetic response of the nervous system to a noxious stimulus after a spinal cord injury at T7 or above.

Defining Characteristics

- Blurred vision
- Bradycardia
- Chest pain
- Chilling
- Conjunctival congestion
- Diaphoresis (above the injury)
- Headache (diffuse pain in different areas of the head and not confined to any nerve distribution area)
- Horner's syndrome
- Metallic taste in mouth
- Nasal congestion
- Pallor (below injury)
- Paresthesia
- Paroxysmal hypertension
- Pilomotor reflex
- Red blotches on skin (above the injury)
- Tachycardia

Related Factors

- Bladder distention
- Bowel distention
- Insufficient caregiver knowledge of disease process
- Insufficient knowledge of disease process
- Skin irritation

00010

Risk for **autonomic dysreflexia**
(1998, 2000, 2013)

Definition

Vulnerable to life-threatening, uninhibited response of the sympathetic nervous system post-spinal shock, in an individual with spinal cord injury or lesion at T6 or above (has been demonstrated in patients with injuries at T7 and T8), which may compromise health.

Risk Factors

Cardiopulmonary Stimuli
  Deep vein thrombosis   Pulmonary emboli

Gastrointestinal Stimuli
  Bowel distention   Gallstones
  Constipation   Gastric ulcer
  Difficult passage of feces   Gastrointestinal system
  Digital stimulation   pathology
  Enemas   Hemorrhoids
  Esophageal reflux disease   Suppositories
  Fecal impaction

Musculoskeletal-Integumentary Stimuli
  Cutaneous stimulation   Pressure over genitalia
  (e.g., pressure ulcer, ingrown   Range of motion exercises
  toenail, dressings, burns, rash)   Spasm
  Fracture   Sunburn
  Heterotopic bone   Wound
  Pressure over bony
  prominence

Neurological Stimuli
  Irritating stimuli below level   Painful stimuli below level
  of injury   of injury

Regulatory Stimuli
- Extremes of environmental temperature
- Temperature fluctuations

Reproductive Stimuli
- Ejaculation
- Labor and delivery period
- Menstruation
- Ovarian cyst
- Pregnancy
- Sexual intercourse

Situational Stimuli
- Constrictive clothing (e.g., straps, stockings, shoes)
- Pharmaceutical agent
- Positioning
- Substance withdrawal (e.g., narcotic, opiate)
- Surgical procedure

Urological Stimuli
- Bladder distention
- Bladder spasm
- Cystitis
- Detrusor sphincter dyssynergia
- Epididymitis
- Instrumentation
- Renal calculi
- Surgical procedure
- Urethritis
- Urinary catheterization
- Urinary tract infection

00116

Disorganized infant behavior
(1994, 1998)

Definition
Disintegrated physiological and neurobehavioral responses of infant to the environment.

Defining Characteristics

Attention-Interaction System
- Impaired response to sensory stimuli (e.g., difficult to soothe, unable to sustain alertness)

Motor System
- Alteration in primitive reflexes
- Exaggerated startle response
- Finger splaying
- Fisting
- Hands to face
- Hyperextension of extremities
- Impaired motor tone
- Jitteriness
- Tremor
- Twitching
- Uncoordinated movement

Physiological
- Abnormal skin color (e.g., pale, dusky, cyanosis)
- Arrhythmia
- Bradycardia
- Desaturation
- Feeding intolerance
- Tachycardia
- Time-out signals (e.g., gaze, hiccough, sneeze, slack jaw, open mouth, tongue thrust)

Regulatory Problems
- Inability to inhibit startle reflex
- Irritability

State-Organization System
- Active-awake (e.g., fussy, worried gaze)
- Diffuse alpha EEG activity with eyes closed
- Irritable crying
- Quiet-awake (e.g., staring, gaze aversion)
- State oscillation

Related Factors

Caregiver
- Cue misreading
- Environmental overstimulation
- Insufficient knowledge of behavioral cues

Environmental
- Inadequate physical environment
- Insufficient containment within environment
- Insufficient sensory stimulation
- Sensory deprivation
- Sensory overstimulation

Individual
- Illness
- Immature neurological functioning
- Low postconceptual age
- Prematurity

Postnatal
- Feeding intolerance
- Impaired motor functioning
- Invasive procedure
- Malnutrition
- Oral impairment
- Pain

Prenatal
- Congenital disorder
- Exposure to teratogen
- Genetic disorder

00117

Readiness for enhanced **organized** infant **behavior**
(1994, 2013)

Definition
A pattern of modulation of the physiological and behavioral systems of functioning (i.e., autonomic, motor, state-organization, self-regulatory, and attentional-interactional systems) in an infant, which can be strengthened.

Defining Characteristics

- Parent expresses desire to enhance cue recognition

- Parent expresses desire to enhance recognition of infant's self-regulatory behaviors

00115

Risk for **disorganized** infant **behavior**
(1994, 2013)

Definition
Vulnerable to alteration in integration and modulation of the physiological and behavioral systems of functioning (i.e., autonomic, motor, state-organization, self-regulatory, and attentional-interactional systems), which may compromise health.

Risk Factors

- Impaired motor functioning
- Insufficient containment within environment
- Invasive procedure
- Oral impairment
- Pain
- Parent expresses desire to enhance environmental conditions
- Prematurity
- Procedure

Domain 10
Life Principles

DOMAIN 10. LIFE PRINCIPLES		
Principles underlying conduct, thought, and behavior about acts, customs, or institutions viewed as being true or having intrinsic worth		
Class 1. Values *The identification and ranking of preferred modes of conduct or end states*		
Code	**Diagnosis**	**Page**
None at this time		
Class 2. Beliefs *Opinions, expectations, or judgments about acts, customs, or institutions viewed as being true or having intrinsic worth*		
Code	**Diagnosis**	**Page**
00068	Readiness for enhanced **spiritual well-being**	361
Class 3. Value/Belief/Action Congruence *The correspondence or balance achieved among values, beliefs, and actions*		
Code	**Diagnosis**	**Page**
00184	Readiness for enhanced **decision-making**	363
00083	**Decisional conflict**	364
00242	Impaired **emancipated decision-making**	365

NANDA International, Inc. Nursing Diagnoses: Definitions & Classification 2015–2017, Tenth Edition. Edited by T. Heather Herdman and Shigemi Kamitsuru.
© 2014 NANDA International, Inc. Published 2014 by John Wiley & Sons, Ltd.
Companion website: www.wiley.com/go/nursingdiagnoses

Class 3. Value/Belief/Action Congruence (continued)		
Code	**Diagnosis**	**Page**
00243	Readiness for enhanced **emancipated decision-making**	366
00244	Risk for impaired **emancipated decision-making**	367
00175	**Moral distress**	368
00169	Impaired **religiosity**	369
00171	Readiness for enhanced **religiosity**	370
00170	Risk for impaired **religiosity**	371
00066	**Spiritual** distress	372
00067	Risk for **spiritual** distress	374

00068

Readiness for enhanced **spiritual well-being**
(1994, 2002, 2013; LOE 2.1)

Definition
A pattern of experiencing and integrating meaning and purpose in life through connectedness with self, others, art, music, literature, nature, and/or a power greater than oneself, which can be strengthened.

Defining Characteristics

Connections to Self
- Expresses desire to enhance acceptance
- Expresses desire to enhance coping
- Expresses desire to enhance courage
- Expresses desire to enhance hope
- Expresses desire to enhance joy
- Expresses desire to enhance love
- Expresses desire to enhance meaning in life
- Expresses desire to enhance meditative practice
- Expresses desire to enhance purpose in life
- Expresses desire to enhance satisfaction with philosophy of life
- Expresses desire to enhance self-forgiveness
- Expresses desire to enhance serenity (e.g., peace)
- Expresses desire to enhance surrender

Connections with Others
- Expresses desire to enhance forgiveness from others
- Expresses desire to enhance interaction with significant other
- Expresses desire to enhance interaction with spiritual leaders
- Expresses desire to enhance service to others

Connections with Art, Music, Literature, and Nature
- Expresses desire to enhance creative energy (e.g., writing, poetry, music)
- Expresses desire to enhance spiritual reading
- Expresses desire to enhance time outdoors

10. Life Principles

Connections with Power Greater than Self

- Expresses desire to enhance mystical experiences
- Expresses desire to enhance participation in religious activity

- Expresses desire to enhance prayerfulness
- Expresses desire to enhance reverence

00184

Readiness for enhanced **decision-making**
(2006, 2013; LOE 2.1)

Definition
A pattern of choosing a course of action for meeting short- and long-term health-related goals, which can be strengthened.

Defining Characteristics

- Expresses desire to enhance congruency of decisions with sociocultural goal
- Expresses desire to enhance congruency of decisions with sociocultural values
- Expresses desire to enhance congruency of decisions with goal
- Expresses desire to enhance congruency of decisions with values
- Expresses desire to enhance decision-making
- Expresses desire to enhance risk-benefit analysis of decisions
- Expresses desire to enhance understanding of choices for decision-making
- Expresses desire to enhance understanding of meaning of choices
- Expresses desire to enhance use of reliable evidence for decisions

Original literature support available at www.nanda.org

10. Life Principles

00083

Decisional conflict
(1988, 2006; LOE 2.1)

Definition

Uncertainty about course of action to be taken when choice among competing actions involves risk, loss, or challenge to values and beliefs.

Defining Characteristics

- Delay in decision-making
- Distress while attempting a decision
- Physical sign of distress (e.g., increase in heart rate, restlessness)
- Physical sign of tension
- Questioning of moral principle while attempting a decision
- Questioning of moral rule while attempting a decision
- Questioning of moral values while attempting a decision
- Questioning of personal beliefs while attempting a decision
- Questioning of personal values while attempting a decision
- Recognizes undesired consequences of actions being considered
- Self-focused
- Uncertainty about choices
- Vacillating among choices

Related Factors

- Conflict with moral obligation
- Conflicting information sources
- Inexperience with decision-making
- Insufficient information
- Insufficient support system
- Interference in decision-making
- Moral principle supports mutually inconsistent actions
- Moral rule supports mutually inconsistent actions
- Moral value supports mutually inconsistent actions
- Perceived threat to value system
- Unclear personal beliefs
- Unclear personal values

Original literature support available at www.nanda.org

00242

Impaired emancipated decision-making
(2013; LOE 2.1)

Definition
A process of choosing a healthcare decision that does not include personal knowledge and/or consideration of social norms, or does not occur in a flexible environment, resulting in decisional dissatisfaction.

Defining Characteristics

- Delay in enacting chosen healthcare option
- Distress when listening to other's opinion
- Excessive concern about what others think is the best decision
- Excessive fear of what others think about a decision
- Feeling constrained in describing own opinion
- Inability to choose a healthcare option that best fits current lifestyle
- Inability to describe how option will fit into current lifestyle
- Limited verbalization about healthcare option in other's presence

Related Factors

- Decrease in understanding of all available healthcare options
- Inability to adequately verbalize perceptions about healthcare options
- Inadequate time to discuss healthcare options
- Insufficient privacy to openly discuss healthcare options
- Limited decision-making experience
- Traditional hierarchical family
- Traditional hierarchical healthcare system

Original literature support available at www.nanda.org

10. Life Principles

00243

Readiness for enhanced **emancipated decision-making**
(2013; LOE 2.1)

Definition

A process of choosing a healthcare decision that includes personal knowledge and/or consideration of social norms, which can be strengthened.

Defining Characteristics

- Expresses desire to enhance ability to choose healthcare options that best fit current lifestyle
- Expresses desire to enhance ability to enact chosen healthcare option
- Expresses desire to enhance ability to understand all available healthcare options
- Expresses desire to enhance ability to verbalize own opinion without constraint
- Expresses desire to enhance comfort to verbalize healthcare options in the presence of others
- Expresses desire to enhance confidence in decision-making
- Expresses desire to enhance confidence to discuss healthcare options openly
- Expresses desire to enhance decision-making
- Expresses desire to enhance privacy to discuss healthcare options

Original literature support available at www.nanda.org

00244

Risk for impaired **emancipated decision-making**
(2013; LOE 2.1)

Definition
Vulnerable to a process of choosing a healthcare decision that does not include personal knowledge and/or consideration of social norms, or does not occur in a flexible environment resulting in decisional dissatisfaction.

Risk Factors

- Inadequate time to discuss healthcare options
- Insufficient confidence to openly discuss healthcare options
- Insufficient information regarding healthcare options
- Insufficient privacy to openly discuss healthcare options
- Insufficient self-confidence in decision-making
- Limited decision-making experience
- Traditional hierarchical family
- Traditional hierarchical healthcare systems

Original literature support available at www.nanda.org

10. Life Principles

00175

Moral distress
(2006; LOE 2.1)

Definition
Response to the inability to carry out one's chosen ethical/moral decision/action.

Defining Characteristics

- Anguish about acting on one's moral choice (e.g., powerlessness, anxiety, fear)

Related Factors

- Conflict among decision-makers
- Conflicting information available for ethical decision-making
- Conflicting information available for moral decision-making
- Cultural incongruence
- End-of-life decisions
- Loss of autonomy
- Physical distance of decision-maker
- Time constraint for decision-making
- Treatment decision

Original literature support available at www.nanda.org

00169

Impaired religiosity
(2004; LOE 2.1)

Definition
Impaired ability to exercise reliance on beliefs and/or participate in rituals of a particular faith tradition.

Defining Characteristics

- Desire to reconnect with previous belief pattern
- Desire to reconnect with previous customs
- Difficulty adhering to prescribed religious beliefs
- Difficulty adhering to prescribed religious rituals (e.g., ceremonies, regulations, clothing, prayer, services, holiday observances)
- Distress about separation from faith community
- Questioning of religious belief patterns
- Questioning of religious customs

Related Factors

Developmental and Situational
- Aging
- End-stage life crisis
- Life transition

Physical
- Illness
- Pain

Psychological
- Anxiety
- Fear of death
- History of religious manipulation
- Ineffective coping strategies
- Insecurity
- Insufficient social support
- Personal crisis

Sociocultural
- Cultural barrier to practicing religion
- Environmental barrier to practicing religion
- Insufficient social integration
- Insufficient sociocultural interaction

Spiritual
- Spiritual crises
- Suffering

Original literature support available at www.nanda.org

00171

Readiness for enhanced **religiosity**
(2004, 2013; LOE 2.1)

Definition

A pattern of reliance on religious beliefs and/or participation in rituals of a particular faith tradition, which can be strengthened.

Defining Characteristics

- Expresses desire to enhance belief patterns used in the past
- Expresses desire to enhance connection with a religious leader
- Expresses desire to enhance forgiveness
- Expresses desire to enhance participation in religious experiences
- Expresses desire to enhance participation in religious practices (e.g., ceremonies, regulations, clothing, prayer, services, holiday observances)
- Expresses desire to enhance religious customs used in the past
- Expresses desire to enhance religious options
- Expresses desire to enhance use of religious material

Original literature support available at www.nanda.org

10. Life Principles

00170

Risk for impaired **religiosity**
(2004, 2013; LOE 2.1)

Definition
Vulnerable to an impaired ability to exercise reliance on religious beliefs and/or participate in rituals of a particular faith tradition, which may compromise health.

Risk Factors

Developmental
- Life transition

Environmental
- Barrier to practicing religion
- Insufficient transportation

Physical
- Hospitalization
- Illness
- Pain

Psychological
- Depression
- Ineffective caregiving
- Ineffective coping strategies
- Insecurity
- Insufficient social support

Sociocultural
- Cultural barrier to practicing religion
- Insufficient social interaction

Spiritual
- Suffering

Original literature support available at www.nanda.org

00066

Spiritual distress
(1978, 2002, 2013; LOE 2.1)

Definition

A state of suffering related to the impaired ability to experience meaning in life through connections with self, others, the world, or a superior being.

Defining Characteristics

- Anxiety
- Crying
- Fatigue
- Fear
- Insomnia

- Questioning identity
- Questioning meaning of life
- Questioning meaning of suffering

Connections to Self
- Anger
- Decrease in serenity
- Feeling of being unloved
- Guilt
- Inadequate acceptance

- Ineffective coping strategies
- Insufficient courage
- Perceived insufficient meaning in life

Connections with Others
- Alienation
- Refuses to interact with spiritual leader

- Refuses to interact with significant other
- Separation from support system

Connections with Art, Music, Literature, and Nature
- Decrease in expression of previous pattern of creativity

- Disinterest in nature
- Disinterest in reading spiritual literature

Connections with Power Greater than Self
- Anger toward power greater than self

- Feeling abandoned
- Hopelessness

- Inability for introspection
- Inability to experience the transcendent
- Inability to participate in religious activities
- Inability to pray
- Perceived suffering
- Request for a spiritual leader
- Sudden change in spiritual practice

Related Factors

- Actively dying
- Aging
- Birth of a child
- Death of significant other
- Exposure to death
- Illness
- Imminent death
- Increasing dependence on another
- Life transition
- Loneliness
- Loss of a body part
- Loss of function of a body part
- Pain
- Perception of having unfinished business
- Receiving bad news
- Self-alienation
- Social alienation
- Sociocultural deprivation
- Treatment regimen
- Unexpected life event

10. Life Principles

00067

Risk for **spiritual** distress
(1998, 2004, 2013; LOE 2.1)

Definition
Vulnerable to an impaired ability to experience and integrate meaning and purpose in life through connectedness within self, literature, nature, and/or a power greater than oneself, which may compromise health.

Risk Factors

Developmental
- Life transition

Environmental
- Environmental change
- Natural disaster

Physical
- Chronic illness
- Physical illness
- Substance abuse

Psychosocial
- Anxiety
- Barrier to experiencing love
- Change in religious ritual
- Change in spiritual practice
- Cultural conflict
- Depression
- Inability to forgive
- Ineffective relationships
- Loss
- Low self-esteem
- Racial conflict
- Separation from support system
- Stressors

Original literature support available at www.nanda.org

DOMAIN 11. Safety/Protection		
Freedom from danger, physical injury, or immune system damage; preservation from loss; and protection of safety and security		
Class 1. Infection *Host responses following pathogenic invasion*		
Code	**Diagnosis**	**Page**
00004	Risk for **infection**	379
Class 2. Physical injury *Bodily harm or hurt*		
Code	**Diagnosis**	**Page**
00031	Ineffective **airway clearance**	380
00039	Risk for **aspiration**	381
00206	Risk for **bleeding**	382
00219	Risk for **dry eye**	383
00155	Risk for **falls**	384
00035	Risk for **injury***	386
00245	Risk for corneal **injury***	387
00087	Risk for perioperative **positioning injury***	388

* The editors acknowledge these concepts are not in alphabetical order, but a decision was made to maintain all "Risk for injury" diagnoses in sequential order.

NANDA International, Inc. Nursing Diagnoses: Definitions & Classification 2015–2017,
Tenth Edition. Edited by T. Heather Herdman and Shigemi Kamitsuru.
© 2014 NANDA International, Inc. Published 2014 by John Wiley & Sons, Ltd.
Companion website: www.wiley.com/go/nursingdiagnoses

Class 2. Physical injury (continued)

Code	Diagnosis	Page
00220	Risk for **thermal injury***	389
00250	Risk for urinary tract **injury***	390
00048	Impaired **dentition**	391
00045	Impaired oral **mucous membrane**	392
00247	Risk for impaired oral **mucous membrane**	394
00086	Risk for peripheral neurovascular **dysfunction**	395
00249	Risk for **pressure ulcer**	396
00205	Risk for **shock**	398
00046	Impaired **skin integrity**	399
00047	Risk for impaired **skin integrity**	400
00156	Risk for **sudden infant death syndrome**	401
00036	Risk for **suffocation**	402
00100	Delayed **surgical recovery**	403
00246	Risk for delayed **surgical recovery**	404
00044	Impaired **tissue integrity**	405
00248	Risk for impaired **tissue integrity**	406
00038	Risk for **trauma**	407
00213	Risk for vascular **trauma**	409

Class 3. Violence
The exertion of excessive force or power so as to cause injury or abuse

Code	Diagnosis	Page
00138	Risk for **other-directed violence**	410
00140	Risk for **self-directed violence**	411
00151	**Self-mutilation**	412
00139	Risk for **self-mutilation**	414
00150	Risk for **suicide**	416

Class 4. Environmental hazards
Sources of danger in the surroundings

Code	Diagnosis	Page
00181	**Contamination**	418
00180	Risk for **contamination**	420
00037	Risk for **poisoning**	421

Class 5. Defensive processes		
The processes by which the self protects itself from the nonself		
Code	Diagnosis	Page
00218	Risk for adverse **reaction to iodinated contrast media**	422
00217	Risk for **allergy response**	423
00041	**Latex allergy response**	424
00042	Risk for **latex allergy response**	425

Class 6. Thermoregulation		
The physiological process of regulating heat and energy within the body for purposes of protecting the organism		
Code	Diagnosis	Page
00005	Risk for imbalanced **body temperature**	426
00007	**Hyperthermia**	427
00006	**Hypothermia**	428
00253	Risk for **hypothermia**	430
00254	Risk for perioperative **hypothermia**	432
00008	Ineffective **thermoregulation**	433

00004

Risk for **infection**
(1986, 2010, 2013; LOE 2.1)

Definition

Vulnerable to invasion and multiplication of pathogenic organisms, which may compromise health.

Risk Factors

- Chronic Illness (e.g., Diabetes Mellitus)
- Inadequate vaccination
- Insufficient knowledge to avoid exposure to pathogens

- Invasive procedure
- Malnutrition
- Obesity

Inadequate Primary Defenses
- Alteration in peristalsis
- Alteration in pH of secretions
- Alteration in skin integrity
- Decrease in ciliary action

- Premature rupture of amniotic membrane
- Prolonged rupture of amniotic membrane
- Smoking
- Stasis of body fluids

Inadequate Secondary Defenses
- Decrease in hemoglobin
- Immunosuppression
- Leukopenia

- Suppressed inflammatory response (e.g., IL-6, CRP)
- Inadequate vaccination

Increased Environmental Exposure to Pathogens
- Exposure to disease outbreak

Original literature support available at www.nanda.org

00031

Ineffective **airway clearance**
(1980, 1996, 1998)

> ### Definition
> Inability to clear secretions or obstructions from the respiratory tract to maintain a clear airway.

Defining Characteristics

- Absence of cough
- Adventitious breath sounds
- Alteration in respiratory pattern
- Alteration in respiratory rate
- Cyanosis
- Difficulty verbalizing

- Diminished breath sounds
- Dyspnea
- Excessive sputum
- Ineffective cough
- Orthopnea
- Restlessness
- Wide-eyed look

Related Factors

Environmental
- Exposure to smoke
- Second-hand smoke

- Smoking

Obstructed Airway
- Airway spasm
- Chronic obstructive pulmonary disease
- Exudate in the alveoli
- Excessive mucus

- Foreign body in airway
- Hyperplasia of the bronchial walls
- Presence of artificial airway
- Retained secretions

Physiological
- Allergic airway
- Asthma

- Infection
- Neuromuscular impairment

00039

Risk for **aspiration**
(1988, 2013)

Definition
Vulnerable to entry of gastrointestinal secretions, oropharyngeal secretions, solids, or fluids to the tracheobronchial passages, which may compromise health.

Risk Factors

- Barrier to elevating upper body
- Decrease in gastrointestinal motility
- Decrease in level of consciousness
- Delayed gastric emptying
- Depressed gag reflex
- Enteral feedings
- Facial surgery
- Facial trauma
- Impaired ability to swallow
- Incompetent lower esophageal sphincter
- Increase in gastric residual
- Increase in intragastric pressure
- Ineffective cough
- Neck surgery
- Neck trauma
- Oral surgery
- Oral trauma
- Presence of oral/nasal tube (e.g., tracheal, feeding)
- Treatment regimen
- Wired jaw

11. Safety/Protection

00206

Risk for **bleeding**
(2008, 2013; LOE 2.1)

Definition
Vulnerable to a decrease in blood volume, which may compromise health.

Risk Factors

- Aneurysm
- Circumcision
- Disseminated intravascular coagulopathy
- Gastrointestinal condition (e.g., ulcer, polyps, varices)
- History of falls
- Impaired liver function (e.g., cirrhosis, hepatitis)
- Inherent coagulopathy (e.g., thrombocytopenia)
- Insufficient knowledge of bleeding precautions
- Postpartum complications (e.g., uterine atony, retained placenta)
- Pregnancy complication (e.g., premature rupture of membranes, placenta previa/ abruption, multiple gestation)
- Trauma
- Treatment regimen

Original literature support available at www.nanda.org

00219

Risk for **dry eye**
(2010, 2013; LOE 2.1)

Definition
Vulnerable to eye discomfort or damage to the cornea and conjunctiva due to reduced quantity or quality of tears to moisten the eye, which may compromise health.

Risk Factors

- Aging
- Autoimmune disease (e.g., rheumatoid arthritis, diabetes mellitus, thyroid disease)
- Contact lens wearer
- Environmental factor (e.g., air conditioning, excessive wind, sunlight exposure, air pollution, low humidity)
- Female gender
- History of allergy
- Hormonal change
- Lifestyle choice (e.g., smoking, caffeine use, prolonged reading)
- Mechanical ventilation
- Neurological lesion with sensory or motor reflex loss (e.g., lagophthalmos, lack of spontaneous blink reflex)
- Ocular surface damage
- Treatment regimen
- Vitamin A deficiency

Original literature support available at www.nanda.org

11. Safety/Protection

00155

Risk for **falls**
(2000, 2013)

Definition
Vulnerable to increased susceptibility to falling, which may cause physical harm and compromise health.

Risk Factors

Adults
- Age ≥ 65 years
- History of falls
- Living alone

- Lower limb prosthesis
- Use of assistive device (e.g., walker, cane, wheelchair)

Children
- Absence of stairway gate
- Absence of window guard
- Age ≤ 2 years
- Inadequate supervision

- Insufficient automobile restraints
- Male gender when < 1 year of age

Cognitive
- Alteration in cognitive functioning

Environment
- Cluttered environment
- Exposure to unsafe weather-related condition (e.g., wet floors, ice)
- Insufficient lighting

- Insufficient anti-slip material in bathroom
- Unfamiliar setting
- Use of restraints
- Use of throw rugs

Pharmaceutical Agents
- Alcohol consumption

- Pharmaceutical agent

Physiological
- Acute illness
- Alteration in blood glucose level

- Anemia
- Arthritis
- Condition affecting the foot

- Decrease in lower extremity strength
- Diarrhea
- Difficulty with gait
- Faintness when extending neck
- Faintness when turning neck
- Hearing impairment
- Impaired balance
- Impaired mobility
- Incontinence
- Neoplasm
- Neuropathy
- Orthostatic hypotension
- Postoperative recovery period
- Proprioceptive deficit
- Sleeplessness
- Urinary urgency
- Vascular disease
- Visual impairment

00035

Risk for **injury**
(1978, 2013)

Definition
Vulnerable to physical damage due to environmental conditions inter-acting with the individual's adaptive and defensive resources, which may compromise health.

Risk Factors

External
- Alteration in cognitive functioning
- Alteration in psychomotor functioning
- Compromised nutritional source (e.g., vitamins, food types)
- Exposure to pathogen
- Exposure to toxic chemical
- Immunization level within community
- Nosocomial agent
- Physical barrier (e.g., design, structure, arrangement of community, building, equipment)
- Unsafe mode of transport

Internal
- Abnormal blood profile
- Alteration in affective orientation
- Alteration in sensation (result-ing from spinal cord injury, diabetes mellitus, etc.)
- Autoimmune dysfunction
- Biochemical dysfunction
- Effector dysfunction
- Extremes of age
- Immune dysfunction
- Impaired primary defense mechanisms (e.g., broken skin)
- Malnutrition
- Sensory integration dysfunction
- Tissue hypoxia

00245

Risk for corneal **injury**
(2013; LOE 2.1)

Definition
Vulnerable to infection or inflammatory lesion in the corneal tissue that can affect superficial or deep layers, which may compromise health.

Risk Factors

- Blinking <5 times per minute
- Exposure of the eyeball
- Glasgow Coma Scale score <7
- Intubation
- Mechanical ventilation
- Periorbital edema
- Pharmaceutical agent
- Prolonged hospitalization
- Tracheostomy
- Use of supplemental oxygen

Original literature support available at www.nanda.org

11. Safety/Protection

00087

Risk for perioperative **positioning injury**
(1994, 2006, 2013; LOE 2.1)

Definition
Vulnerable to inadvertent anatomical and physical changes as a result of posture or equipment used during an invasive/surgical procedure, which may compromise health.

Risk Factors

- Disorientation
- Edema
- Emaciation
- Immobilization
- Muscle weakness
- Obesity
- Sensoriperceptual disturbance from anesthesia

Original literature support available at www.nanda.org

11. Safety/Protection

00220

Risk for **thermal injury**
(2010, 2013; LOE 2.1)

Definition
Vulnerable to extreme temperature damage to skin and mucous membranes, which may compromise health.

Risk Factors

- Alteration in cognitive functioning
- Extremes of age
- Extremes of environmental temperature
- Fatigue
- Inadequate protective clothing (e.g., flame-retardant sleepwear, gloves, ear covering)
- Inadequate supervision
- Inattentiveness
- Insufficient knowledge of safety precautions (patient, caregiver)
- Intoxication (alcohol, drug)
- Neuromuscular impairment
- Neuropathy
- Smoking
- Treatment regimen
- Unsafe environment

Original literature support available at www.nanda.org

11. Safety/Protection

00250

Risk for urinary tract **injury**
(2013; LOE 2.1)

Definition
Vulnerable to damage of the urinary tract structures from use of catheters, which may compromise health.

Risk Factors

- Condition preventing ability to secure catheter (e.g., burn, trauma, amputation)
- Long-term use of urinary catheter
- Multiple catheterizations
- Retention balloon inflated to ≥30 ml
- Use of large caliber urinary catheter

Original literature support available at www.nanda.org

11. Safety/Protection

00048

Impaired **dentition**
(1998)

Definition
Disruption in tooth development/eruption patterns or structural integrity of individual teeth.

Defining Characteristics

- Abraded teeth
- Absence of teeth
- Dental caries
- Enamel discoloration
- Erosion of enamel
- Excessive oral calculus
- Excessive oral plaque
- Facial asymmetry
- Halitosis
- Incomplete tooth eruption for age
- Loose tooth
- Malocclusion
- Premature loss of primary teeth
- Root caries
- Tooth fracture
- Tooth misalignment
- Toothache

Related Factors

- Barrier to self-care
- Bruxism
- Chronic vomiting
- Difficulty accessing dental care
- Economically disadvantaged
- Excessive intake of fluoride
- Excessive use of abrasive oral cleaning agents
- Genetic predisposition
- Habitual use of staining substance (e.g., coffee, red wine, tea, tobacco)
- Insufficient dietary habits
- Insufficient knowledge of dental health
- Insufficient oral hygiene
- Malnutrition
- Oral temperature sensitivity
- Pharmaceutical agent

11. Safety/Protection

00045

Impaired oral **mucous membrane**
(1982, 1998, 2013)

Definition
Injury to the lips, soft tissue, buccal cavity, and/or oropharynx.

Defining Characteristics

- Bad taste in mouth
- Bleeding
- Cheilitis
- Coated tongue
- Decrease in taste sensation
- Desquamation
- Difficulty eating
- Difficulty speaking
- Enlarged tonsils
- Exposure to pathogen
- Geographic tongue
- Gingival hyperplasia
- Gingival pallor
- Gingival pocketing deeper than 4 mm
- Gingival recession
- Halitosis
- Hyperemia
- Impaired ability to swallow
- Macroplasia
- Mucosal denudation
- Oral discomfort
- Oral edema
- Oral fissure
- Oral lesion
- Oral mucosal pallor
- Oral nodule
- Oral pain
- Oral papule
- Oral ulcer
- Oral vesicles
- Presence of mass (e.g., hemangioma)
- Purulent oral-nasal drainage
- Purulent oral-nasal exudates
- Smooth atrophic tongue
- Spongy patches in mouth
- Stomatitis
- White patches in mouth
- White plaque in mouth
- White, curd-like oral exudate
- Xerostomia

Related Factors

- Alcohol consumption
- Allergy
- Alteration in cognitive functioning
- Autoimmune disease
- Autosomal disorder
- Barrier to dental care
- Barrier to oral self-care

- Behavior disorder (e.g., attention deficit, oppositional defiant)
- Chemical injury agent (e.g., burn, capsaicin, methylene chloride, mustard agent)
- Cleft lip
- Cleft palate
- Decrease in hormone level in women
- Decrease in platelets
- Decrease in salivation
- Dehydration
- Depression
- Immunodeficiency
- Immunosuppression
- Infection
- Insufficient knowledge of oral hygiene
- Insufficient oral hygiene
- Loss of oral support structure
- Malnutrition
- Mechanical factor (e.g., ill-fitting dentures, braces, endotracheal/nasogastric tube, oral surgery)
- Mouth breathing
- Nil per os (NPO) >24 hours
- Oral trauma
- Smoking
- Stressors
- Syndrome (e.g., Sjögren's)
- Treatment regimen

Original literature support available at www.nanda.org

00247

Risk for impaired oral **mucous membrane**
(2013; LOE 2.1)

Definition
Vulnerable to injury to the lips, soft tissues, buccal cavity, and/or oropharynx, which may compromise health.

Risk Factors

- Alcohol consumption
- Allergy
- Alteration in cognitive functioning
- Autoimmune disease
- Autosomal disorder
- Barrier to dental care
- Barrier to oral self-care
- Behavior disorder (e.g., attention deficit, oppositional defiant)
- Chemotherapy
- Decrease in hormone level in women
- Economically disadvantaged
- Immunodeficiency
- Immunosuppression
- Inadequate nutrition
- Infection
- Insufficient knowledge of oral hygiene
- Insufficient oral hygiene
- Mechanical factor (e.g., orthodontic appliance, device for ventilation or food, ill-fitting dentures)
- Radiation therapy
- Smoking
- Stressors
- Surgical procedure
- Syndrome (e.g., Sjögren's)
- Trauma

Original literature support available at www.nanda.org

00086

Risk for peripheral neurovascular **dysfunction**
(1992, 2013)

Definition

Vulnerable to disruption in the circulation, sensation, and motion of an extremity, which may compromise health.

Risk Factors

- Burns
- Fracture
- Immobilization
- Mechanical compression (e.g., tourniquet, cast, brace, dressing, restraint)

- Orthopedic surgery
- Trauma
- Vascular obstruction

00249

Risk for **pressure ulcer**
(2013; LOE 2.2)

Definition
Vulnerable to localized injury to the skin and/or underlying tissue usually over a bony prominence as a result of pressure, or pressure in combination with shear (NPUAP, 2007).

Risk Factors

- ADULT: Braden Scale score of <18
- Alteration in cognitive functioning
- Alteration in sensation
- American Society of Anesthesiologists (ASA) Physical Status classification score ≥2
- Anemia
- Cardiovascular disease
- CHILD: Braden Q Scale of ≤16
- Decrease in mobility
- Decrease in serum albumin level
- Decrease in tissue oxygenation
- Decrease in tissue perfusion
- Dehydration
- Dry skin
- Edema
- Elevated skin temperature by 1-2 °C
- Extended period of immobility on hard surface (e.g., surgical procedure ≥2 hours)
- Extremes of age
- Extremes of weight
- Female gender
- Hip fracture
- History of cerebral vascular accident
- History of pressure ulcer
- History of trauma
- Hyperthermia
- Impaired circulation
- Inadequate nutrition
- Incontinence
- Insufficient caregiver knowledge of pressure ulcer prevention
- Low score on Risk Assessment Pressure Sore (RAPS) scale
- Lymphopenia
- New York Heart Association (NYHA) Functional Classification ≥2
- Non-blanchable erythema
- Pharmaceutical agents (e.g., general anesthesia, vasopressors, antidepressant, norepinephrine)
- Physical immobilization
- Pressure over bony prominence

- Reduced triceps skin fold thickness
- Scaly skin
- Self-care deficit
- Shearing forces
- Skin moisture
- Smoking
- Surface friction
- Use of linen with insufficient moisture wicking property

National Pressure Ulcer Advisory Panel (NPUAP). (2007). Updated Pressure Ulcer Stages. Available at: http://www.npuap.org/resources/educational-and-clinical-resources/pressure-ulcer-categorystaging-illustrations/, accessed on March 20, 2014.

Original literature support available at www.nanda.org

00205

Risk for **shock**
(2008, 2013; LOE 2.1)

Definition
Vulnerable to an inadequate blood flow to the body's tissues that may lead to life-threatening cellular dysfunction, which may compromise health.

Risk Factors

- Hypotension
- Hypovolemia
- Hypoxemia
- Hypoxia

- Infection
- Sepsis
- Systemic inflammatory response syndrome (SIRS)

Original literature support available at www.nanda.org

00046

Impaired **skin integrity**
(1975, 1998)

Definition
Altered epidermis and/or dermis.

Defining Characteristics

- Alteration in skin integrity
- Foreign matter piercing skin

Related Factors

External

- Chemical injury agent (e.g., burn, capsaicin, methylene chloride, mustard agent)
- Extremes of age
- Humidity
- Hyperthermia
- Hypothermia

- Mechanical factor (e.g., shearing forces, pressure, physical immobility)
- Moisture
- Pharmaceutical agent
- Radiation therapy

Internal

- Alteration in fluid volume
- Alteration in metabolism
- Alteration in pigmentation
- Alteration in sensation (resulting from spinal cord injury, diabetes mellitus, etc.)
- Alteration in skin turgor

- Hormonal change
- Immunodeficiency
- Impaired circulation
- Inadequate nutrition
- Pressure over bony prominence

11. Safety/Protection

00047

Risk for impaired **skin integrity**
(1975, 1998, 2010, 2013; LOE 2.1)

Definition
Vulnerable to alteration in epidermis and/or dermis, which may compromise health.

Risk Factors

External
- Chemical injury agent (e.g., burn, capsaicin, methylene chloride, mustard agent)
- Excretions
- Extremes of age
- Humidity
- Hyperthermia
- Hypothermia
- Mechanical factor (e.g., shearing forces, pressure, physical immobility)
- Moisture
- Radiation therapy
- Secretions

Internal
- Alteration in metabolism
- Alteration in pigmentation
- Alteration in sensation (resulting from spinal cord injury, diabetes mellitus, etc.)
- Alteration in skin turgor
- Hormonal change
- Immunodeficiency
- Impaired circulation
- Inadequate nutrition
- Pharmaceutical agent
- Pressure over bony prominence
- Psychogenetic factor

00156

Risk for **sudden infant death syndrome**
(2002, 2013; LOE 3.2)

Definition
Vulnerable to unpredicted death of an infant.

Risk Factors

Modifiable
- Delay in prenatal care
- Exposure to smoke
- Infant overheating
- Infant overwrapping
- Infant placed in prone position to sleep
- Infant placed in side-lying position to sleep
- Insufficient prenatal care
- Soft underlayment (e.g., loose items placed near infant)

Potentially Modifiable
- Low birth weight
- Prematurity
- Young parental age

Nonmodifiable
- Age 2-4 months
- Ethnicity (e.g., African American or Native American)
- Male gender
- Season of the year (i.e., winter and fall)

11. Safety/Protection

00036

Risk for **suffocation**
(1980, 2013)

Definition
Vulnerable to inadequate air availability for inhalation, which may compromise health.

Risk Factors

External

- Access to empty refrigerator/ freezer
- Eating large mouthfuls of food
- Gas leak
- Low-strung clothesline
- Pacifier around infant's neck
- Playing with plastic bag
- Propped bottle in infant's crib
- Small object in airway
- Smoking in bed
- Soft underlayment (e.g., loose items placed near infant)
- Unattended in water
- Unvented fuel-burning heater
- Vehicle running in closed garage

Internal

- Alteration in cognitive functioning
- Alteration in olfactory function
- Emotional disturbance
- Face/neck disease
- Face/neck injury
- Impaired motor functioning
- Insufficient knowledge of safety precautions

00100

Delayed **surgical recovery**
(1998, 2006, 2013; LOE 2.1)

Definition
Extension of the number of postoperative days required to initiate and perform activities that maintain life, health, and well-being.

Defining Characteristics

- Discomfort
- Evidence of interrupted healing of surgical area
- Excessive time required for recuperation
- Impaired mobility
- Inability to resume employment
- Loss of appetite
- Postpones resumption of work
- Requires assistance for self-care

Related Factors

- American Society of Anesthesiologists (ASA) Physical Status classification score ≥3
- Diabetes mellitus
- Edema at surgical site
- Extensive surgical procedure
- Extremes of age
- History of delayed wound healing
- Impaired mobility
- Malnutrition
- Obesity
- Pain
- Perioperative surgical site infection
- Persistent nausea
- Persistent vomiting
- Pharmaceutical agent
- Postoperative emotional response
- Prolonged surgical procedure
- Psychological disorder in postoperative period
- Surgical site contamination
- Trauma at surgical site

Original literature support available at www.nanda.org

11. Safety/Protection

00246

Risk for delayed **surgical recovery**
(2013; LOE 2.1)

> **Definition**
> Vulnerable to an extension of the number of postoperative days required to initiate and perform activities that maintain life, health, and well-being, which may compromise health.

Risk Factors

- American Society of Anesthesiologists (ASA) Physical Status classification score ≥ 3
- Diabetes mellitus
- Edema at surgical site
- Extensive surgical procedure
- Extremes of age
- History of delayed wound healing
- Impaired mobility
- Malnutrition
- Obesity
- Pain
- Perioperative surgical site infection
- Persistent nausea
- Persistent vomiting
- Pharmaceutical agent
- Postoperative emotional response
- Prolonged surgical procedure
- Psychological disorder in postoperative period
- Surgical site contamination
- Trauma at surgical site

Original literature support available at www.nanda.org

00044

Impaired **tissue integrity**
(1986, 1998, 2013; LOE 2.1)

Definition
Damage to the mucous membrane, cornea, integumentary system, muscular fascia, muscle, tendon, bone, cartilage, joint capsule, and/or ligament.

Defining Characteristics

- Damaged tissue
- Destroyed tissue

Related Factors

- Alteration in metabolism
- Alteration in sensation
- Chemical injury agent (e.g., burn, capsaicin, methylene chloride, mustard agent)
- Excessive fluid volume
- Extremes of age
- Extremes of environmental temperature
- High voltage power supply
- Humidity
- Imbalanced nutritional state (e.g., obesity, malnutrition)
- Impaired circulation
- Impaired mobility
- Insufficient fluid volume
- Insufficient knowledge about maintaining tissue integrity
- Insufficient knowledge about protecting tissue integrity
- Mechanical factor
- Peripheral neuropathy
- Pharmaceutical agent
- Radiation
- Surgical procedure

11. Safety/Protection

00248

Risk for impaired **tissue integrity**
(2013; LOE 2.1)

Definition
Vulnerable to damage to the mucous membrane, cornea, integumentary system, muscular fascia, muscle, tendon, bone, cartilage, joint capsule, and/or ligament, which may compromise health.

Risk Factors

- Alteration in metabolism
- Alteration in sensation
- Chemical injury agent (e.g., burn, capsaicin, methylene chloride, mustard agent)
- Excessive fluid volume
- Extremes of age
- Extremes of environmental temperature
- High voltage power supply
- Humidity
- Imbalanced nutritional state (e.g., obesity, malnutrition)
- Impaired circulation
- Impaired mobility
- Insufficient fluid volume
- Insufficient knowledge about maintaining tissue integrity
- Insufficient knowledge about protecting tissue integrity
- Mechanical factor
- Peripheral neuropathy
- Pharmaceutical agent
- Radiation therapy
- Surgical procedure

00038

Risk for **trauma**
(1980, 2013)

Definition
Vulnerable to accidental tissue injury (e.g., wound, burn, fracture), which may compromise health.

Risk Factors

External

- Absence of call-for-aid device
- Absence of stairway gate
- Absence of window guard
- Access to weapon
- Bathing in very hot water
- Bed in high position
- Children riding in front seat of car
- Defective appliance
- Delay in ignition of gas appliance
- Dysfunctional call-for-aid device
- Electrical hazard (e.g., faulty plug, frayed wire, overloaded outlet/fuse box)
- Exposure to corrosive product
- Exposure to dangerous machinery
- Exposure to radiation
- Exposure to toxic chemical
- Extremes of environmental temperature
- Flammable object (e.g., clothing, toys)
- Gas leak

- Grease on stove
- High crime neighborhood
- Icicles hanging from roof
- Inadequate stair rails
- Inadequately stored combustible (e.g., matches, oily rags)
- Inadequately stored corrosive (e.g., lye)
- Insufficient lighting
- Insufficient protection from heat source
- Misuse of headgear (e.g., hard hat, motorcycle helmet)
- Misuse of seat restraint
- Insufficient anti-slip material in bathroom
- Nonuse of seat restraints
- Obstructed passageway
- Playing with dangerous object
- Playing with explosive
- Pot handle facing front of stove
- Proximity to vehicle pathway (e.g., driveway, railroad track)
- Slippery floor
- Smoking in bed
- Smoking near oxygen
- Struggling with restraints

- Unanchored electric wires
- Unsafe operation of heavy equipment (e.g., excessive speed, while intoxicated, without required eyewear)
- Unsafe road
- Unsafe walkway

- Use of cracked dishware
- Use of throw rugs
- Use of unstable chair
- Use of unstable ladder
- Wearing loose clothing around open flame

Internal
- Alteration in cognitive functioning
- Alteration in sensation (resulting from spinal cord injury, diabetes mellitus, etc.)
- Decrease in eye-hand coordination
- Decrease in muscle coordination

- Economically disadvantaged
- Emotional disturbance
- History of trauma (e.g., physical, psychological, sexual)
- Impaired balance
- Insufficient knowledge of safety precautions
- Insufficient vision
- Weakness

00213

Risk for vascular **trauma**
(2008, 2013; LOE 2.1)

Definition
Vulnerable to damage to vein and its surrounding tissues related to the presence of a catheter and/or infused solutions, which may compromise health.

Risk Factors

- Difficulty visualizing artery or vein
- Inadequate anchoring of catheter
- Inappropriate catheter type
- Inappropriate catheter width
- Insertion site
- Irritating solution (e.g., concentration, temperature, pH)
- Length of time catheter is in place
- Rapid infusion rate

Original literature support available at www.nanda.org

00138

Risk for **other-directed violence**
(1980, 1996, 2013)

Definition
Vulnerable to behaviors in which an individual demonstrates that he or she can be physically, emotionally, and/or sexually harmful to others.

Risk Factors

- Access to weapon
- Alteration in cognitive functioning
- Cruelty to animals
- Fire-setting
- History of childhood abuse (e.g., physical, psychological, sexual)
- History of substance abuse
- History of witnessing family violence
- Impulsiveness
- Motor vehicle offense (e.g., traffic violations, use of a motor vehicle to release anger)
- Negative body language (e.g., rigid posture, clenching of fists/jaw, hyperactivity, pacing, threatening stances)
- Neurological impairment (e.g., positive EEG, head trauma, seizure disorders)
- Pathological intoxication
- Pattern of indirect violence (e.g., tearing objects off walls, urinating/defecating on floor, stamping feet, temper tantrum,

  throwing objects, breaking a window, slamming doors, sexual advances)
- Pattern of other-directed violence (e.g., hitting/kicking/spitting/scratching others, throwing objects/biting someone, attempted rape, rape, sexual molestation, urinating/defecating on a person)
- Pattern of threatening violence (e.g., verbal threats against property/people, social threats, cursing, threatening notes/gestures, sexual threats)
- Pattern of violent anti-social behavior (e.g., stealing, insistent borrowing, insistent demands for privileges, insistent interrupting, refusal to eat/take medication, ignoring instructions)
- Perinatal complications
- Prenatal complications
- Psychotic disorder
- Suicidal behavior

11. Safety/Protection

00140

Risk for **self-directed violence**
(1994, 2013; LOE)

> **Definition**
> Vulnerable to behaviors in which an individual demonstrates that he or she can be physically, emotionally, and/or sexually harmful to self.

Risk Factors

- Age ≥ 45 years
- Age 15-19 years
- Behavioral cues (e.g., writing forlorn love notes, directing angry messages at a significant other who has rejected the person, giving away personal items, taking out a large life insurance policy)
- Conflict about sexual orientation
- Conflict in interpersonal relationship(s)
- Employment concern (e.g., unemployed, recent job loss/failure)
- Engagement in autoerotic sexual acts
- History of multiple suicide attempts
- Insufficient personal resources (e.g., achievement, insight, affect unavailable and poorly controlled)
- Marital status (e.g., single, widowed, divorced)
- Mental health issue (e.g., depression, psychosis, personality disorder, substance abuse)
- Occupation (e.g., executive, administrator/owner of business, professional, semi-skilled worker)
- Pattern of difficulties in family background (e.g., chaotic or conflictual, history of suicide)
- Physical health issue
- Psychological disorder
- Social isolation
- Suicidal ideation
- Suicidal plan
- Verbal cues (e.g., talking about death, "better off without me," asking about lethal dosage of medication)

00151

Self-mutilation
(2000)

Definition
Deliberate self-injurious behavior causing tissue damage with the intent of causing nonfatal injury to attain relief of tension.

Defining Characteristics

- Abrading
- Biting
- Constricting a body part
- Cuts on body
- Hitting
- Ingestion of harmful substance
- Inhalation of harmful substance
- Insertion of object into body orifice
- Picking at wound
- Scratches on body
- Self-inflicted burn
- Severing of a body part

Related Factors

- Absence of family confidant
- Adolescence
- Alteration in body image
- Autism
- Borderline personality disorder
- Character disorder
- Childhood illness
- Childhood surgery
- Depersonalization
- Developmental delay
- Dissociation
- Disturbance in interpersonal relationships
- Eating disorder
- Emotional disorder
- Family divorce
- Family history of self-destructive behavior
- Family substance abuse
- Feeling threatened with loss of significant relationship
- History of childhood abuse (e.g., physical, psychological, sexual)
- History of self-directed violence
- Impaired self-esteem
- Impulsiveness
- Inability to express tension verbally
- Incarceration

- Ineffective communication between parent and adolescent
- Ineffective coping strategies
- Irresistible urge for self-directed violence
- Irresistible urge to cut self
- Isolation from peers
- Labile behavior
- Living in nontraditional setting (e.g., foster, group, or institutional care)
- Low self-esteem
- Mounting tension that is intolerable
- Negative feeling (e.g., depression, rejection, self-hatred, separation anxiety, guilt, depersonalization)
- Pattern of inability to plan solutions
- Pattern of inability to see long-term consequences
- Peers who self-mutilate
- Perfectionism
- Psychotic disorder
- Requires rapid stress reduction
- Sexual identity crisis
- Substance abuse
- Use of manipulation to obtain nurturing relationship with others
- Violence between parental figures

00139

Risk for **self-mutilation**
(1992, 2000, 2013)

Definition
Vulnerable to deliberate self-injurious behavior causing tissue damage
with the intent of causing nonfatal injury to attain relief of tension.

Risk Factors

- Adolescence
- Alteration in body image
- Autism
- Battered child
- Borderline personality disorder
- Character disorder
- Childhood illness
- Childhood surgery
- Depersonalization
- Developmental delay
- Dissociation
- Disturbance in interpersonal relationships
- Eating disorder
- Emotional disorder
- Family divorce
- Family history of self-destructive behavior
- Family substance abuse
- Feeling threatened with loss of significant relationship
- History of childhood abuse (e.g., physical, psychological, sexual)
- History of self-directed violence
- Impaired self-esteem
- Impulsiveness
- Inability to express tension verbally
- Incarceration
- Ineffective coping strategies
- Irresistible urge for self-directed violence
- Isolation from peers
- Living in nontraditional setting (e.g., foster, group, or institutional care)
- Loss of control over problem-solving situation
- Loss of significant relationship(s)
- Low self-esteem
- Mounting tension that is intolerable
- Negative feelings (e.g., depression, rejection, self-hatred, separation anxiety, guilt, depersonalization)
- Pattern of inability to plan solutions
- Pattern of inability to see long-term consequences
- Peers who self-mutilate

11. Safety/Protection

- Perfectionism
- Psychotic disorder
- Requires rapid stress reduction
- Sexual identity crisis
- Substance abuse
- Use of manipulation to obtain nurturing relationship with others
- Violence between parental figures

00150

Risk for **suicide**
(2000, 2013)

Definition
Vulnerable to self-inflicted, life-threatening injury.

Risk Factors

Behavioral
- Changing a will
- Giving away possessions
- History of suicide attempt
- Impulsiveness
- Making a will
- Marked change in attitude
- Marked change in behavior
- Marked change in school performance
- Purchase of a gun
- Stockpiling medication
- Sudden euphoric recovery from major depression

Demographic
- Age (e.g., elderly people, young adult males, adolescents)
- Divorced status
- Ethnicity (e.g., white, Native American)
- Male gender
- Widowed

Physical
- Chronic pain
- Physical illness
- Terminal illness

Psychological
- Family history of suicide
- Guilt
- History of childhood abuse (e.g., physical, psychological, sexual)
- Homosexual youth
- Psychiatric disorder
- Substance abuse

Situational
- Access to weapon
- Adolescents living in nontraditional settings (e.g., juvenile detention center, prison, halfway house, group home)
- Economically disadvantaged
- Institutionalization
- Living alone
- Loss of autonomy
- Loss of independence
- Relocation
- Retired

Social
- Cluster suicides
- Disciplinary problems
- Disruptive family life
- Grieving
- Helplessness
- Hopelessness
- Insufficient social support
- Legal difficulty
- Loneliness
- Loss of important relationship
- Social isolation

Verbal
- Reports desire to die
- Threat of killing self

00181

Contamination
(2006; LOE 2.1)

Definition
Exposure to environmental contaminants in doses sufficient to cause adverse health effects.

Defining Characteristics

Pesticides
- Dermatological effects of pesticide exposure
- Gastrointestinal effects of pesticide exposure
- Neurological effects of pesticide exposure
- Pulmonary effects of pesticide exposure
- Renal effects of pesticide exposure

Chemicals
- Dermatological effects of chemical exposure
- Gastrointestinal effects of chemical exposure
- Immunological effects of chemical exposure
- Neurological effects of chemical exposure
- Pulmonary effects of chemical exposure
- Renal effects of chemical exposure

Biologicals
- Dermatological effects of exposure to biologicals
- Gastrointestinal effects of biological exposure
- Neurological effects of biological exposure
- Pulmonary effects of biological exposure
- Renal effects of biological exposure

Pollution
- Neurological effects of pollution exposure
- Pulmonary effects of pollution exposure

Waste
- Dermatological effects of waste exposure
- Gastrointestinal effects of waste exposure
- Hepatic effects of waste exposure
- Pulmonary effects of waste exposure

11. Safety/Protection

Radiation

- Exposure to radioactive material
- Genetic effects of radiation exposure
- Immunological effects of radiation exposure
- Neurological effects of radiation exposure
- Oncological effects of radiation exposure

Related Factors

External

- Carpeted flooring
- Chemical contamination of food
- Chemical contamination of water
- Economically disadvantaged
- Exposure to areas with high contaminant level
- Exposure to atmospheric pollutants
- Exposure to bioterrorism
- Exposure to disaster (natural or man-made)
- Exposure to radiation
- Flaking, peeling surface in presence of young children (e.g., paint, plaster)
- Household hygiene practices
- Inadequate breakdown of contaminant
- Inadequate municipal services (e.g., trash removal, sewage treatment facilities)
- Inadequate protective clothing
- Inappropriate use of protective clothing
- Ingestion of contaminated material (e.g., radioactive, food, water)
- Personal hygiene practices
- Playing where environmental contaminants are used
- Unprotected exposure to chemical (e.g., arsenic)
- Use of environmental contaminant in the home
- Use of noxious material in insufficiently ventilated area (e.g., lacquer, paint)
- Use of noxious material without effective protection (e.g., lacquer, paint)

Internal

- Age (e.g., children <5 years, older adults)
- Concomitant exposure
- Developmental characteristics of children
- Female gender
- Gestational age during exposure
- Inadequate nutrition
- Pre-existing disease
- Pregnancy
- Previous exposure to contaminant
- Smoking

Original literature support available at www.nanda.org

11. Safety/Protection

00180

Risk for **contamination**
(2006, 2013; LOE 2.1)

Definition

Vulnerable to exposure to environmental contaminants which may compromise health.

Risk Factors

External

- Carpeted flooring
- Chemical contamination of food
- Chemical contamination of water
- Economically disadvantaged
- Exposure to areas with high contaminant level
- Exposure to atmospheric pollutants
- Exposure to bioterrorism
- Exposure to disaster (natural or man-made)
- Exposure to radiation
- Flaking, peeling surface in presence of young children (e.g., paint, plaster)
- Inadequate breakdown of contaminant
- Inadequate household hygiene practices
- Inadequate municipal services (e.g., trash removal, sewage treatment facilities)
- Inadequate personal hygiene practices
- Inadequate protective clothing
- Inappropriate use of protective clothing
- Playing where environmental contaminants are used
- Unprotected exposure to chemical (e.g., arsenic)
- Unprotected exposure to heavy metal (e.g., chromium, lead)
- Use of environmental contaminant in the home
- Use of noxious material in insufficiently ventilated area (e.g., lacquer, paint)
- Use of noxious material without effective protection (e.g., lacquer, paint)

Internal

- Concomitant exposure
- Developmental characteristics of children
- Extremes of age
- Female gender
- Gestational age during exposure
- Inadequate nutrition
- Pre-existing disease
- Pregnancy
- Previous exposure to contaminant
- Smoking

Original literature support available at www.nanda.org

00037

Risk for **poisoning**
(1980, 2006, 2013; LOE 2.1)

Definition
Vulnerable to accidental exposure to, or ingestion of, drugs or dangerous products in sufficient doses, which may compromise health.

Risk Factors

External

- Access to dangerous product
- Access to illicit drugs potentially contaminated by poisonous additives
- Access to large supply of pharmaceutical agents in house
- Access to pharmaceutical agent

Internal

- Alteration in cognitive functioning
- Emotional disturbance
- Inadequate precautions against poisoning
- Insufficient knowledge of pharmacological agents
- Insufficient knowledge of poisoning prevention
- Occupational setting without adequate safeguards
- Reduced vision

Original literature support available at www.nanda.org

11. Safety/Protection

00218

Risk for adverse reaction to iodinated contrast media
(2010, 2013; LOE 2.1)

> **Definition**
> Vulnerable to noxious or unintended reaction associated with the use of iodinated contrast media that can occur within seven days after contrast agent injection, which may compromise health.

Risk Factors

- Anxiety
- Chronic illness
- Concurrent use of pharmaceutical agents (e.g., beta-blockers, interleukin-2, metformin, nephrotoxins)
- Contrast media precipitates adverse event (e.g., iodine concentration, viscosity, high osmolality, ion toxicity)
- Dehydration
- Extremes of age
- Fragile vein (e.g., chemotherapy/radiation in limb to be injected, indwelling line for >24 hours, axillary lymph node dissection in limb to be injected, distal intravenous access site)
- Generalized debilitation
- History of allergy
- History of previous adverse effect from iodinated contrast media
- Unconsciousness

Original literature support available at www.nanda.org

00217

Risk for **allergy response**
(2010, 2013; LOE 2.1)

Definition
Vulnerable to an exaggerated immune response or reaction to substances, which may compromise health.

Risk Factors

- Allergy to insect sting
- Exposure to allergen (e.g., pharmaceutical agent)
- Exposure to environmental allergen (e.g., dander, dust, mold, pollen)
- Exposure to toxic chemical
- Food allergy (e.g., avocado, banana, chestnut, kiwi, peanut, shellfish, mushroom, tropical fruit)
- Repeated exposure to allergen-producing environmental substance

Original literature support available at www.nanda.org

00041

Latex allergy response
(1998, 2006; LOE 2.1)

Definition
A hypersensitive reaction to natural latex rubber products.

Defining Characteristics

Life-Threatening Reactions within 1 Hour of Exposure
- Bronchospasm
- Chest tightness
- Contact urticaria progressing to generalized symptoms
- Dyspnea
- Edema (i.e., lips, throat, tongue, uvula)
- Hypotension
- Myocardial infarction
- Respiratory arrest
- Syncope
- Wheezing

Type IV Reactions Occurring ≥1 Hour after Exposure
- Discomfort reaction to additives (e.g., thiurams and carbamates)
- Eczema
- Skin irritation
- Skin redness

Generalized Characteristics
- Generalized discomfort
- Generalized edema
- Reports total body warmth
- Restlessness
- Skin flushing

Gastrointestinal Characteristics
- Abdominal pain
- Nausea

Orofacial Characteristics
- Erythema (e.g., eyes, facial, nasal)
- Itching (e.g., eyes, facial, nasal, oral)
- Nasal congestion
- Periorbital edema
- Rhinorrhea
- Tearing of the eyes

Related Factors

- Hypersensitivity to natural latex rubber protein

Original literature support available at www.nanda.org

00042

Risk for **latex allergy response**
(1998, 2006, 2013; LOE 2.1)

Definition
Vulnerable to a hypersensitive reaction to natural latex rubber products, which may compromise health.

Risk Factors

- Allergy to poinsettia plant
- Food allergy (e.g., avocado, banana, chestnut, kiwi, peanut, shellfish, mushroom, tropical fruit)
- Frequent exposure to latex product
- History of allergy
- History of asthma
- History of latex reaction
- History of surgery during infancy
- Multiple surgical procedures

Original literature support available at www.nanda.org

11. Safety/Protection

00005

Risk for imbalanced **body temperature**
(1986, 2000, 2013; LOE 2.1)

Definition
Vulnerable to failure to maintain body temperature within normal parameters, which may compromise health.

Risk Factors

- Acute brain injury
- Alteration in metabolic rate
- Condition affecting temperature regulation
- Decreased sweat response
- Dehydration
- Extremes of age
- Extremes of environmental temperature
- Extremes of weight
- Inactivity
- Inappropriate clothing for environmental temperature
- Increase in oxygen demand
- Increased body surface area to weight ratio
- Inefficient nonshivering thermogenesis
- Insufficient supply of subcutaneous fat
- Pharmaceutical agent
- Sedation
- Sepsis
- Vigorous activity

11. Safety/Protection

00007

Hyperthermia
(1986, 2013; LOE 2.2)

Definition
Core body temperature above the normal diurnal range due to failure of thermoregulation.

Defining Characteristics

- Abnormal posturing
- Apnea
- Coma
- Convulsions
- Flushed skin
- Hypotension
- Infant does not maintain suck
- Irritability
- Lethargy
- Seizure
- Skin warm to touch
- Stupor
- Tachycardia
- Tachypnea
- Vasodilation

Related Factors

- Decreased sweat response
- Dehydration
- High environmental temperature
- Illness
- Inappropriate clothing
- Increase in metabolic rate
- Ischemia
- Pharmaceutical agent
- Sepsis
- Trauma
- Vigorous activity

Original literature support available at www.nanda.org

00006

Hypothermia
(1986, 1988, 2013; LOE 2.2)

Definition
Core body temperature below the normal diurnal range due to failure of thermoregulation.

Defining Characteristics

- Acrocyanosis
- Bradycardia
- Cyanotic nail beds
- Decrease in blood glucose level
- Decrease in ventilation
- Hypertension
- Hypoglycemia
- Hypoxia
- Increase in metabolic rate
- Increase in oxygen consumption
- Peripheral vasoconstriction
- Piloerection
- Shivering
- Skin cool to touch
- Slow capillary refill
- Tachycardia

Accidental Low Body Temperature in Children and Adults
- Mild hypothermia, core temperature 32-35 °C
- Moderate hypothermia, core temperature 30-32 °C
- Severe hypothermia, core temperature <30 °C

Injured Adults and Children
- Hypothermia, core temperature <35 °C
- Severe hypothermia, core temperature <32 °C

Neonates
- Grade 1 hypothermia, core temperature 36-36.5 °C
- Grade 2 hypothermia, core temperature 35-35.9 °C
- Grade 3 hypothermia, core temperature 34-34.9 °C
- Grade 4 hypothermia, core temperature <34 °C
- Infant with insufficient energy to maintain sucking
- Infant with insufficient weight gain (<30 g/d)
- Irritability
- Jaundice
- Metabolic acidosis
- Pallor
- Respiratory distress

Related Factors

- Alcohol consumption
- Damage to hypothalamus
- Decrease in metabolic rate
- Economically disadvantaged
- Extremes of age
- Extremes of weight
- Heat transfer (e.g., conduction, convection, evaporation, radiation)
- Inactivity
- Insufficient caregiver knowledge of hypothermia prevention
- Insufficient clothing
- Insufficient supply of subcutaneous fat
- Low environmental temperature
- Malnutrition
- Pharmaceutical agent
- Radiation
- Trauma

Neonates

- Delay in breastfeeding
- Early bathing of newborn
- High risk out of hospital birth
- Immature stratum corneum
- Increased body surface area to weight ratio
- Increase in oxygen demand
- Increase in pulmonary vascular resistance (PVR)
- Ineffective vascular control
- Inefficient nonshivering thermogenesis
- Unplanned out-of-hospital birth

Original literature support available at www.nanda.org

00253

Risk for **hypothermia**
(2013; LOE 2.1)

Definition

Vulnerable to a failure of thermoregulation that may result in a core body temperature below the normal diurnal range, which may compromise health.

Risk Factors

- Alcohol consumption
- Damage to hypothalamus
- Economically disadvantaged
- Extremes of age
- Extremes of weight
- Heat transfer (e.g., conduction, convection, evaporation, radiation)
- Inactivity
- Insufficient caregiver knowledge of hypothermia prevention

- Insufficient clothing
- Insufficient supply of subcutaneous fat
- Low environmental temperature
- Malnutrition
- Pharmaceutical agent
- Radiation
- Trauma

Children and Adults: Accidental

- Mild hypothermia, core temperature approaching 35 °C
- Moderate hypothermia, core temperature approaching 32 °C

- Severe hypothermia, core temperature approaching 30 °C

Children and Adults: Injured Patients

- Hypothermia, core temperature approaching 35 °C

- Severe hypothermia, core temperature approaching 32 °C

Neonates

- Decrease in metabolic rate
- Delay in breastfeeding
- Early bathing of newborn
- Grade 1 hypothermia, core temperature approaching 36.5 °C

- Grade 2 hypothermia, core temperature approaching 36.0 °C
- Grade 3 hypothermia, core temperature approaching 35.0 °C

- Grade 4 hypothermia, core temperature approaching 34.0 °C
- High-risk out-of-hospital birth
- Immature stratum corneum
- Increased body surface area to weight ratio
- Increase in oxygen demand
- Increase in pulmonary vascular resistance (PVR)
- Ineffective vascular control
- Inefficient nonshivering thermogenesis
- Unplanned out-of-hospital birth

Original literature support available at www.nanda.org

00254

Risk for perioperative **hypothermia**
(2013; LOE 2.1)

Definition
Vulnerable to an inadvertent drop in core body temperature below 36 °C/96.8 °F occuring one hour before to 24 hours after surgery, which may compromise health.

Risk Factors

- American Society of Anesthesiologists (ASA) Physical Status classification score >1
- Cardiovascular complications
- Combined regional and general anesthesia
- Diabetic neuropathy
- Heat transfer (e.g., high volume of unwarmed infusion, unwarmed irrigation >20 liters)
- Low body weight
- Low environmental temperature
- Low preoperative temperature (<36 °C/96.8 °F)
- Surgical procedure

Original literature support available at www.nanda.org

00008

Ineffective **thermoregulation**
(1986)

Definition
Temperature fluctuation between hypothermia and hyperthermia.

Defining Characteristics

- Cyanotic nail beds
- Fluctuations in body temperature above and below the normal range
- Flushed skin
- Hypertension
- Increase in body temperature above normal range
- Increase in respiratory rate
- Mild shivering
- Moderate pallor
- Piloerection
- Reduction in body temperature below normal range
- Seizures
- Skin cool to touch
- Skin warm to touch
- Slow capillary refill
- Tachycardia

Related Factors

- Extremes of age
- Fluctuating environmental temperature
- Illness
- Trauma

Domain 12
Comfort

DOMAIN 12. COMFORT		
Sense of mental, physical, or social well-being or ease		
Class 1. Physical comfort *Sense of well-being or ease and/or freedom from pain*		
Code	**Diagnosis**	**Page**
00214	Impaired **comfort**	437
00183	Readiness for enhanced **comfort**	438
00134	**Nausea**	439
00132	Acute **pain**	440
00133	Chronic **pain**	442
00256	Labor **pain**	444
00255	Chronic **pain syndrome**	445
Class 2. Environmental comfort *Sense of well-being or ease in/with one's environment*		
Code	**Diagnosis**	**Page**
00214	Impaired **comfort**	437
00183	Readiness for enhanced **comfort**	438

NANDA International, Inc. Nursing Diagnoses: Definitions & Classification 2015–2017,
Tenth Edition. Edited by T. Heather Herdman and Shigemi Kamitsuru.
© 2014 NANDA International, Inc. Published 2014 by John Wiley & Sons, Ltd.
Companion website: www.wiley.com/go/nursingdiagnoses

3. Social comfort *Sense of well-being or ease with one's social situation*		
Code	**Diagnosis**	**Page**
00214	Impaired **comfort**	437
00183	Readiness for enhanced **comfort**	438
00054	Risk for **loneliness**	446
00053	**Social isolation**	447

Domain 12. *Comfort*

Class 1. *Physical Comfort*
Class 2. *Environmental Comfort*
Class 3. *Social Comfort*

00214

Impaired **comfort**
(2008, 2010; LOE 2.1)

Definition
Perceived lack of ease, relief, and transcendence in physical, psychospiritual, environmental, cultural, and/or social dimensions.

Defining Characteristics

- Alteration in sleep pattern
- Anxiety
- Crying
- Discontent with situation
- Distressing symptoms
- Fear
- Feeling cold
- Feeling hot
- Feeling of discomfort
- Feeling of hunger
- Inability to relax
- Irritability
- Itching
- Moaning
- Restlessness
- Sighing
- Uneasy in situation

Related Factors

- Illness-related symptoms
- Insufficient environmental control
- Insufficient privacy
- Insufficient resources (e.g., financial, social, knowledge)
- Insufficient situational control
- Noxious environmental stimuli
- Treatment regimen

Original literature support available at www.nanda.org

12. Comfort

Class 1: Physical Comfort 437

00183

Readiness for enhanced **comfort**
(2006, 2013; LOE 2.1)

Definition

A pattern of ease, relief, and transcendence in physical, psychospiritual, environmental, and/or social dimensions, which can be strengthened.

Defining Characteristics

- Expresses desire to enhance comfort
- Expresses desire to enhance feeling of contentment
- Expresses desire to enhance relaxation
- Expresses desire to enhance resolution of complaints

Original literature support available at www.nanda.org

00134

Nausea
(1998, 2002, 2010; LOE 2.1)

Definition
A subjective phenomenon of an unpleasant feeling in the back of the throat and stomach, which may or may not result in vomiting.

Defining Characteristics

- Aversion toward food
- Gagging sensation
- Increase in salivation
- Increase in swallowing
- Nausea
- Sour taste

Related Factors

Biophysical
- Biochemical dysfunction (e.g., uremia, diabetic ketoacidosis)
- Esophageal disease
- Exposure to toxin
- Gastric distention
- Gastrointestinal irritation
- Increase in intracranial pressure (ICP)
- Intra-abdominal tumors
- Labyrinthitis
- Liver capsule stretch
- Localized tumor (e.g., acoustic neuroma, brain tumor, bone metastasis)
- Menière's disease
- Meningitis
- Motion sickness
- Pancreatic disease
- Pregnancy
- Splenic capsule stretch
- Treatment regimen

Situational
- Anxiety
- Fear
- Noxious environmental stimuli
- Noxious taste
- Psychological disorder
- Unpleasant visual stimuli

Original literature support available at www.nanda.org

12. Comfort

00132

Acute **pain**
(1996, 2013; LOE 2.2)

Definition

An unpleasant sensory and emotional experience associated with actual or potential tissue damage, or described in terms of such damage (International Association for the Study of Pain); sudden or slow onset of any intensity from mild to severe with an anticipated or predictable end.

Defining Characteristics

- Appetite change
- Change in physiological parameter (e.g., blood pressure, heart rate, respiratory rate, oxygen saturation, and end-tidal CO_2)
- Diaphoresis
- Distraction behavior
- Evidence of pain using standardized pain behavior checklist for those unable to communicate verbally (e.g., Neonatal Infant Pain Scale, Pain Assessment Checklist for Seniors with Limited Ability to Communicate)
- Expressive behavior (e.g., restlessness, crying, vigilance)
- Facial expression of pain (e.g., eyes lack luster, beaten look, fixed or scattered movement, grimace)
- Guarding behavior
- Hopelessness
- Narrowed focus (e.g., time perception, thought processes, interaction with people and environment)
- Positioning to ease pain
- Protective behavior
- Proxy report of pain behavior/ activity changes (e.g., family member, caregiver)
- Pupil dilation
- Self-focused
- Self-report of intensity using standardized pain scale (e.g., Wong-Baker FACES scale, visual analogue scale, numeric rating scale)
- Self-report of pain characteristics using standardized pain instrument (e.g., McGill Pain Questionnaire, Brief Pain Inventory)

Related Factors

- Biological injury agent (e.g., infection, ischemia, neoplasm)
- Chemical injury agent (e.g., burn, capsaicin, methylene chloride, mustard agent)
- Physical injury agent (e.g., abscess, amputation, burn, cut, heavy lifting, operative procedure, trauma, overtraining)

Original literature support available at www.nanda.org

00133

Chronic **pain**
(1986, 1996, 2013; LOE 2.2)

Definition
Unpleasant sensory and emotional experience associated with actual or potential tissue damage, or described in terms of such damage (International Association for the Study of Pain); sudden or slow onset of any intensity from mild to severe, constant or recurring without an anticipated or predictable end and a duration of greater than three (>3) months.

Defining Characteristics

- Alteration in ability to continue previous activities
- Alteration in sleep pattern
- Anorexia
- Evidence of pain using standardized pain behavior checklist for those unable to communicate verbally (e.g., Neonatal Infant Pain Scale, Pain Assessment Checklist for Seniors with Limited Ability to Communicate)
- Facial expression of pain (e.g., eyes lack luster, beaten look, fixed or scattered movement, grimace)

- Proxy report of pain behavior/activity changes (e.g., family member, caregiver)
- Self-focused
- Self-report of intensity using standardized pain scale (e.g., Wong-Baker FACES scale, visual analogue scale, numeric rating scale)
- Self-report of pain characteristics using standardized pain instrument (e.g., McGill Pain Questionnaire, Brief Pain Inventory)

Related Factors

- Age >50 years
- Alteration in sleep pattern
- Chronic musculoskeletal condition
- Contusion
- Crush injury

- Damage to the nervous system
- Emotional distress
- Fatigue
- Female gender
- Fracture
- Genetic disorder

- History of abuse (e.g., physical, psychological, sexual)
- History of genital mutilation
- History of overindebtedness
- History of static work postures
- History of substance abuse
- History of vigorous exercise
- Imbalance of neurotransmitters, neuromodulators, and receptors
- Immune disorder (e.g., HIV-associated neuropathy, varicella-zoster virus)
- Impaired metabolic functioning
- Increase in body mass index
- Ineffective sexuality pattern
- Injury agent*
- Ischemic condition
- Malnutrition
- Muscle injury
- Nerve compression
- Post-trauma related condition (e.g., infection, inflammation)
- Prolonged computer use (>20 hours/week)
- Prolonged increase in cortisol level
- Repeated handling of heavy loads
- Social isolation
- Spinal cord injury
- Tumor infiltration
- Whole-body vibration

Original literature support available at www.nanda.org

*May be present, but is not required; pain may be of unknown etiology

00256

Labor pain
(2013; LOE 2.1)

Definition
Sensory and emotional experience that varies from pleasant to unpleasant, associated with labor and childbirth.

Defining Characteristics

- Alteration in blood pressure
- Alteration in heart rate
- Alteration in muscle tension
- Alteration in neuroendocrine functioning
- Alteration in respiratory rate
- Alteration in sleep pattern
- Alteration in urinary functioning
- Decrease in appetite
- Diaphoresis
- Distraction behavior
- Expressive behavior
- Facial expression of pain (e.g., eyes lack luster, beaten look, fixed or scattered movement, grimace)

- Increase in appetite
- Narrowed focus
- Nausea
- Pain
- Perineal pressure
- Positioning to ease pain
- Protective behavior
- Pupil dilation
- Self-focused
- Uterine contraction
- Vomiting

Related Factors

- Cervical dilation

- Fetal expulsion

Original literature support available at www.nanda.org

00255

Chronic **pain syndrome**
(2013; LOE 2.2)

Definition
Recurrent or persistent pain that has lasted at least three months, and that significantly affects daily functioning or well-being.

Defining Characteristics

- Anxiety (00146)
- Constipation (00011)
- Deficient knowledge (000126)
- Disturbed sleep pattern (00198)
- Fatigue (00093)
- Fear (00148)
- Impaired mood regulation (00241)
- Impaired physical mobility (00085)
- Insomnia (00095)
- Obesity (00232)
- Social isolation (00053)
- Stress overload (00177)

Original literature support available at www.nanda.org

00054

Risk for **loneliness**
(1994, 2006, 2013; LOE 2.1)

Definition
Vulnerable to experiencing discomfort associated with a desire or need for more contact with others, which may compromise health.

Risk Factors

- Affectional deprivation
- Emotional deprivation
- Physical isolation
- Social isolation

Original literature support available at www.nanda.org

00053

Social isolation
(1982)

Definition
Aloneness experienced by the individual and perceived as imposed by others and as a negative or threatening state.

Defining Characteristics

- Absence of support system
- Aloneness imposed by others
- Cultural incongruence
- Desire to be alone
- Developmental delay
- Developmentally inappropriate interests
- Disabling condition
- Feeling different from others
- Flat affect
- History of rejection
- Hostility
- Illness
- Inability to meet expectations of others
- Insecurity in public
- Meaningless actions
- Member of a subculture
- Poor eye contact
- Preoccupation with own thoughts
- Purposelessness
- Repetitive actions
- Sad affect
- Values incongruent with cultural norms
- Withdrawn

Related Factors

- Alteration in mental status
- Alteration in physical appearance
- Alteration in wellness
- Developmentally inappropriate interests
- Factors impacting satisfying personal relationships (e.g., developmental delay)
- Inability to engage in satisfying personal relationships
- Insufficient personal resources (e.g., poor achievement, poor insight, affect unavailable and poorly controlled)
- Social behavior incongruent with norms
- Values incongruent with cultural norms

12. Comfort

Domain 13
Growth/Development

DOMAIN 13. GROWTH/DEVELOPMENT		
Age-appropriate increases in physical dimensions, maturation of organ systems, and/or progression through the developmental milestones		
Class 1. Growth *Increases in physical dimensions or maturity of organ systems*		
Code	**Diagnosis**	**Page**
00113	Risk for disproportionate **growth**	451
Class 2. Development *Progress or regression through a sequence of recognized milestones in life*		
Code	**Diagnosis**	**Page**
00112	Risk for delayed **development**	452

NANDA International, Inc. Nursing Diagnoses: Definitions & Classification 2015–2017,
Tenth Edition. Edited by T. Heather Herdman and Shigemi Kamitsuru.
© 2014 NANDA International, Inc. Published 2014 by John Wiley & Sons, Ltd.
Companion website: www.wiley.com/go/nursingdiagnoses

00113

Risk for disproportionate **growth**
(1998, 2013)

Definition

Vulnerable to growth above the 97th percentile or below the 3rd percentile for age, crossing two percentile channels, which may compromise health.

Risk Factors

Caregiver

- Alteration in cognitive functioning
- Learning disability
- Mental health issue (e.g., depression, psychosis, personality disorder, substance abuse)
- Presence of abuse (e.g., physical, psychological, sexual)

Environmental

- Deprivation
- Economically disadvantaged
- Exposure to teratogen
- Exposure to violence
- Lead poisoning
- Natural disaster

Individual

- Anorexia
- Chronic illness
- Infection
- Insatiable appetite
- Maladaptive feeding behavior by caregiver
- Maladaptive self-feeding behavior
- Malnutrition
- Prematurity
- Substance abuse

Prenatal

- Congenital disorder
- Exposure to teratogen
- Genetic disorder
- Inadequate maternal nutrition
- Maternal infection
- Multiple gestation
- Substance abuse

*Note: This diagnosis will retire from the NANDA-I Taxonomy in the **2018–2020** edition unless additional work is completed to separate the focus of (1) growth that is above the 97th percentile, and (2) growth that is below the 3rd percentile into separate diagnostic concepts.*

13. Growth/Development

00112

Risk for delayed **development**
(1998, 2013)

Definition
Vulnerable to delay of 25% or more in one or more of the areas of social or self-regulatory behavior, or in cognitive, language, gross, or fine motor skills, which may compromise health.

Risk Factors

Prenatal
- Economically disadvantaged
- Endocrine disorder
- Functional illiteracy
- Genetic disorder
- Infection
- Inadequate nutrition
- Insufficient prenatal care
- Late-term prenatal care
- Maternal age ≤15 years
- Maternal age ≥35 years
- Substance abuse
- Unplanned pregnancy
- Unwanted pregnancy

Individual
- Behavior disorder (e.g., attention deficit, oppositional defiant)
- Brain injury (e.g., abuse, accident, hemorrhage, shaken baby syndrome)
- Chronic illness
- Congenital disorder
- Failure to thrive
- Genetic disorder
- Hearing impairment
- History of adoption
- Inadequate nutrition
- Involvement with the foster care system
- Lead poisoning
- Natural disaster
- Positive drug screen
- Prematurity
- Recurrent otitis media
- Seizure disorder
- Substance abuse
- Technology dependence (e.g., ventilator, augmentative communication)
- Treatment regimen
- Visual impairment

Environmental
- Economically disadvantaged
- Exposure to violence

Caregiver
- Learning disability
- Mental health issue (e.g., depression, psychosis, personality disorder, substance abuse)

- Presence of abuse (e.g., physical, psychological, sexual)

Nursing Diagnoses Accepted for Development and Clinical Validation 2015–2017

One diagnosis, *Disturbed energy field* (00050), was reslotted to a new level of evidence: Theoretical Level (1.2). The rationale for this move, which removed the diagnosis from the taxonomy, is that all of the literature used to support this diagnosis was related to interventions, and not to the concept of energy field itself, nor of the concept of disturbed energy field.

To be considered at this level of evidence, the definition, defining characteristics, and related factors, or risk factors, must be provided with theoretical references cited, if available. Expert opinion may be used to substantiate the need for a diagnosis. The intention of diagnoses received at this level is to enable discussion of the concept, testing for clinical usefulness and applicability, and to stimulate research. At this stage, the label and its component parts are categorized as "Received for Development and Clinical Validation," and identified as such on the NANDA-I website (www.nanda.org) and a separate section in the Definitions and Classification text.

Disturbed **energy field** (formerly held the code 00050) – Removed from the taxonomy, categorized as LOE 1.2
2013 (1994, 2004)

Definition
Disruption of the flow of energy surrounding a person's being that results in disharmony of the body, mind, and/or spirit

Defining Characteristics

Perception of changes in patterns of energy flow, such as:
- ☐ Movement (wave, spike, tingling, dense, flowing)
- ☐ Sounds (tone, words)
- ☐ Temperature change (warmth, coolness)

NANDA International, Inc. Nursing Diagnoses: Definitions & Classification 2015–2017, Tenth Edition. Edited by T. Heather Herdman and Shigemi Kamitsuru.
© 2014 NANDA International, Inc. Published 2014 by John Wiley & Sons, Ltd.
Companion website: www.wiley.com/go/nursingdiagnoses

- ☐ Visual changes (image, color)
- ☐ Disruption of the field (deficit, hole, spike, bulge, obstruction, congestion, diminished flow in energy field)

Related Factors

- Slowing or blocking of energy flows secondary to:
  - ☐ Maturational factors
    - Age-related developmental crisis
    - Age-related developmental difficulties
  - ☐ Pathophysiological factors
    - Illness
    - Injury
    - Pregnancy
  - ☐ Situational factors
    - Anxiety
    - Fear
    - Grieving
    - Pain
  - ☐ Treatment-related factors
    - Chemotherapy
    - Immobility
    - Labor and delivery
    - Perioperative experiences

Part 4
NANDA International, Inc.
2015–2017

NANDA International Position Statements	**459**
NANDA International Processes and Procedures for Diagnosis Submission and Review	**461**
Glossary of Terms	**464**
An Invitation to Join NANDA International	**470**

NANDA International, Inc. Nursing Diagnoses: Definitions & Classification 2015–2017,
Tenth Edition. Edited by T. Heather Herdman and Shigemi Kamitsuru.
© 2014 NANDA International, Inc. Published 2014 by John Wiley & Sons, Ltd.
Companion website: www.wiley.com/go/nursingdiagnoses

NANDA International Position Statements

From time to time, the NANDA International Board of Directors provides position statements as a result of requests from members or users of the NANDA-I taxonomy. Currently, there are two position statements: one addresses the use of the NANDA-I taxonomy as an assessment framework, and the other addresses the structure of the nursing diagnosis statement when included in a care plan. NANDA-I publishes these statements in an attempt to prevent others from interpreting NANDA-I's stance on important issues, and to prevent misunderstandings or misinterpretations.

NANDA INTERNATIONAL Position Statement #1
The Use of Taxonomy II as an Assessment
Framework

Nursing assessments provide the starting point for determining nursing diagnoses. It is vital that a recognized nursing assessment framework is used in practice to identify the patient's* problems, risks, and outcomes for enhancing health.

NANDA International does not endorse one single assessment method or tool. The use of an evidence-based nursing framework such as Gordon's Functional Health Pattern Assessment should guide assessments that support nurses in determination of NANDA-I nursing diagnoses.

For accurate determination of nursing diagnoses, a useful, evidence-based assessment framework is best practice.

NANDA INTERNATIONAL Position Statement #2
The Structure of the Nursing Diagnosis Statement
When Included in a Care Plan

NANDA International believes that the structure of a Nursing Diagnosis as a statement including the diagnosis label and the related factors as exhibited by defining characteristics is best clinical practice, and may be an effective teaching strategy.

NANDA International, Inc. Nursing Diagnoses: Definitions & Classification 2015–2017, Tenth Edition. Edited by T. Heather Herdman and Shigemi Kamitsuru.
© 2014 NANDA International, Inc. Published 2014 by John Wiley & Sons, Ltd.
Companion website: www.wiley.com/go/nursingdiagnoses

The accuracy of the nursing diagnosis is validated when a nurse is able to clearly identify and link to the defining characteristics, related factors, and/or risk factors found within the patient's* assessment.

While this is recognized as best practice, it may be that some information systems do not provide this opportunity. Nurse leaders and nurse informaticists must work together to ensure that vendor solutions are available that allow the nurse to validate accurate diagnoses through clear identification of the diagnostic statement, related and/or risk factors, and defining characteristics.

*NANDA International defines patient as "individual, family, group or community."
Updated October 2010 by NANDA International Board of Directors.

NANDA International Processes and Procedures for Diagnosis Submission and Review

Proposed diagnoses and revisions of diagnoses undergo a systematic review to determine consistency with the established criteria for a nursing diagnosis. All submissions are subsequently staged according to evidence supporting either the level of development or validation.

Diagnoses may be submitted at various levels of development (e.g., label and definition; label, definition, defining characteristics, or risk factors; theoretical level for development and clinical validation; or label, definition, defining characteristics, and related factors).

NANDA-I Diagnosis Submission Guidelines are available on the NANDA-I website (www.nanda.org). Diagnoses should be submitted electronically using the form available on the NANDA-I website.

On receipt, the diagnosis will be assigned to a primary reviewer from the Diagnosis Development Committee (DDC). This person will work with the submitter as the DDC reviews the submission.

Information on the *full review process* and *expedited review process* for all new and revised diagnosis submissions is available on our website (www.nanda.org) in the section on diagnosis development. All potential submitters are strongly recommended to review this information prior to submitting.

Information is also available on our website regarding the *procedure to appeal a DDC decision on diagnosis review*. This process explains the recourse available to a submitter if a submission is not accepted.

NANDA-I Diagnosis Submission: Level of Evidence Criteria

The NANDA-I Education and Research Committee has been tasked to review and revise, as appropriate, these criteria to better reflect the state of the science related to evidence-based nursing. Individuals interested in submitting a diagnosis are advised to refer to the NANDA-I website for updates, as they come available (www.nanda.org).

NANDA International, Inc. Nursing Diagnoses: Definitions & Classification 2015–2017,
Tenth Edition. Edited by T. Heather Herdman and Shigemi Kamitsuru.
© 2014 NANDA International, Inc. Published 2014 by John Wiley & Sons, Ltd.
Companion website: www.wiley.com/go/nursingdiagnoses

1.1 Label Only

The label is clear, stated at a basic level, and supported by literature references, and these are identified. The DDC will consult with the submitter and provide education related to diagnostic development through printed guidelines and workshops. At this stage, the label is categorized as "Received for Development" and identified as such on the NANDA-I website.

1.2 Label and Definition

The label is clear and stated at a basic level. The definition is consistent with the label. The label and definition are distinct from other NANDA-I diagnoses and definitions. The definition differs from the defining characteristics and label, and these components are not included in the definition. At this stage, the diagnosis must be consistent with the current NANDA-I definition of nursing diagnosis (see the "Glossary of Terms"). The label and definition are supported by literature references, and these are identified. At this stage, the label and its definition are categorized as "Received for Development" and identified as such on the NANDA-I website.

1.3 Theoretical Level

The definition, defining characteristics, and related factors, or risk factors, are provided with theoretical references cited, if available. Expert opinion may be used to substantiate the need for a diagnosis. The intention of diagnoses received at this level is to enable discussion of the concept, testing for clinical usefulness and applicability, and to stimulate research. At this stage, the label and its component parts are categorized as "Received for Development and Clinical Validation," and identified as such on the NANDA-I website and a separate section in this book.

2.1 Label, Definition, Defining Characteristics and Related Factors, or Risk Factors, and References

References are cited for the definition, each defining characteristic, and each related factor, or for each risk factor. In addition, it is required that nursing outcomes and nursing interventions from a standardized nursing terminology (e.g., NOC, NIC) be provided for each diagnosis.

2.2 Concept Analysis

The criteria in 2.1 are met. In addition, a narrative review of relevant literature, culminating in a written concept analysis, is required to demonstrate the existence of a substantive body of knowledge under-lying the diagnosis. The literature review/concept analysis supports the label and definition, and includes discussion and support of the defin-ing characteristics and related factors (for problem-focused diagnoses), risk factors (for risk diagnoses), or defining characteristics (for health promotion diagnoses).

2.3 Consensus Studies Related to Diagnosis Using Experts

The criteria in 2.1 are met. Studies include those soliciting expert opin-ion, Delphi, and similar studies of diagnostic components in which nurses are the subjects.

3. Clinically Supported (Validation and Testing)

3.1 Literature Synthesis

The criteria in 2.2 are met. The synthesis is in the form of an integrated review of the literature. Search terms/MESH terms used in the review are provided to assist future researchers.

3.2 Clinical Studies Related to Diagnosis, but Not Generalizable to the Population

The criteria in 2.2 are met. The narrative includes a description of stud-ies related to the diagnosis, which includes defining characteristics and related factors, or risk factors. Studies may be qualitative in nature, or quantitative studies using nonrandom samples, in which patients are subjects.

3.3 Well-Designed Clinical Studies with Small Sample Sizes

The criteria in 2.2 are met. The narrative includes a description of studies related to the diagnosis, which includes defining characteristics or risk factors, and related factors. Random sampling is used in these studies, but the sample size is limited.

3.4 Well-designed Clinical Studies with Random Sample of Sufficient Size to Allow for Generalizability to the Overall Population

The criteria in 2.2 are met. The narrative includes a description of stud-ies related to the diagnosis, which includes defining characteristics and related factors, or risk factors. Random sampling is used in these stud-ies, and the sample size is sufficient to allow for generalizability of results to the overall population.

Glossary of Terms

Nursing Diagnosis

A nursing diagnosis is a clinical judgment concerning a human response to health conditions/life processes, or a vulnerability for that response, by an individual, family, group, or community. A nursing diagnosis provides the basis for selection of nursing interventions to achieve outcomes for which the nurse has accountability. (Approved at the Ninth NANDA Conference; amended in 2009 and 2013.)

Problem-Focused Nursing Diagnosis

A clinical judgment concerning an undesirable human response to health conditions/life processes that exists in an individual, family, group, or community.

Health Promotion Nursing Diagnosis

A clinical judgment concerning motivation and desire to increase well-being and to actualize human health potential. These responses are expressed by a readiness to enhance specific health behaviors, and can be used in any health state. Health promotion responses may exist in an individual, family, group, or community.

Risk Nursing Diagnosis

A clinical judgment concerning the vulnerability of an individual, family, group, or community for developing an undesirable human response to health conditions/life processes.

Syndrome

A clinical judgment concerning a specific cluster of nursing diagnoses that occur together, and are best addressed together and through similar interventions.

NANDA International, Inc. Nursing Diagnoses: Definitions & Classification 2015–2017, Tenth Edition. Edited by T. Heather Herdman and Shigemi Kamitsuru.
© 2014 NANDA International, Inc. Published 2014 by John Wiley & Sons, Ltd.
Companion website: www.wiley.com/go/nursingdiagnoses

Diagnostic Axes

Axis

An axis is operationally defined as a dimension of the human response that is considered in the diagnostic process. There are seven axes that parallel the International Standards Reference Model for a Nursing Diagnosis:

- Axis 1: the focus of the diagnosis
- Axis 2: subject of the diagnosis (individual, caregiver, family, group, community)
- Axis 3: judgment (impaired, ineffective, etc.)
- Axis 4: location (bladder, auditory, cerebral, etc.)
- Axis 5: age (infant, child, adult, etc.)
- Axis 6: time (chronic, acute, intermittent)
- Axis 7: status of the diagnosis (problem-focused, risk, health promotion)

The axes are represented in the labels of the nursing diagnoses through their values. In some cases, they are named explicitly, such as with the diagnoses *Ineffective Community Coping* and *Compromised Family Coping*, in which the subject of the diagnosis (in the first instance "community" and in the second instance "family") is named using the two values "community" and "family" taken from Axis 2 (subject of the diagnosis). *"Ineffective"* and *"compromised"* are two of the values contained in Axis 3 (judgment).

In some cases, the axis is implicit, as is the case with the diagnosis *Activity intolerance*, in which the subject of the diagnosis (Axis 2) is always the patient. In some instances an axis may not be pertinent to a particular diagnosis and therefore is not part of the nursing diagnosis label. For example, the time axis may not be relevant to every diagnosis. In the case of diagnoses without explicit identification of the subject of the diagnosis, it may be helpful to remember that NANDA-I defines patient as *"an individual, family, group or community."*

Axis 1 (the focus) and Axis 3 (judgment) are essential components of a nursing diagnosis. In some cases, however, the focus contains the judgment (for example, *Nausea*); in these cases the judgment is not explicitly separated out in the diagnosis label. Axis 2 (subject of the diagnosis) is also essential, although, as described above, it may be implied and therefore not included in the label. The Diagnosis Development Committee requires these axes for submission; the other axes may be used where relevant for clarity.

Axis 1 The Focus of the Diagnosis

The focus is the principal element or the fundamental and essential part, the root, of the nursing diagnosis. It describes the "human response" that is the core of the diagnosis.

The focus of the diagnosis may consist of one or more nouns. When more than one noun is used (for example, *Activity intolerance*), each one contributes a unique meaning to the diagnosis, as if the two were a single noun; the meaning of the combined term, however, is different from when the nouns are stated separately. Frequently, an adjective (*Spiritual*) may be used with a noun (*Distress*) to denote the focus *Spiritual Distress*. (see Chapter 4, Table 1, p. 95)

Axis 2 Subject of the Diagnosis

The person(s) for whom a nursing diagnosis is determined. The values in Axis 2 that represent the NANDA-I definition of "patient" are:

- *Individual:* a single human being distinct from others, a person
- *Caregiver:* a family member or helper who regularly looks after a child or a sick, elderly, or disabled person
- *Family:* two or more people having continuous or sustained relationships, perceiving reciprocal obligations, sensing common meaning, and sharing certain obligations toward others; related by blood and/or choice
- *Group:* a number of people with shared characteristics
- *Community:* a group of people living in the same locale under the same governance. Examples include neighborhoods and cities

Axis 3 Judgment

A descriptor or modifier that limits or specifies the meaning of the focus of the diagnosis. The focus together with the nurse's judgment about it forms the diagnosis. The values in Axis 3 are found in Chapter 4, Table 2, p. 98.

Axis 4 Location

Describes the parts/regions of the body and/or their related functions – all tissues, organs, anatomical sites, or structures. For the locations in Axis 4, see Chapter 4, Table 3, p. 100.

Axis 5 Age

Refers to the age of the person who is the subject of the diagnosis (Axis 2). The values in Axis 5 are noted below, with all definitions *except* that of older adult being drawn from the World Health Organization (2013):

- **Fetus**: an unborn human more than 8 weeks after conception, until birth
- **Neonate**: a child< 28 days of age
- **Infant**: a child >28 days and < 1 year of age
- **Child**: person aged 1 to 9 years, inclusive
- **Adolescent**: person aged 10 to 19 years, inclusive
- **Adult**: a person older than 19 years of age unless national law defines a person as being an adult at an earlier age
- **Older adult**: a person >65 years of age

Axis 6 Time

Describes the duration of the nursing diagnosis (Axis 1). The values in Axis 6 are:

- *Acute:* lasting <3 months
- *Chronic:* lasting ≥3 months
- *Intermittent:* stopping or starting again at intervals, periodic, cyclic
- *Continuous:* uninterrupted, going on without stop
- *Perioperative:* occurring or performed at or around the time of an operation

Axis 7 Status of the Diagnosis

Refers to the actuality or potentiality of the problem/syndrome or to the categorization of the diagnosis as a health promotion diagnosis. The values in Axis 7 are *Problem-focused*, *Health Promotion*, and *Risk*.

Components of a Nursing Diagnosis

Diagnosis Label

Provides a name for a diagnosis that reflects, at a minimum, the focus of the diagnosis (from Axis 1) and the nursing judgment (from Axis 3). It is a concise term or phrase that represents a pattern of related cues. It may include modifiers.

Definition

Provides a clear, precise description; delineates its meaning and helps differentiate it from similar diagnoses.

Defining Characteristics

Observable cues/inferences that cluster as manifestations of a problem-focused, health promotion diagnosis or syndrome. This does not only imply those things that the nurse can see, but things that are seen, heard (e.g., the patient/family tells us), touched, or smelled.

Risk Factors

Environmental factors and physiological, psychological, genetic, or chemical elements that increase the vulnerability of an individual, family, group, or community to an unhealthy event. Only risk diagnoses have risk factors.

Related Factors

Factors that appear to show some type of patterned relationship with the nursing diagnosis. Such factors may be described as antecedent to, associated with, related to, contributing to, or abetting. Only problem-focused nursing diagnoses and problem-focused syndromes must have related factors; health promotion diagnoses may have related factors, if they help to clarify the diagnosis.

Definitions for Classification of Nursing Diagnoses

Classification

Systematic arrangement of related phenomena in groups or classes based on characteristics that objects have in common.

Level of Abstraction

Describes the concreteness/abstractness of a concept:

- Very abstract concepts are theoretical, may not be directly measurable, are defined by concrete concepts, are inclusive of concrete concepts, are disassociated from any specific instance, are independent of time and space, have more general descriptors, and may not be clinically useful for planning treatment
- Concrete concepts are observable and measurable, limited by time and space, constitute a specific category, are more exclusive, name

a real thing or class of things, are restricted by nature, and may be clinically useful for planning treatment

Nomenclature

A system or set of terms or symbols especially in a particular science, discipline, or art; the act or process or an instance of naming (Merriam-Webster, 2009).

Taxonomy

"Classification: especially orderly classification of plants and animals according to their presumed natural relationships"; the word is derived from the root word, taxon – "the name applied to a taxonomic group in a formal system of nomenclature" (Merriam-Webster, 2009).

References

Merriam-Webster, Inc. (2009). *Merriam-Webster's Collegiate Dictionary* (11th ed.) Springfield, MA: Author.

Oxford Dictionary On-Line, British and World Version. (2013). Oxford University Press. Available at: http://www.oxforddictionaries.com/

Pender, N.J., Murdaugh, C.L., & Parsons, M.A. (2006). *Health promotion in nursing practice* (5th ed.). Upper Saddle River, NJ: Pearson Prentice-Hall.

World Health Organization (2013). Health topics: Infant, newborn. Available at: http://www.who.int/topics/infant_newborn/en/.

World Health Organization (2013). Definition of key terms. Available at: http://www.who.int/hiv/pub/guidelines/arv2013/intro/keyterms/en/.

An Invitation to Join NANDA International

Words are powerful. They allow us to communicate ideas and experiences to others so that they may share our understanding. Nursing diagnoses are an example of a powerful and precise terminology that highlights and renders visible the unique contribution of nursing to global health. Nursing diagnoses communicate the professional judgments that nurses make every day – to our patients, our colleagues, members of other disciplines, and the public. They are our words.

NANDA International: A Member-Driven Organization

Our Vision

NANDA International, Inc. (NANDA-I) will be a global force for the development and use of nursing's standardized diagnostic terminology to improve the healthcare of all people.

Our Mission

To facilitate the development, refinement, dissemination, and use of standardized nursing diagnostic terminology.

- We provide the world's leading evidence-based nursing diagnoses for use in practice and to determine interventions and outcomes
- We fund research through the NANDA-I Foundation
- We are a supportive and energetic global network of nurses who are committed to improving the quality of nursing care through evidence-based practice

Our Purpose

Implementation of nursing diagnosis enhances every aspect of nursing practice, from garnering professional respect to assuring accurate documentation for reimbursement.

NANDA International, Inc. Nursing Diagnoses: Definitions & Classification 2015–2017, Tenth Edition. Edited by T. Heather Herdman and Shigemi Kamitsuru.
© 2014 NANDA International, Inc. Published 2014 by John Wiley & Sons, Ltd.
Companion website: www.wiley.com/go/nursingdiagnoses

NANDA International exists to develop, refine, and promote terminology that accurately reflects nurses' clinical judgments. This unique, evidence-based perspective includes social, physiological, psychological, and spiritual dimensions of care.

Our History

NANDA International, Inc. was originally named the North American Nursing Diagnosis Association (NANDA), and was founded in 1982. The organization grew out of the National Conference Group, a task force established at the First National Conference on the Classification of Nursing Diagnoses, held in St. Louis, Missouri, USA, in 1973. This conference and the ensuing task force ignited interest in the concept of standardizing nursing terminology. In 2002, NANDA was relaunched as NANDA International to reflect increasing worldwide interest in the field of nursing terminology development. Although we no longer use the name "North American Nursing Diagnosis Association," and it is not appropriate to refer to the organization by this name unless quoting it prior to 2002, (nor is *North American Nursing Diagnosis Association, International* correct to use), we did maintain "NANDA" as a brand name or trademark within our name, because of its international recognition as the leader in nursing diagnostic terminology.

As of this edition, NANDA-I has approved 235 diagnoses for clinical use, testing, and refinement. A dynamic, international process of diagnosis review and classification approves and updates terms and definitions for identified human responses.

NANDA-I has international networks in Brazil, Colombia, Ecuador, Mexico, Nigeria–Ghana, Peru, and Portugal, as well as a German-language group; other country, specialty, and/or language groups interested in forming a NANDA-I Network should contact the CEO/Executive Director of NANDA-I at execdir@nanda.org. NANDA-I also has collaborative links with nursing terminology societies around the world, including: the Japanese Society of Nursing Diagnoses (JSND), the Association for Common European Nursing Diagnoses, Interventions and Outcomes (ACENDIO), the Asociacíon Española de Nomenclatura, Taxonomia y Diagnóstico de Enfermeria (AENTDE), the Association Francophone Européenne des Diagnostics Interventions Résultats Infirmiers (AFEDI), the Nursing Intervention Classification (NIC), and the Nursing Outcomes Classification (NOC).

NANDA International's Commitment

NANDA-I is a member-driven, grassroots organization committed to the development of nursing diagnostic terminology. The desired outcome of the Association's work is to provide nurses at all levels and in all areas of practice with a standardized nursing terminology with which to:

- name actual or potential human responses to health problems, and life processes
- develop, refine, and disseminate evidence-based terminology representing clinical judgments made by professional nurses
- facilitate study of the phenomena of concern to nurses for the purpose of improving patient care, patient safety, and patient outcomes for which nurses have accountability
- document care for reimbursement of nursing services
- contribute to the development of informatics and information standards, ensuring the inclusion of nursing terminology in electronic healthcare records.

Nursing terminology is the key to defining the future of nursing practice and ensuring the knowledge of nursing is represented in the patient record – NANDA-I is the global leader in this effort. Join us and become a part of this exciting process.

Involvement Opportunities

The participation of NANDA-I members is critical to the growth and development of nursing terminology. Many opportunities exist for participation on committees, as well as in the development, use, and refinement of diagnoses, and in research. Opportunities also exist for international liaison work and networking with nursing leaders.

Why Join NANDA-I?

Professional Networking

- Professional relationships are built through serving on committees, attending our various conferences, participation in the Nursing Diagnosis Discussion Forum, reaching out through the Online Membership Directory, and participating in our Social Media feeds (e.g., Facebook and Twitter)
- NANDA-I Membership Network Groups connect colleagues within a specific country, region, language, or nursing specialty
- Professional contribution and achievement are recognized through our Founders, Mentors, Unique Contribution, and Editor's Awards. Research grant awards are offered through the NANDA-I Foundation
- Fellows are identified by NANDA-I as nursing leaders with standardized nursing language expertise in the areas of education, administration, clinical practice, informatics, and research

- Members receive a complimentary subscription to our online scientific journal, *The International Journal of Nursing Knowledge* (IJNK). IJNK communicates efforts to develop and implement standardized nursing language across the globe. The NANDA-I website offers resources for nursing diagnosis development, refinement, and submission, NANDA-I taxonomy updates, and an Online Membership Directory

Member Benefits

- Members receive discounts on NANDA-I taxonomy publications, including print, electronic, and summary list versions of *NANDA-I Nursing Diagnoses & Classification*
- We partner with organizations offering products/services of interest to the nursing community, with a price advantage for members. Member discounts apply to our biennial conference and NANDA-I products, such as our T-shirts and tote bags
- Our Regular Membership fees are based on the World Health Organization's classification of countries. It is our hope this will enable more individuals with interest in the work of NANDA-I to participate in setting the future direction of the organization

How to Join

Go to www.nanda.org for more information and instructions for membership registration.

Who Is Using the NANDA International Taxonomy?

- International Standards Organization compatible
- Health Level 7 International registered
- SNOMED-CT available
- Unified Medical Language System compatible
- American Nurses' Association recognized terminology

The NANDA-I taxonomy is currently available in Bahasa Indonesian, Basque, Orthodox Chinese, Czech, Dutch, English, Estonian, French, German, Italian, Japanese, Portuguese, Spanish (European and Hispanoamerican editions), and Swedish.

For more information, and to apply for membership online, please visit: www. nanda.org

Index

Note: Page numbers in *italics* refer to Figures; those in **bold** to Tables

absorption, 154
activity/exercise
  disuse syndrome, 214
  impaired bed mobility, 215
  impaired physical mobility,
    216–17
  impaired sitting, 219
  impaired standing, 220
  impaired transfer ability, 221
  impaired walking, 222
  impaired wheelchair mobility, 218
activity intolerance, 225–6
activity planning, ineffective, 321–2
activity/rest
  activity/exercise, 214–22
  cardiovascular/pulmonary
    responses, 223–39
  domains, 60, *61*, 62–5, **69–70**
  energy balance, 223–4
  self-care, 241–7
  sleep/rest, 209–13
airway clearance, ineffective, 380
allergy response, 423–5
American Nurses Association (ANA),
    92, 105
anxiety, 323–4
aspiration, 381
assessment
  data collection, 31
  defining characteristics, 110
  domains, 124–5
  evidence-based, 35
  human responses, 32–3
  in-depth, 32, 41, 43–4
  medical diagnoses, 33
  NANDA-I Taxonomy, 35

nursing disciplines, 32, 125–6
potential diagnoses, 31–2
preoperative teaching, 33
"real" diagnoses, 125
screening, 34
steps, diagnosis, 31–2, *32*
attention, 251–9
autonomic dysreflexia, 350–352
axes
  age, 92, 100
  diagnostic focus, 92–3, 94
  judgment, 92–3, 97, **98–9**
  location, 92, 97, **100**
  status of diagnosis, 92, 100–101
  subject of diagnosis, 92–3, 97
  time, 92, 100

bed mobility, impaired, 215
bleeding, 382
blood glucose level, unstable, 171
body image, disturbed, 275–6
bowel incontinence, 192
breastfeeding
  ineffective, 156–7
  interrupted, 158
  readiness for enhanced, 159
breast milk, insufficient, 155
breathing pattern, ineffective, 227

cardiac output, decreased, 228–30
cardiac tissue perfusion, decreased,
    235
cardiovascular function, impaired, 231
cardiovascular/pulmonary responses
  activity intolerance, 225–6
  decreased cardiac output, 228–9

NANDA International, Inc. Nursing Diagnoses: Definitions & Classification 2015–2017,
Tenth Edition. Edited by T. Heather Herdman and Shigemi Kamitsuru.
© 2014 NANDA International, Inc. Published 2014 by John Wiley & Sons, Ltd.
Companion website: www.wiley.com/go/nursingdiagnoses

cardiovascular/pulmonary
  responses (cont'd)
  decreased cardiac tissue perfusion,
    234
  dysfunctional ventilatory weaning
    response, 238–9
  impaired cardiovascular function,
    230
  impaired spontaneous ventilation,
    233
  ineffective breathing pattern, 227
  ineffective cerebral tissue
    perfusion, 235
  ineffective gastrointestinal
    perfusion, 231
  ineffective peripheral tissue
    perfusion, 236–7
  ineffective renal perfusion, 232
caregiving roles
  impaired parenting, 283–5,
    287–8
  readiness for enhanced parenting,
    286
  strain, 279–82
cerebral tissue perfusion, ineffective,
  236
childbearing process
  ineffective, 307–8, 310
  readiness for enhanced, 309
classification
  healthcare knowledge, 57
  health promotion (domain),
    57, 60
  NANDA-I Taxonomy, functions,
    57, 60
  Taxonomy II, 57, 58–9
cognition
  acute confusion, 252, 253
  chronic confusion, 254
  deficient knowledge, 257
  impaired memory, 259
  ineffective impulse control, 256
  labile emotional control, 255
  readiness for enhanced
    knowledge, 258
comfort
  domains, 65, **78**
  physical, 439–45
  social, 446–7

Committee for Nursing Practice
  Information Infrastructure
  (CNPII), 91–2
communication
  impaired verbal, 261–2
  readiness for enhanced, 260
community coping
  ineffective, 328
  readiness for enhanced, 329
confusion
  acute, 252, 253
  chronic, 254
constipation
  chronic functional, 199–200
  gastrointestinal function, 193–7
  perceived, 195
coping responses
  anxiety, 323–4
  chronic sorrow, 348
  complicated grieving, 339–40
  compromised family coping,
    330–331
  death anxiety, 334
  defensive coping, 325
  disabled family coping, 332
  fear, 336–7
  grieving, 338
  impaired mood regulation, 341
  impaired resilience, 345, 347
  ineffective activity planning, 321–2
  ineffective community coping, 328
  ineffective coping, 326
  ineffective denial, 335
  powerlessness, 343–4
  readiness for enhanced community
    coping, 329
  readiness for enhanced coping, 327
  readiness for enhanced family
    coping, 333
  readiness for enhanced power, 342
  readiness for enhanced resilience,
    346
  stress overload, 349
coping/stress tolerance
  coping responses, 321–49
  domains, 65, **74**
  neurobehavioral stress, 351–7
  post-trauma responses, 315–20
corneal injury, 387

data analysis
  conversion to information, 35,
    36, 37
  documentation, 37
  modified nursing process, 39, *39*
  nursing concepts, 39
  nursing knowledge, 37
  objective and subjective data, *36*, 37
  patient's human responses, 38–9
data collection, 31
death anxiety, 334
decisional conflict, 364
decision-making
  impaired emancipated, 365, 367
  readiness for enhanced, 363
  readiness for enhanced
    emancipated, 366
defensive processes
  allergy response, 423
  iodinated contrast media, adverse
    reaction, 422
  latex allergy response, 423–5
defining characteristics
  assessment, 117
  definition, 117
  human response, 117
denial, ineffective, 335
dentition, impaired, 391
development, delayed, 452–3
Diagnostic and Statistical Manual of
  Mental Disorders (DSM-IV), 21
diarrhea, 198
digestion, 154
disturbed energy field, 455–6
disuse syndrome, 214
dry eye, 383

electrolyte imbalance, 175
elimination and exchange
  domains, 65, **68**
  gastrointestinal function, 193–203
  respiratory function, 203
  urinary function, 183–91
energy balance
  fatigue, 223
  wandering, 224
environmental hazards
  contamination, 418–20
  poisoning, 421

falls, 384–5
family coping
  compromised, 330–331
  disabled, 332
  readiness for enhanced, 333
family health management,
  ineffective, 149
family relationships
  dysfunctional, 290–292
  impaired attachment, 289
  interrupted, 293
  readiness for enhanced, 294
fear, 336–7
fluid balance, readiness for
  enhanced, 176
fluid volume
  deficient, 177, 178
  excess, 179
  imbalanced, 180
frail elderly syndrome, 141–3

gastrointestinal function
  bowel incontinence, 192
  chronic functional constipation,
    199–200
  constipation, 193–4, 196–7
  diarrhea, 198
  dysfunctional, 201–2
  perceived constipation, 195
gastrointestinal motility,
  dysfunctional, 201–2
gastrointestinal perfusion,
  ineffective, 232
Gordon's Functional Health Patterns
  (FHP) assessment, 35
grieving, 338
growth
  development, 65, 78, 452–3
  disproportionate, 451

health awareness
  deficient diversional activity, 139
  sedentary lifestyle, 140
health management
  deficient community, 144
  frail elderly syndrome, 141–3
  ineffective, 147
  ineffective family, 149
  ineffective health maintenance, 146

health management (*cont'd*)
  ineffective protection, 152
  noncompliance, 150–151
  readiness for enhanced, 148
  risk-prone health behavior, 145
health promotion
  domains, 65, **66**
  health awareness, 139–40
  health management, 141–52
hope, readiness for enhanced, 265
human dignity, compromised, 267
hydration
  deficient fluid volume, 177, 178
  electrolyte imbalance, 175
  excess fluid volume, 179
  imbalanced fluid volume, 180
  readiness for enhanced fluid
    balance, 176
hyperthermia, 427
hypothermia, 428–30

impaired gas exchange, 203
impulse control, ineffective, 256
infant behavior
  disorganized, 354–5, 357
  readiness for enhanced
    organized, 356
infant feeding pattern, ineffective, 160
infection, 379
ingestion
  imbalanced nutrition, 170
  impaired swallowing, 168–9
  ineffective breastfeeding, 156–7
  ineffective infant feeding
    pattern, 160
  insufficient breast milk, 155
  interrupted breastfeeding, 158
  obesity, 163–4
  overweight, 165–8
  readiness for enhanced
    breastfeeding, 159
  readiness for enhanced nutrition,
    162
injury, 388
insomnia, 209
International Classification of Disease
  Taxonomy, ICD-10, 21
*International Considerations on the Use of
  the NANDA-I Nursing Diagnoses,* 116

International Standards Organization
  (ISO) terminology model, 92, *92*
intracranial adaptive capacity,
  decreased, 350
iodinated contrast media, adverse
  reaction, 422

knowledge
  deficient, 257
  readiness for enhanced, 258

labile emotional control, 255
level of evidence (LOE) criteria
  diagnoses, 128–9
  publication and inclusion, 462–4
  received for development, 462
  validation and testing, 463
life principles
  beliefs, 361–2
  domain, 65, **75**
  value/belief/action congruence,
    363–74
liver function, impaired, 174
loneliness, 446

maternal–fetal dyad, disturbed, 311
memory, impaired, 259
metabolism
  impaired liver function, 174
  neonatal jaundice, 172–3
  unstable blood glucose level, 171
mood regulation, impaired, 341
moral distress, 368

NANDA International (NANDA-I)
    Taxonomy
  axes, definitions, 94–101
  case study, 64–5
  certain diagnoses, 127
  classification, 56–60
  clinical reasoning, 63–4
  cognitive map, 63
  definition, 52, 106
  development and revision, 127
  diagnosis submission and review,
    461–3
  diagnostic concepts, 28–9, 92–3
  domains and classes, 21–2
  Electronic Health Records, 126

expenses, 107
and Gordon's FHP, 35
grocery taxonomy, 53, *54, 55,* 56
new nursing diagnoses, 2015–2017,
    5–6, **6–7**
nursing knowledge, terminology, 52
official translation rights holders,
    107
patient's human response, 64
perinatal nursing practice, 62–3
revisions to labels, 11, **12**
slotting changes, nursing diagnosis,
    10, **10**
structure, 52–6
taxonomy, definition, 106
Taxonomy I, 65, 91
Taxonomy II *see* Taxonomy II,
    domains
Taxonomy III *see* Taxonomy III,
    domains (von Krogh's model)
tissue perfusion, 62
NANDA-I nursing diagnosis model
developing and submitting, 101–3
diagnostic foci, 91, **95–6,** 102
disorganized infant behavior,
    101, *102*
individual impaired standing,
    101, *101*
ISO Reference Terminology Model,
    91, *92*
outcome or intervention studies, 103
readiness for enhanced family
    coping, 101, *102*
NANDA-I's Diagnosis Development
    Committee (DDC), 127
nausea, 439
neonatal jaundice, 172–3
neurobehavioral stress
autonomic dysreflexia, 350–352
decreased intracranial adaptive
    capacity, 350
disorganized infant behavior,
    354–5, 357
readiness for enhanced organized
    infant behavior, 356
neurovascular dysfunction,
    peripheral, 395
NIC *see* Nursing Interventions
    Classification (NIC)

NOC *see* Nursing Outcome
    Classification (NOC)
noncompliance, 150–151
nursing assessment framework, 107
nursing diagnosis
assessment, 24–5
care plan, 114–15, 122–3
clinical reasoning, 115
collaborative healthcare team, 21, *22*
concepts, 24
critical care unit, nurses, 110–111
defining characteristics, 26, **26**
diabetes mellitus, 27–8
diagnostic indicators, benefits,
    13, 14–15
domains and classes, 22
electronic health record, 27
evaluation, 28
health promotion diagnosis, 22, 26
interventions and outcomes, 23,
    23, 27–8, 62, 111–12, 122
label, parts, 25, *25,* 112–14
LOE criteria, 128
and medical diagnosis, 112
missing codes, 128
new diagnosis, 127
nurse (or nursing student), 23–4
operating room and outpatient
    clinics, 110
outcome setting, 23, *23,* 27, 29, *39*
patient chart, 116
patient record, documentation,
    116
potential *see* potential nursing
    diagnosis
problem-focused, 22
process, *23,* 23–4
references, 129
removed from NANDA-I
    Taxonomy II, 2015–2017,
    11–12, **13**
revised, 2015–2017, 7, **8–10,**
    11, **128**
revisions to labels, NANDA-I,
    11, **12**
risk factors, 22, 26, **26**
slotting changes, NANDA-I, 10, **10**
SNAPPS diagnostic aid, 119–20, *120*
syndrome, 23

nursing diagnosis (*cont'd*)
  teaching/learning, 123–6
  types, NANDA-I classification, 111
  uses, 28–9
Nursing Interventions Classification
    (NIC), 27
Nursing Outcome Classification
    (NOC), 27
nutrition
  absorption, 154
  digestion, 154
  hydration, 175–80
  imbalanced, 49, 161
  ingestion, 155–71
  metabolism, 172–4
  readiness for enhanced, 162

obesity, 163–4
oral mucous membrane, impaired,
    392–4
overweight, 165–8

parental role conflict, 298
parenting
  impaired, 283–5, 287–8
  readiness for enhanced, 286
perception/cognition
  attention, 251–9
  communication, 260–262
  domains, 65, **70–71**
performance, 295–301
perioperative positioning injury, 388
peripheral tissue perfusion,
    ineffective, 237–8
personal identity, disturbed, 268–9
physical comfort
  acute pain, 440–441
  chronic pain, 442–3
  chronic pain syndrome, 445
  impaired comfort, 437
  labor pain, 446
  nausea, 439
  readiness for enhanced comfort,
    438
physical injury
  aspiration, 381
  bleeding, 382
  corneal injury, 387
  delayed surgical recovery, 403–4

dry eye, 383
falls, 384–5
impaired dentition, 391
impaired oral mucous membrane,
    392–4
impaired skin integrity,
    399–400
impaired tissue integrity, 405–6
ineffective airway clearance, 380
infection, 379
injury, 386
perioperative positioning injury, 388
peripheral neurovascular
    dysfunction, 395
pressure ulcer, 396–7
shock, 398
sudden infant death syndrome, 401
suffocation, 402
thermal injury, 389
trauma, 406–8
urinary tract injury, 390
vascular trauma, 409
physical mobility, impaired, 216–17
post-trauma syndrome, 315–17
potential nursing diagnosis *see also*
    nursing diagnosis
  conceptual nursing knowledge, 40
  data patterns, 40
  defining characteristics and related
    factors, comparison, **45–6,** 47
  differentiation process, 44, 47
  domains and classes, comparison,
    47, **47**
  expert nurse, 39–40
  interventions, 40
  NANDA-I nursing diagnoses, 43
  new diagnoses, 44
  previous diagnoses, 43
  SEA TOW, *48,* 48–9
  stress and coping, 47–8
powerlessness, 343–4
power, readiness for enhanced, 342
pressure ulcer, 396–7
problem, etiology (related factors)
    and signs/symptoms (defining
    characteristics) (PES), 107
problem-focused diagnosis, 109,
    120–121
protection, ineffective, 152

rape-trauma syndrome, 318
RAPS *see* Risk Assessment Pressure
    Sore (RAPS) Scale
related factors
    definition, 117
    nursing diagnosis, 118
    PES statement, 118
relationship
    ineffective, 295, 297
    readiness for enhanced, 296
religiosity
    impaired, 369, 371
    readiness for enhanced, 370
relocation stress syndrome,
    319–20
renal perfusion, ineffective, 233
reproduction
    disturbed maternal–fetal
        dyad, 311
    ineffective childbearing process,
        307–8, 310
    readiness for enhanced
        childbearing process, 309
resilience
    impaired, 345, 347
    readiness for enhanced, 346
respiratory function, 203
Risk Assessment Pressure Sore
    (RAPS) Scale, 119
risk diagnosis
    definition, 117
    medical diagnosis, 120–121
    PES format, 109
    RAPS Scale, 119
risk-prone health behavior, 145
role performance
    impaired social interaction, 301
    ineffective, 299–300
    ineffective relationship, 295,
        297
    parental role conflict, 298
    readiness for enhanced
        relationship, 296
role relationships
    caregiving roles, 279–88
    domains, 65, **72**
    family relationships, 289–94
    role performance, 295–301
Roy Adaptation Model, 34

safety/protection
    defensive processes, 422–5
    domains, 65, **76–7**
    environmental hazards, 418–21
    infection, 379
    physical injury, 380–409
    thermoregulation, 426–33
    violence, 410–417
SEA TOW, *48*, 48–9
self-care
    bathing self-care deficit, 242
    dressing self-care deficit, 243
    feeding self-care deficit, 244
    impaired home maintenance, 241
    readiness for enhanced, 246
    self-neglect, 247
    toileting self-care deficit, 245
self-concept
    compromised human dignity, 267
    disturbed personal identity,
        268–9
    hopelessness, 266
    readiness for enhanced, 270
    readiness for enhanced hope, 265
self-esteem
    chronic low, 271–2
    situational low, 273–4
self-mutilation, 412–14
self-neglect, 247
self-perception
    body image, 275–6
    domains, 65, **71**
    self-concept, 265–70
    self-esteem, 271–4
sexual identity
    ineffective sexuality pattern, 306
    sexual dysfunction, 305
sexuality
    domains, 65, **73**
    reproduction, 307–11
    sexual function, 305–6
shock, 398
sitting, impaired, 219
skin integrity, impaired, 399–400
sleep/rest
    disturbed sleep pattern, 213
    enhanced sleep, 212
    insomnia, 209
    sleep deprivation, 210–211

SNL *see* standardized nursing
language (SNL)
social comfort
isolation, 447
loneliness, 446
social interaction, impaired, 301
sorrow, chronic, 348
spiritual distress, 372–4
spiritual well-being, readiness for
enhanced, 361–2
spontaneous ventilation, impaired,
234
standardized nursing language (SNL)
American Nurses Association
(ANA), 105
definition, 105
differences, 105–6
standing, impaired, 220
strain, 279–82
stressors, 47–8, 49
stress overload, 349
subjective *vs.* objective data, 37–8
sudden infant death syndrome, 401
suffocation, 402
suicide, 416–17
surgical recovery, delayed, 403–4
swallowing, impaired, 169–70

Taxonomy I *see* NANDA International
(NANDA-I) Taxonomy
Taxonomy II, domains *see also*
NANDA International
(NANDA-I) Taxonomy
activity/rest, 60, *61*, 62, 65,
69–70
comfort, 65, **78**
coping/stress tolerance, 65, **74**
definition, 91
elimination and exchange, 65, **68**
growth/development, 65, **78**
health promotion, 65, **66**
life principles, 65, **75**
nursing assessment framework, 107
nutrition, 65, **67**
perception/cognition, 65, **70–71**
role relationships, 65, **72**
safety/protection, 65, **76–7**
self-perception, 65, **71**
sexuality, 65, **73**

structure, 91–2
Taxonomy III, domains (von Krogh's
model) *see also* NANDA
International (NANDA-I)
Taxonomy
and classes, 79, *79*, *80*
environmental, 79, **90**
existential, 79, **84–6**
family, 79, **89**
functional, 79, **86–7**
mental, 79, **83–4**
physiological, 79, **80–83**
safety, 79, **88**
thermal injury, 389
thermoregulation
hyperthermia, 427
hypothermia, 428–31
imbalanced body temperature,
426
ineffective, 433
perioperative hypothermia, 432
tissue integrity, impaired, 405–6
transfer ability, impaired, 221
trauma, 407–8
Tripartite Model of Nursing Practice
(2008), *121*, 121–2

urinary elimination
impaired, 183
readiness for enhanced, 184
urinary incontinence
functional, 185
overflow, 186
reflex, 187
stress, 188
urge, 189–90
urinary retention, 191
urinary tract injury, 390

value/belief/action congruence
decisional conflict, 364
impaired emancipated decision-
making, 365, 367
impaired religiosity, 369, 371
moral distress, 368
readiness for enhanced decision-
making, 363
readiness for enhanced emancipated
decision-making, 366

readiness for enhanced religiosity, 370

readiness for enhanced spiritual well-being, 361–2

spiritual distress, 372–4

vascular trauma, 409

ventilatory weaning response, dysfunctional, 239–40

violence
other-directed, 410
self-directed, 411
self-mutilation, 412–14
suicide, 416–17

walking, impaired, 222

wheelchair mobility, impaired, 218